Essentials in Ophthalmology

Series Editors
Arun D. Singh

More information about this series at http://www.springer.com/series/5332

Andreas Stahl

Editor

Anti-Angiogenic Therapy in Ophthalmology

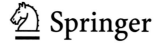
Springer

Editor
Andreas Stahl, MD
Eye Center at the Medical Center
University of Freiburg
Freiburg, Germany

ISSN 1612-3212   ISSN 2196-890X   (electronic)
Essentials in Ophthalmology
ISBN 978-3-319-24095-4   ISBN 978-3-319-24097-8   (eBook)
DOI 10.1007/978-3-319-24097-8

Library of Congress Control Number: 2016937532

Springer Cham Heidelberg New York Dordrecht London

Printed on acid-free paper

Springer International Publishing AG Switzerland is part of Springer Science+Business Media (www.springer.com)

Preface

In 2006, intraocular anti-VEGF therapy for exudative age-related macular degeneration (AMD) was ranked among the top 10 breakthroughs of the year by Science Magazine. Since then, antiangiogenic therapy has broadened its impact from AMD treatment to various other diseases of the eye like macular oedema in diabetic retinopathy or retinal vein occlusion. In other areas, for example, retinopathy of prematurity (ROP), antiangiogenic therapy is just beginning to find its place and is currently being evaluated in clinical studies that weigh its benefit against potential risks. As a third category, there are indications like macular telangiectasia where antiangiogenic therapy has after initial hopeful use become to be seen as potentially unfavourable in the long run.

Due to the broad use of antiangiogenic therapies in these fundamentally different ocular diseases, it is crucial for the treating physician to understand both the underlying principles of angiogenic eye diseases and the available clinical data on therapies and outcome. This book therefore combines an overview over retinal vascular physiology with a detailed analysis of the available clinical data on antiangiogenic therapy in various ocular disorders. The authors are all experts in their respective fields and have achieved to combine concise but crucial pathophysiologic background information with detailed clinical data reflecting our current state of knowledge on antiangiogenic therapy in ophthalmology.

Freiburg, Germany   Andreas Stahl, MD

Contents

Contributors

Hansjürgen T. Agostini, MD Eye Center, Albert-Ludwigs-University Freiburg, Freiburg im Breisgau, Germany

Björn Bachmann, MD Department of Ophthalmology, University of Cologne, Cologne, Germany

James Bainbridge, PhD, FRCOphth Department of Genetics, UCL Institute of Ophthalmology, London, UK

Felix Bock, PhD Department of Ophthalmology, University of Cologne, Cologne, Cologne, Germany

Jing Chen, PhD Department of Ophthalmology, Boston Children's Hospital, Harvard Medical School, Boston, MA, USA

Emily Y. Chew, MD National Institutes of Health, National Eye Institute, Bethesda, MD, USA

Claus Cursiefen, MD Department of Ophthalmology, University of Cologne, Cologne, Germany

Nicolas Feltgen Universitätsmedizin Göttingen, University Eye Hospital, Göttingen, Germany

Robert P. Finger, MD, MIH, PhD Department of Ophthalmology, Centre for Eye Research Australia, Royal Victorian Eye and Ear Hospital, University of Melbourne, East Melbourne, VIC, Australia

Dujon Fuzzard, MBBS/BMedSc Department of Ophthalmology, Centre for Eye Research Australia, Royal Victorian Eye and Ear Hospital, University of Melbourne, East Melbourne, VIC, Australia

Salvatore Grisanti, MD Department of Ophthalmology, University of Lübeck, Lübeck, Schleswig-Holstein, Germany

Robyn H. Guymer, MBBS, PhD, FRANZCO Department of Ophthalmology, Centre for Eye Research Australia, Royal Victorian Eye and Ear Hospital, University of Melbourne, East Melbourne, VIC, Australia

Ann Hellström, MD, PhD Department of Ophthalmology, Institute of Neuroscience and Physiology, The Queen Silvia Children's Hospital, The Sahlgrenska Academy at University of Gothenburg, Gothenburg, Sweden

Frank G. Holz, MD Department of Ophthalmology, University of Bonn, Bonn, Germany

Deniz Hos, MD Department of Ophthalmology, University of Cologne, Cologne, Cologne, Germany

Peter Charbel Issa, MD, DPhil Department of Ophthalmology, University of Bonn, Bonn, Germany

Bernd Junker, MD Hannover Medical School, University Eye Hospital, Hannover, Germany

Tim U. Krohne, MD, FEBO Department of Ophthalmology, University of Bonn, Bonn, Germany

Clemens Lange, MD, PhD Eye Center, University Hospital Freiburg, Freiburg, Germany

Chi-Hsiu Liu, PhD Department of Ophthalmology, Boston Children's Hospital, Harvard Medical School, Boston, MA, USA

Julia Lüke, MD, PD Department of Ophthalmology, University of Lübeck, Lübeck, Schleswig-Holstein, Germany

Matthias Lüke, MD, PD Department of Ophthalmology, University of Lübeck, Lübeck, Schleswig-Holstein, Germany

Carsten H. Meyer, MD, FEBO, FMH Department of Ophthalmology, Pallas Clinic, Aargau, Switzerland

Amelie Pielen, MD Hannover Medical School, University Eye Hospital, Hannover, Germany

Przemyslaw Sapieha, PhD Departments of Ophthalmology and Biochemistry, Maisonneuve-Rosemont Hospital Research Center, Maisonneuve-Rosemont Hospital, University of Montreal, Montreal, QC, Canada

Lois E.H. Smith, MD, PhD Department of Ophthalmology, Harvard Medical School, Boston Children's Hospital, Boston, MA, USA

Andreas Stahl, MD Eye Center at the Medical Center, University of Freiburg, Freiburg, Germany

David J. Valent, DO National Institutes of Health, National Eye Institute, Bethesda, MD, USA

Focke Ziemssen, MD Center for Ophthalmology, Eberhard-Karl University Tübingen, Tübingen, Germany

Retinal Vascular Development

Jing Chen, Chi-Hsiu Liu, and Przemyslaw Sapieha

1.1 Anatomy of Blood Vessel Networks in the Eye

To aid in understanding retinal vascular development, we will first describe the origins of ocular blood vessels. The orbital vascular anatomy is highly complex in human. The ophthalmic artery, the first major branch of the internal carotid artery, is the main source of the arterial supply to the orbit and its derived arterial structures. It passes beneath the optic nerve and accompanies the nerve through the optic canal into the inner wall of the orbit. The central retinal artery, the first branch of the ophthalmic artery, pierces the optic nerve sheath inferiorly about 8–15 mm (in humans) behind the globe, and occupies a central position within the optic nerve when entering the retina. Other branches of ophthalmic artery, including the poste-

rior ciliary arteries, serve the optic nerve head, choroid, ciliary body, and iris (Gray 2008; Paul Riordan-Eva 2011; Hayreh 2006).

1.1.1 Retinal Vessels

The retina is one of the most structurally intricate and metabolically active tissues in the body. It receives its blood supply from two sources: (1) the central retinal artery and its three branched plexi, which supplies the inner two-thirds of the retina; and (2) the choriocapillaris (choriocapillary layer) adjacent to the Bruch's membrane which supplies the outer retina. The central retinal artery and its accompanying vein run along the inferior margin of the optic nerve sheath and enter the eye through the optic disk. The vessel branches then immediately bifurcate into the superior nasal and temporal, or the inferior nasal and temporal branches, each supplying a distinct quadrant of the retina. The branching pattern of the vessels is either dichotomous or at right angles to the original vessel (Gray 2008; Paul Riordan-Eva 2011; Netter 2006). Branches from the central retinal artery then dive into the retina towards photoreceptors forming a capillary plexus which provides nutrients to the inner retinal layers. The overall structure of retinal vessels is composed of three distinct capillary layers, one in the nerve fiber layer and the other two along each sides of the inner nuclear layer (Fig. 1.1).

J. Chen (✉) • C.-H. Liu
Department of Ophthalmology, Boston Children's Hospital, Harvard Medical School, 300 Longwood Avenue, Boston, Boston, MA 02115, USA
e-mail: Jing.Chen@childrens.harvard.edu; Chi-Hsiu.Liu@childrens.harvard.edu

P. Sapieha
Departments of Ophthalmology and Biochemistry, Maisonneuve-Rosemont Hospital Research Centre, Maisonneuve-Rosemont Hospital, University of Montreal, 5415 Assomption Boulvard, Montreal, QC, Canada, H1T 2M4
e-mail: Mike.Sapieha@umontreal.ca

© Springer International Publishing Switzerland 2016
A. Stahl (ed.), *Anti-Angiogenic Therapy in Ophthalmology*, Essentials in Ophthalmology, DOI 10.1007/978-3-319-24097-8_1

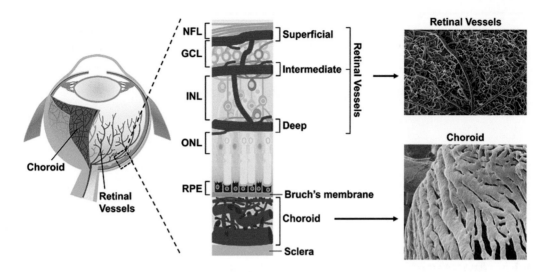

Fig. 1.1 A schematic illustration of the ocular vasculature. *Left*: A schematic cross-section through an eye showing the retinal vasculature lining the inner surface of the retina and the choroid vessels. *Right*: An enlarged cross-sectional illustration of the eye showing detailed structure of the retinal and choroidal vasculature. Three layers of retinal vessels are embedded among retinal neurons: the superficial retinal vasculature lies in the NFL; the intermediate and deep retinal vascular networks align along each sides of the INL. The choroidal vessels between RPE and sclera serve to supply blood to the outer portion of the retina. *GCL* ganglion cell layer, *INL* inner nuclear layer, *NFL* nerve fiber layer, *ONL* outer nuclear layer, *RPE* retinal pigment epithelium. Enlarged images on the *right* depict retinal and choroidal vascular cast from mouse eyes

Retinal vessels have a non-fenestrated endothelium forming the inner blood–retinal barrier. In addition, branches of the central retinal artery are terminal arteries that do not anastomose with each other (Gray 2008; Netter 2006). Contrary to the inner retinal layers, the photoreceptor layer is avascular without blood vessels from the central retinal artery. Thus, it relies on the choriocapillaris to supply oxygen and nutrient by diffusion from choroidal vessels.

1.1.2 Choroidal Vessels

The choroid, a thin highly vascular membrane, lies between the retina and the sclera and invests the posterior five-sixths of the globe in human. The choroid vessels originate from two groups of branches of the ophthalmic artery: (1) the short posterior ciliary arteries, which supply the posterior portion of choroid; (2) the long posterior ciliary arteries, which supply the anterior choroid, ciliary body, and iris. They are distinguished in three layers of choroidal vasculature: the innermost choriocapillaris, the intermediate Sattler's

layer, and the outermost Haller's layer (Hartnett 2013). The more outer the vessels are located in the choroid, the bigger the size of their lumens. While the outermost choroidal layer is composed mainly of small arteries and veins, the innermost choriocapillaris is characterized by an exceedingly fine capillary plexus adjacent to the Bruch's membrane (Fig. 1.1) (Paul Riordan-Eva 2011; Ross and Pawlina 2005). In humans, the capillaries of the choriocapillaris are approximately 3–18 μm in diameter and oval shaped in the posterior eye, becoming gradually wider (approximately 6–36 μm in diameter) and longer (36–400 μm in length) as they move towards the equatorial region. The choriocapillaris is a sinusoidal vascular plexus with highly fenestrated endothelium, and as the site of the greatest blood flow in the body (Henkind et al. 1979), it provides 65–85 % of the blood volume in the eye. Through diffusion, it nourishes the cells in the outer portion of the retina (Bela et al. 2011), including the retinal pigment epithelium (RPE) and photoreceptors, as well as the fovea, which contains only photoreceptors for high acuity central vision and is devoid of other retinal neurons.

Interestingly, some mammalian species such as echidnas, guinea pigs, and rabbits lack retinal vasculature, with their oxygen and nutrient supply to the retina being solely provided by diffusion from the choriocapillaris. It appears that the thickness of the retina is directly related to their evolutionary vascularization state. These avascular retinas are typically thinner than the theoretical oxygen diffusion maximum of 143 μm, whereas vascularized retinas are approximately twice as thick, yet their avascular portion are still within the oxygen diffusion limit (Chase 1982; Buttery et al. 1991; Dreher et al. 1992).

1.1.3 Hyaloidal Vessels

The hyaloid vasculature is a transient embryonic vascular bed which develops during embryonic and fetal stages to provide blood supply to the developing eye. The hyaloid artery originates from the ophthalmic artery. It enters the embryonic fissure and extends through the vitreous to the lens. In the developing eye, the hyaloid vasculature plays an important role in many aspects. It supplies the inner part of the retina with oxygen and nutrients; it is also involved in the development and maturation of the lens and makes up the primary vitreous (Hartnett 2013; Fruttiger 2007). During human fetal development, the hyaloid vasculature is first seen at the fourth week of gestation and reaches its maximum prominence during the ninth week. During mid-gestation, the hyaloid vasculature regresses and the retinal vasculature contemporaneously develops. Regression of the hyaloid artery leaves a central extension from the optic disk to the posterior lens surface, called the hyaloid canal or Cloquet's canal (Hartnett 2013).

1.2 Development of Retinal Vasculature

Among the three vascular beds in the eye, the retinal vasculature is the most extensively studied. The development of the retinal vasculature has served as an excellent model for elucidating the mechanisms of vascular development, remod-

eling, and maturation. Studies on retinal vasculature over the past several decades have greatly expanded our understanding of the fundamental processes governing normal and pathologic vascularization including the relationship between hypoxia and vessel growth, as well as the contribution of neurovascular interaction in vascular homeostasis.

1.2.1 Angiogenesis Is the Dominant Process in Retinal Vascular Development

Blood vessels are generally composed of several distinct cell layers with a single layer of endothelial cells forming the lumen in the innermost part of the vessel. In large macrovessels such as aortae, the inner endothelial cell layer is covered by a central layer of mural cells/smooth muscle cells, and usually an external layer consisting of connective tissue lined with small vessels and nerves. In microvessels and capillaries, which constitute most of the retinal vessels, the endothelial cell layer is covered externally by a noncontiguous single layer of pericytes/mural cells, allowing close interaction of vascular endothelial cells with surrounding neurons, glia, and inflammatory cells to coordinate the process of vascular growth, remodeling, and repair.

The developmental vascularization process in the retina is mediated primarily via angiogenesis (Fruttiger 2002), similarly as some other tissues such as the kidney and the brain. In angiogenesis, vascular endothelial cells sprout and proliferate from preexisting blood vessels, usually venules, and develop into new vessels with fully functional lumen. During this process, local increases in growth factors destabilize a portion of the preexisting vessels, allowing the activation of pericytes and remodeling of extracellular matrix. Endothelial cell migration and proliferation subsequently occurs to form new vessels. Angiogenesis is also considered the dominant process governing new blood vessel growth during the wound healing process and in pathologic retinal vessel growth such as in tumors and retinopathies (Saint-Geniez and D'Amore 2004).

This mechanism of angiogenic development is in contrast with vasculogenesis where dispersed primitive vascular precursor cells or hemangioblasts cluster together and form into tube-like endothelial structures, in the absence of existing vessels. Vasculogenesis occurs during the embryonic development of the circulatory system and gives rise to the heart and the first primitive vascular plexus such as the yolk sac circulation. It was suggested that the very initial process of vascular development in the retina results from vasculogenesis from resident angioblasts (McLeod et al. 2006), then angiogenesis becomes dominant to form the rest of retinal vasculature. Yet with increasing evidences of circulating endothelial precursor cells from bone marrow modifying developing and injured retinal blood vessels (Grant et al. 2002; Sengupta et al. 2003; Dorrell et al. 2004), the precise distinction between angiogenesis and vasculogenesis is becoming blurry.

1.2.2 Temporal and Spatial Development of Three Layers of Retinal Vasculature

In humans, retinal vascularization starts in utero at about 16 weeks of gestational age and is completed at approximately 40 weeks of gestation, right before birth. Developmental retinal vascularization occurs concurrently as the hyaloid vessels regress. The retina is vascularized first in the most superficial (i.e., innermost) layer on the vitreous side, starting from the optic nerve head and then progressing centrifugally outwards towards the ora serrata, the peripheral edge of the retina. This superficial primary plexus reaches the nasal side of the ora serrata at about 36 weeks gestational age, and the temporal retina at approximately 40 weeks gestational age. As the superficial layer is nearing completion, retinal vessels dive into the retina to form first a deep and then an intermediate layer along with a well-organized network of inter-connecting vessels to complete three vascular layers: a superficial vascular layer which lies in the inner part of the nerve fiber layer, an intermediate

layer in the inner plexiform layer, and a deep layer in the outer plexiform layer (Dorrell et al. 2002) (Fig. 1.1).

In other mammals such as primates and rodents, the conserved pattern of three retinal vascular layers forms over varying timescales (Gariano and Gardner 2005). In mice, one of the most studied model systems of retinal vascular development, the superficial vascular plexus starts to develop during the first week after birth, with radial growth as seen similarly in humans (Fig. 1.2). During the second week, angiogenic sprouts start to form from the superficial layer and grow perpendicular to the primary vascular plexus into the retina to create two deeper layers of capillary networks. A complete vascular system is formed by the end of three weeks after birth (Stahl et al. 2010a). Studies in the mouse retina have shed light on the cross talk among multiple cell types that function together to direct vascular growth in the retina, and identified the important roles of oxygen and oxygen-mediated growth factors in this process.

1.2.3 Oxygen and VEGF in Retinal Vascular Development

1.2.3.1 Lack of Oxygen Drives Blood Vessel Growth in the Eye

A hypothesized role of oxygen in retinal vascular development originates from early observations that capillaries grow more profusely near venules than around arteries (Michaelson 1948; Ashton 1966; Wise 1961). Observed retinal vascular patterns from some eye diseases also support this notion. In retinopathy of prematurity and diabetic retinopathy, an initial lack of retinal vessels with resulting retinal ischemia precedes pathologic vessel growth, supporting the idea of hypoxia as a critical stimulator of new blood vessel growth (Gariano and Gardner 2005). During development, as retinal neurons and glial cells differentiate and mature, their metabolic demands increase, creating a radial wave of hypothesized "physiologic hypoxia" that leads the development of new vessels from the center towards the periphery of the retina (Chan-Ling et al. 1995) (Fig. 1.2).

Development of superficial vascular plexus in mice

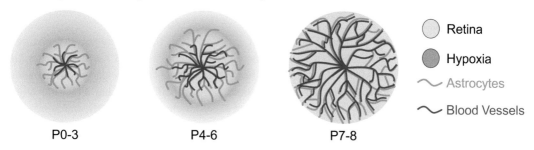

Development of intermediate and deep vascular layers in mice

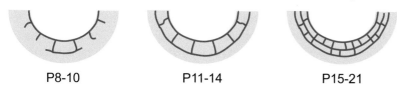

Fig. 1.2 A schematic illustration of the retinal vascular development in mice. *Top panel*: A scheme of retinal vascular growth that originates from the optic nerve head after birth and grows radially towards the peripheral of the retina, and reaches the edge of the retina around postnatal day (P) 8. The growth of the superficial vascular plexus of retinal vessels (*red*) follows a hypothesized physiologic hypoxia wave (*blue*) and an astro-cytic template (*green*). *Bottom panel*: After completion of the superficial vascular layer, blood vessels dive down towards the outer retina during the second week after birth, forming a deeper layer of vessels first, and an intermediate vascular layer last. The whole retinal vascular growth process is completed approximately three weeks after birth in mice. In humans, this process occurs prenatally during in utero development

After new vessels have formed, bringing oxygen and alleviating hypoxia, the vascular growth continues radially towards the peripheral retina.

1.2.3.2 VEGF Is A Dominant Growth Factor Governing Retinal Vascular Growth

The effect of oxygen on vascular growth is mediated in large part by vascular endothelial growth factor (VEGF), a hypoxia-induced growth factor. VEGF is expressed in the developing retina in a pattern that coincides with retinal blood vessel development both temporally and spatially (Stone et al. 1995; Pierce et al. 1995, 1996). VEGF and other hypoxia-induced growth factors are induced through the transcription factor hypoxia-inducible factor (HIF), a global regulator of O_2 homeostasis (Wang et al. 1995; Wang and Semenza 1993a, b), composed of an oxygen-sensitive α unit and a constitutively expressed transcription activating β subunit.

Under normoxic conditions, HIF1α or HIF2α are hydroxylated on a proline residue by the prolyl hydroxylases, enabling its interaction with von Hippel–Lindau protein, resulting in its ubiquitylation and proteasomal degradation (Jaakkola et al. 2001; Ohh et al. 2000; Epstein et al. 2001). Under hypoxic conditions, HIF1α or HIF2α escapes prolyl hydroxylation and interacts with HIF1β to form a heterodimer, which then translocates to the nucleus and activates target genes such as VEGF by binding to a hypoxia-responsive element in their promoter region (Wang et al. 1995). While a gradient of VEGF is found preceding the superficial vascular plexus in the retina, it is also postulated that the relative hypoxia of the deeper retinal layers during development also results in a VEGF gradient that favors sprouting from the superficial layer downwards, resulting in the formation of first the deep and then the intermediate layers of capillary networks (Stone et al. 1995; Pierce et al. 1995).

In addition to VEGF, erythropoietin (Epo) is another hypoxia-induced growth factor that plays an important role during retinal blood vessel homeostasis (Chen et al. 2008, 2009; Watanabe et al. 2005). As a growth hormone that is best known for its role in stimulating erythropoiesis, Epo also has potent neuroprotective and pro-angiogenic effects (Caprara and Grimm 2012), and was suggested important for the formation of the intermediate plexus of retina vessels in an HIF-dependent manner (Caprara et al. 2011). In the vitreous of patients with diabetic retinopathy (Watanabe et al. 2005; Katsura et al. 2005), retinopathy of prematurity (Sato et al. 2009) or retinal vein occlusion (Stahl et al. 2010b), Epo is upregulated along with VEGF. These oxygen-regulated hypoxia-responsive factors are therefore considered as some of the master regulators of both normal retinal vessel development and proliferative retinopathies (Stone et al. 1995; Aiello et al. 1995; Smith et al. 1997).

Besides these hypoxia-regulated growth factors, some other non-oxygen-regulated growth factors are also important for retinal vascular development, in part through modulation of the VEGF response. For example, the Tie1–Tie2 receptors are related tyrosine kinase receptors selectively expressed on vascular endothelial cells and required for embryonic vascular development (Dumont et al. 1994; Sato et al. 1995). Angiopoietin2, a Tie2 ligand, promotes retinal angiogenesis through increasing sensitivity to the angiogenic effects of VEGF in retinal vessels (Hackett et al. 2002; Oshima et al. 2004), and the balance between the counteracting effects of angiopoietin1 and angiopoietin2 dictates the consequent vascular response. In addition, the significant role of insulin-like growth factor-1 (IGF-1) in retinal vascular development was supported by the finding that IGF-1 is required for maximum VEGF activation of vascular endothelial cell proliferation and survival pathways (Smith et al. 1997, 1999). In premature infants, low IGF-1 levels are associated with an increased risk of retinopathy of prematurity (Hellstrom et al. 2001, 2002, 2003; Smith 2005; Lofqvist et al. 2006), characterized by slowed, deficient development of retinal vessels in its initial stage.

1.2.3.3 Retinal Neuroglia Serves as the Template of Retinal Vascular Growth

In order to form the stereotyped and precisely organized pattern of retinal vasculature, the diffused gradients of oxygen and hypoxia alone would be insufficient. Striking structural alignment exists among retinal vessels, astrocytes, and neurons (Fig. 1.3a), suggesting the contribution of cellular guidance mechanisms during retinal angiogenesis. Astrocytes are a type of glial cells formed from precursor cells that migrated into the retina from the optic nerve head during embryonic development (Chu et al. 2001), prior to the formation of retinal blood vessels. Astrocyte growth in the retina follows the radially oriented ganglion cell axons (Dorrell et al. 2002; Gariano et al. 1996), which synthesize platelet-derived growth factor (PDGF) to stimulate the growth and alignment of astrocytes (Fruttiger et al. 1996), that express PDGF receptor alpha (PDGFR-α). A complex interconnected astrocytic network forms at the inner surface of the retina after birth just preceding the vessels. The spatially and temporally overlapping pattern of astrocyte network preceding vascular growth led to the hypothesis that astrocytes secrete VEGF and other growth factors to guide the filopodia of sprouting endothelial cells towards the right direction in an R-cadherin-dependent manner (Dorrell et al. 2002; Gariano et al. 1996; Watanabe and Raff 1988; Gerhardt et al. 2003) (Fig. 1.3b). However, some recent findings challenge this indispensable role of astrocytes in retinal vascular development (Weidemann et al. 2010; Scott et al. 2010), suggesting that astrocytic VEGF is perhaps more critical for vascular maintenance in pathologic conditions. This indicates the possibility that other cells surrounding blood vessels, such as retinal neurons and inflammatory cells, may also be crucial in governing retinal vascular development. Both cell types are capable of secreting angiogenic factors including VEGF and will be discussed in the next sections.

1.2.3.4 Dynamics of Vascular Growth

As described above, retinal vessels elaborate their networks throughout the retina by angio-

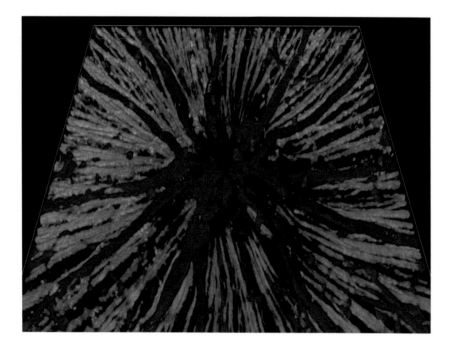

a

b

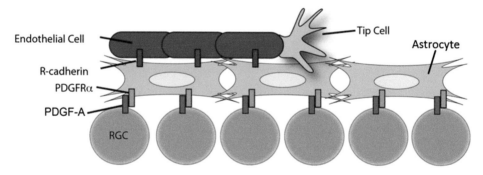

Endothelial Cell

Tip Cell

Astrocyte

R-cadherin

PDGFRα

PDGF-A

RGC

Fig. 1.3 Structural alignment of retinal neuroglia and vessels. (a) Three-dimensional reconstruction of an adult mouse retinal flatmount. The image depicts the inner retinal vascular plexus (*red*; stained with Isolectin B4) interwoven with retinal ganglion neurons and their axons (*green*; stained with β-III tubulin). (b) Model of vascular growth during retinal development. Astrocytes, express platelet-derived growth factor alpha-receptor (PDGFR-α) and invade the developing retina from the optic nerve head, ahead of the vascular front. They travel on top of PDGF-α-expressing retinal ganglion cells (RGCs). Nascent vessels follow the astrocytic template and form R-cadherin junctions with proximal astrocytes. Adapted from Sapieha, Blood, 2012

genesis, a coordinated process involving endothelial cell proliferation, migration, and assembly into tube-like structures containing a lumen (Provis et al. 1997; Dorrell and Friedlander 2006). Typically, vessel growth is stimulated by angiogenic factors such as VEGF, fibroblast growth factors, angiopoietin2, and/or other chemokines, through a process modulated in part by microglia (Fantin et al. 2010; Rymo et al. 2011). As a consequence of angiogenic signaling, angiopoietin2 stimulates pericyte detachment from the vessel walls, leading to basement membrane degradation by matrix metalloproteinases (MMPs). Endothelial cells then slacken their VE-cadherin

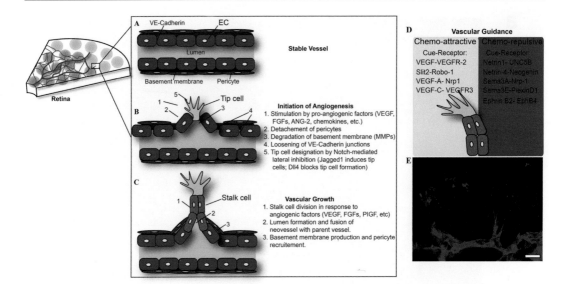

Fig. 1.4 Graphic depiction of the cellular mechanisms governing retinal angiogenesis. (**a**) A stable, quiescent vessel with aligned endothelial cells (ECs), united by VE-cadherin-rich junctions, and covered by pericytes. (**b**) Upon stimulation by angiogenic factors, a cascade of events ensues leading to pericyte detachment, basement membrane degradation and endothelial junction loosening. Determination of stalk versus tip cell phenotypes is achieved through Notch-dependent signaling. VEGF through VEGFR2 induces the Notch ligand Dll4 on tip cells which subsequently activates Notch in adjacent endothelial cells and specifies their stalk cell phenotype. Conversely, the Notch ligand Jagged1 is highly expressed by stalk cells and antagonizes Dll4. This promotes VEGFR2 expression and renders ECs more responsive to VEGF and thus more susceptible to form tip cells. (**c**) Once the vessel has sprouted, stalk cells behind the tip cell divide and assemble to form the lumen of the neovessel. Pericytes are then recruited and basement membrane is laid down. (**d**) To reach its final destination, the growing neovessel must navigate through the tissue by responding to a series of diffusible and membrane-bound attractive and repellent guidance cues. (**e**) Confocal image of sprouting retinal vessels with filopodia-rich tip cells (stained with isolectin B4) from P4 mouse retinas. Scale bar: 10 μm. Adapted from Sapieha, Blood, 2012

and claudin-rich junctions and a leading tip cell protrudes and advances towards the attractant angiogenic gradients (reviewed in (Carmeliet and Jain 2011)) (Fig. 1.4a–c).

Growth of nascent blood vessels occurs via the advancement of leader tip cells (Gerhardt et al. 2003), with the leading tip position sometimes shared by several endothelial cells. Endothelial tip cells, which are induced by VEGF, are non-mitotic and enriched in both receptors for angiogenic factor (such as VEGFR) and other receptors that were initially described to respond to neuronal guidance cues (Huber et al. 2003). The physiological role of tip cells is to probe the tissue environment through their projecting filopodias and guide the nascent vessel towards growth factor gradients or guidance cues to its appropriate final destination. These neuro-

nal guidance receptors include the neuropilins and plexins (for semaphorins), Unc5b, neogenin and DCC (for netrins), the Eph receptors (for ephrins), and roundabouts (for slits) (Adams et al. 1999; Klagsbrun and Eichmann 2005; Wilson et al. 2006) (Fig. 1.4d–e). Once the tip cells come in contact with a given cue, they will respond by either advancing, stalling, turning, or retracting depending on which cell surface receptor predominates and the overall intracellular environment of the tip cells (Larrivee et al. 2009). The role of neuronal guidance cues in vascular growth has been comprehensively reviewed (Larrivee et al. 2009; Carmeliet and Tessier-Lavigne 2005; De Smet et al. 2009; Gelfand et al. 2009). Conversely, the stalk cells, stimulated by Dll4/Jagged1/Notch-mediated later cellular inhibition (Hellstrom et al. 2007; Benedito et al.

2009), are located behind tip cells in the wake of the vascular front, and divide in response to VEGF to form a lumen.

1.2.4 Neurovascular Cross Talk in Retinal Vascular Development

The retina is the most metabolically active tissue of the body, per weight. It is also the most external and accessible portion of the central nervous system (CNS). Central neurons such as those that populate the retina require a steady supply of nutrients and oxygen to ensure appropriate neuronal function and sensory transmission. Consequently, nervous and vascular systems must be adequately paired. In recent years, it has become clear that neurons play an important role in instigating, promoting, and steering angiogenesis within nervous tissue and specifically in the retina (Edwards et al. 2011; Fukushima et al. 2011; Kim et al. 2011; Nakamura-Ishizu et al. 2012; Sapieha et al. 2008).

1.2.4.1 Influence of Retinal Ganglion Cells on Vascular Growth

There is a current debate on whether astrocytes or alternatively, retinal neurons such as retinal ganglion cells are primary drivers of retinal developmental vascular growth, since evidence has been provided for both. One possible interpretation to reconcile the contribution of both cell populations during retinal vascular plexus formation suggests astrocytes contribute to trophic support of vessels through providing a template for growth (Fruttiger et al. 1996; Gerhardt et al. 2003; Uemura et al. 2006) as described above, while retinal neurons may drive vascular growth to ensure their own metabolic support (Sapieha 2012). This view is supported by findings in the human fetus during the formation of the outer vascular plexus of the retina at 25–26 weeks of gestation (Hughes et al. 2000). Interestingly, this time frame coincides with the first appearance of visually evoked potentials and thus functional neurons (Dreher and Robinson 1988) and likely reflects an increase in oxygen consumption and

metabolic activity from the newly operating neurons and their need for fuel (Cringle et al. 2006). In addition, cell-specific ablation of VEGF, HIF-1α, or HIF-2α in astrocytes has no overt defects on developmental retinal vascularization (Weidemann et al. 2010; Scott et al. 2010), while neuroretinal-specific knockout of HIF-1α substantially perturbs retinal vascular development (Caprara et al. 2011; Nakamura-Ishizu et al. 2012) suggesting that a neuronal cell population, rather than astrocytes, likely provides angiogenic factors during retinal development. One such neuronal cell population is retinal ganglion cells (RGCs). Among retinal neuron cell types, RGCs are the most anatomically coupled with the superficial retinal vascular plexus. A specific role for RGCs in vascular development was established using mouse models of genetic ablation of RGCs (Edwards et al. 2011; Sapieha et al. 2008). In transgenic mice which express a toxin in newly formed RGCs and hence eliminate RGCs as they form (Mu et al. 2005), astrocytic networks remain largely intact, yet these mice are completely devoid of a retinal vascular plexus and show persistent hyaloid vasculature (Sapieha et al. 2008). Similarly, *Math 5$^{-/-}$* mice which lack 95 % of RGCs do not form a functional retinal vascular layer (Edwards et al. 2011).

1.2.4.2 Photoreceptors and Retinal Vascular Growth

In addition to RGCs, photoreceptors may also play a significant role in determining retinal energy demand and hence influence vascular growth. Photoreceptors are the most abundant neuronal cell population in the retina and also require very high rates of oxygenation (Wangsa-Wirawan and Linsenmeier 2003). While the direct impact of photoreceptors on retinal vascular development is unclear given their contemporaneous maturation and migration towards the outer retina during retinal vascular formation, evidence for a role of photoreceptor in vascular maintenance comes directly from clinical observations. Patients suffering from both proliferative diabetic retinopathy and retinitis pigmentosa with progressive photoreceptors loss show considerably less pathological retinal angiogenesis than diabetic patients with healthy photoreceptors (Sternberg et al. 1984). Furthermore, preretinal neovascularization associated with late-stage diabetes mellitus has been reported to spontaneously regress with the onset of retinitis pigmentosa (Lahdenranta et al. 2001). Similarly, mice with genetically ablated photoreceptors failed to mount reactive retinal neovascularization in a model of oxygen-induced proliferative retinopathy (Lahdenranta et al. 2001), and diabetic mice that had photoreceptor degeneration showed lower levels of retinal pro-angiogenic VEGF (de Gooyer et al. 2006). These observations likely stem from the high energetic requirements of photoreceptor neurons (Linsenmeier and Padnick-Silver 2000) and hence loss of photoreceptors substantially reduces the energy demand of the retina, reducing the stimuli for angiogenic factors and consequent pathologic neovascularization.

1.2.4.3 Neuronal Energy Metabolism May Underlie Retinal Angiogenesis

One potential mechanism by which the energy status in retinal neuron may modulate vascular network development is likely evolutionarily conserved and directly employs intermediates of energy metabolism, such as those from glucose, the main energy source of CNS including retinas. By activating cognate G-protein-coupled receptors, energy metabolites such as lactate (Ahmed et al. 2010), α-ketoglutarate and succinate (He et al. 2004) have documented physiological roles beyond ATP production. In this regard, cellular signaling events triggered via energy metabolites in response to a compromised energy status in retinal neurons have been proposed as a contributor to both physiological and pathological retinal vascularization (Sapieha et al. 2008; Grant et al. 1999, 2001; Mino et al. 2001). This concept has been elucidated for the Krebs cycle intermediate succinate and its receptor GPR91 (Sapieha et al. 2008). Succinate accumulates under conditions of hypoxic stress by a mechanism involving feedback inhibition of succinate dehydrogenase by nonoxidized flavin and nicotinamide nucleotides and by reactive oxygen species (Gutman et al. 1980; Meixner-

Monori et al. 1985). When succinate levels rise, they activate GPR91 with a half-maximal response of 28–25 μM (He et al. 2004) and prompt release of VEGF and angiopoietins 1 and 2. When succinate levels rise substantially, they can stabilize HIF with a K_i between 350 and 460 μM, further promoting secretion of HIF-dependent angiogenic growth factors. Together this suggests that the succinate-GPR91 axis can act as an early sensor of hypoxic stress and work to enhance regional circulation, and once hypoxia is sustained, succinate levels rise further and stabilize HIF, which then activates a collection of pathways to non-discriminately provoke angiogenesis.

Another potential pathway that retinal neurons may employ to reinstate local circulation is via the metabolically regulated protein deacetylase sirtuin-1 (Sirt-1). Sirt1 is an NAD$^+$-dependent protein deacetylase critical for neuronal function in the CNS (Michan 2013; Michan et al. 2010), and can be activated under stress condition to regulate cell cycle and longevity (Brunet et al. 2004). When retinal ganglion neurons sense tissue ischemia and hypoxia such as during an ischemic retinopathy, they induce increased levels of Sirt1 (Chen et al. 2013). In mice with neuronal deficiency of Sirt1, the reparative angiogenesis that takes place during the mouse model of ischemic retinopathies is significantly attenuated. These effects are likely mediated through Sirt1-mediated deacetylation of HIF which helps maintain elevated levels of HIF and its consequent reparative angiogenic growth factors (Chen et al. 2013). Together, these studies, underscore the propensity of retinal neurons to govern their vascular environment and reciprocally regulate their metabolic supply.

1.2.5 Immune Influence on Retinal Vessel Development

As blood vessels develop throughout the inner retina, they are accompanied by microglia, the primary resident immune cells of the retina (Fig. 1.5). Microglia are myeloid-derived tissue macrophages of the CNS which populate the

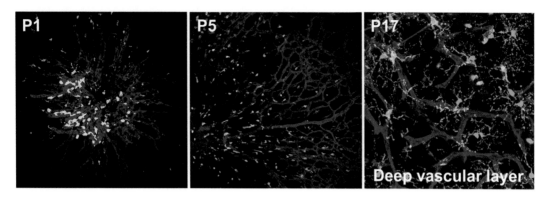

Fig. 1.5 Microglia and retinal vascular development. Immunohistochemistry on developing mouse retinas demonstrates that microglial cells (stained in *green*) are associated with nascent vasculature. This relationship between vessels (stained in *red*) and microglia lasts throughout development of the various vascular layers that make up the retina. *P* postnatal day

mammalian retina before it becomes vascularized and become activated in response to injury (Dejda et al. 2014). Retinal microglia are rapidly activated after an inflammatory insult (Santos et al. 2008; Chen et al. 2002), yet during development, there is increasing evidence that they associate with growing vessels and play a key role in promoting normal vascularization.

Evidence for the major contribution of microglia to retinal vascular growth is severalfold. Microglia associate directly with nascent vessels at the vascular front and modulate angiogenesis (Checchin et al. 2006; Kubota et al. 2009; Stefater Iii et al. 2011). They are found apposed to developing vessels during human fetal development, and pharmacologic depletion of retinal microglia slowed retinal vessel development (Checchin et al. 2006). Similarly, osteopetrotic *csf-1*$^{op/op}$ mice, which harbor an inactivation mutation in the *csf-1* gene and are deficient in retinal microglia in the first week of postnatal development, show significantly sparser retinal vessel networks when compared to wild-type controls (Rymo et al. 2011). This may be partially attributed to the vascular anastomosis-promoting properties of microglia (Smith et al. 1997) and their ability to regulate vessel branching (Stefater Iii et al. 2011).

Given the inherent role of microglia in defending the retina against foreign intrusion, they may also partake in perturbing vascular development during bouts of systemic inflam-

mation in preterm infants (Tremblay et al. 2013). In this regard, neonatal sepsis is being recognized as a major risk factor for developing severe retinopathy of prematurity (Klinger et al. 2010; Tolsma et al. 2011; Lee and Dammann 2012). Experimentally induced systemic inflammation mimicking a sepsis-like state in mice provokes a profound increase in the number of activated microglia in intimate association with the nascent vascular plexuses of the retina, and leads to compromised vascular development and formation of dense, almost neovascular membrane-like structures on the retina (Tremblay et al. 2013). This aberrant vascular development leads to compromised retinal function in later life in mice as determined by electroretinograms (Tremblay et al. 2013). Hence, while required for normal stereotyped vascular development, over-activation of retinal microglia may perturb retinal angiogenesis and lead to vascular sequelae similar to those observed in patients with ROP.

1.2.6 Remodeling of Retinal Vascular Growth

Once fully formed, the superficial layer of retinal vessels is remodeled before sprouting to the deeper layer (Ishida et al. 2003) as regulated by the specific needs of the local tissue for oxygen and nutrients. Maturation and pruning of the superficial plexus leads to a less dense network with finer vessels compared to the structures formed during early development. Relative hyperoxia around arteries is considered an important factor for pruning of existing vasculature. Local hyperoxia would lead to local suppression of VEGF, which is an endothelial survival factor for immature capillaries. Reduction of VEGF leads to regression of these immature capillaries in areas with excess vasculature (Claxton and Fruttiger 2003; Alon et al. 1995). Leukocytes from the circulation also participate in vessel remodeling through induction of endothelial cell apoptosis, a process considered most relevant in the context of early vessel loss in diabetic retinopathy (Ishida et al. 2003).

1.3 Development of Choroid and Hyaloid Vessels

1.3.1 Choroidal Development

In humans, a definitive choriocapillaris layer appears at around 8–12 weeks of gestational age, prior to the formation of retinal vessels. The primitive choroidal vascular system arises from the surrounding mesoderm during optic cup development. Following the development of RPE, this primitive choroidal vascular layer continues to expand (Saint-Geniez and D'Amore 2004), until the capillaries completely encircle the optic cup.

The mechanisms of choroidal vascular development overall are less well studied and understood than those related to the development of the retinal vasculature. Clinically, the retinal vasculature can be clearly observed funduscopically in humans, while visualization of the choroidal plexus is blocked by a dense layer of RPE. In animal models, retinal vasculature development can be easily studied due to the postnatal development of retinal vessels in rodents and advanced imaging techniques on retinal flat mounts which expose retinal vessels. In contrast, choroidal vasculature is less readily quantifiable during development. Nevertheless, the formation and

maturation of the choroidal vasculature appears to be tightly associated with signals produced by RPE cells (Zhao and Overbeek 2001). In particular, VEGF and its receptor are highly expressed by RPE cells at the time of choriocapillaris formation (Gogat et al. 2004; Yi et al. 1998), suggesting involvement of RPE-derived VEGF in the choroidal vascular development. Furthermore, in colobomas, failure of RPE differentiation results in defective development of the choroid and sclera (Torczynski 1982). In addition, in patients with exudative age-related macular degeneration, degeneration of RPE cells and associated overproduction of VEGF leads to pathological activation and sprouting of the normally quiescent choriocapillaris; all pointing towards an essential role of VEGF in mediating choroidal vessels growth during development and in pathologies.

1.3.2 Hyaloidal Regression

During early eye development, the hyaloid artery penetrates into the optic cup and extends through the vitreous to form branches which envelop the developing lens. As retinal vasculature forms, the hyaloid vessel regresses (Saint-Geniez and D'Amore 2004; Zhu et al. 2000), and eventually disappears upon completion of eye development, usually before 34 weeks of gestation in humans.

The mechanisms governing both formation and regression of hyaloid vessels are still incompletely defined. VEGF was suggested to trigger the growth of hyaloid vessels because VEGF is expressed in the portion of the lens closest to the forming vessels (Gogat et al. 2004; Mitchell et al. 1998; Shui et al. 2003). In addition, patients with VEGF-induced endothelial cell hyperplasia also have disorganized and persistent hyaloid vessels, further supporting a role of VEGF in hyaloid formation (Ash and Overbeek 2000).

Recently, an entirely different process has been uncovered for hyaloid regression and retinal vascular formation from studies investigating a group of rare hereditary eye diseases: Norrie disease and familial exudative vitreoretinopathy

(FEVR). A common feature in these diseases is that hyaloid vasculature fails to regress, resulting in persistent fetal vasculature. This is associated with incomplete formation of retinal vasculature with a lack of deep retinal plexus growth (Rehm et al. 2002), as well as a poorly developed neural retina and impaired vision. These genetic diseases arise from a number of mutations in an interrelated Wnt/β-catenin signaling pathway: Wnt ligands Norrin or Wnt receptors Frizzled4 and Lrp5. These works suggest a critical role for Wnt signaling in hyaloid regression in part through macrophage-mediated endothelial cell apoptosis (Xu et al. 2004; Niehrs 2004; Lobov et al. 2005). Yet development of retinal vessels also depends in part on Wnt signaling as lack of Wnt activation results in delayed development of primary vascular plexus and deficient intermediate and deep layer vessel formation in the retina (Xu et al. 2004; Ye et al. 2011; Chen et al. 2011, 2012). Beyond development, a pathological role for Wnt signaling is suggested in destructive neovascular growth in retinopathies (Chen et al. 2011; Ohlmann et al. 2010). In addition, a critical role for Wnt signaling in maintaining the integrity of blood–brain barrier, and potentially blood–retinal barrier was proposed, likely through mediation of tight junction proteins (Chen et al. 2011, 2012; Liebner et al. 2008; Daneman et al. 2009; Wang et al. 2012).

1.4 Formation of Blood–Retinal Barrier

As blood vessels mature in the retina, a functional blood–retinal barrier (BRB) starts to form at 26–34 weeks gestation to prevent toxins, pathogens, and other large molecules from entering and harming the retina (Choi et al. 2007). Similar to the blood–brain barrier, the BRB is vital to preserve the integrity and function of the retina. In the outer retina, the choriocapillaris is highly fenestrated to allow blood flow beneath the basal surface of the RPE, which digests shed photoreceptor outer segments and clears other photoreceptor waste. The RPE with tight junctions on the apical surface adjacent to the photo-

receptors constitute the outer BRB to block leakage from the choroid into the retina (Fig. 1.6a). The inner BRB is formed by tight/adherens junctions among non-fenestrated retinal vascular endothelial cells and the surrounding pericytes and glia end feet (Fig. 1.6a, b). Similar to the outer BRB, the inner BRB maintains barrier integrity (Janzer and Raff 1987) to prevent leakage from retinal blood vessels.

Two types of junctions, tight and adherens junctions, maintain the proper function of BRB (Fig. 1.6c). The tight junctions are the most apically located complexes that restrict intracellular movement of solute and fluid from entering the retina between the vascular endothelial cells in inner BRB, or RPE cells in outer BRB. The three major transmembrane proteins involved in the formation of tight junctions are occludin, claudin, and junctional adhesion molecule (JAM). The extracellular domains of these transmembrane proteins cross-interact to seal the intercellular space between neighboring cells while the cytoplasmic domains of these proteins are linked to actin filaments via zonula occludens proteins (ZOs) (Ross and Pawlina 2005; Runkle and Antonetti 2011) for stable anchoring with the cytoskeleton. The more basally located adherens junctions are composed of cadherins and provide lateral adhesion between cells. The extracellular portions of cadherins interact with similar domains from the neighboring cells; on the cytoplasmic side, cadherins are bound to α, β, or γ-catenins resulting in the formation of cadherin-catenin complexes which are bound to actin filaments by vinculin (Ross and Pawlina 2005; Runkle and Antonetti 2011). Together, the tight and adherens junctions restrict the passage of molecules of a certain size through the cells to reduce permeability and maintain BRB. VEGF is considered a main inducer of vascular permeability, since it was initially identified as a vascular permeability factor (Senger et al. 1983). VEGF may promote breakdown of BRB through downregulating tight junction proteins essential for cellular adhesion (Argaw et al. 2009).

Alteration of BRB plays a crucial role in many vascular eye diseases, where breakdown of BRB can lead to exudate, hemorrhage, and

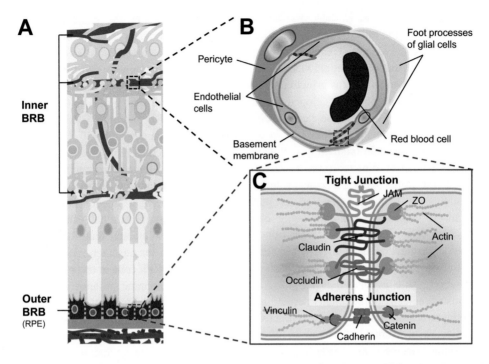

Fig. 1.6 Compositions of blood–retinal barrier (BRB). (**a**) Schematic illustration of the localization of inner and outer BRB in the eye. The inner BRB is mainly composed of retinal vascular endothelial cells (ECs) and the end feet of surrounding pericytes and glia. The outer BRB is established by retinal pigment epithelial (RPE) cells. The BRB plays a fundamental role in maintaining the specialized environment in the neural retina. (**b**) A magnified view showing detailed composition of the inner BRB. The retinal vascular ECs with junction complexes between neighboring ECs form the main structure of the inner BRB, resting on the basement membrane which is surrounded by pericytes and Müller glial cell foot processes. (**c**) An overview of the junction complexes between endothelial cells in the inner BRB, or between RPE cells in the outer BRB. The apical side illustrates the tight junction, including junction adhesion molecules (JAMs), occludin, and claudin, all transmembrane proteins with their extracellular domains on adjacent cells joining each other to form a sealing barrier. The intracellular domain of these tight junction molecules are complexed to the scaffolding adaptor protein zonula occludens (ZO), which is in turn anchored to the actin cytoskeleton. The adherens junction, usually on the more basal side than tight junctions, is mainly composed of cadherin, transmembrane proteins that form dimers on adjacent cells. Cadherin is partnered with α, β, or γ-catenins, the complex of which is again connected to the actin cytoskeleton network via vinculin

retinal detachment. The inner BRB is compromised in diabetic retinopathy, leading to retinal edema and often severe visual impairment. In exudative age-related macular degeneration, in contrast, it is the outer BRB that is compromised when choroidal blood vessels (fenestrated without tight junctions) grow through Bruch's membrane and into the subretinal space, breaking through the RPE's outer BRB. Increased levels of vitreous VEGF in both diseases may play a significant role in inducing vascular permeability in these conditions. Retinal vein occlusion, another common retinal vascular disease, is also associated with plasma leakage and hemorrhage in its initial stage due to increased intraluminal pressure in the obstructed vein; and in later stages due to VEGF-induced proliferation of leaky neovessels and VEGF-induced increased permeability of normal vessels.

While breakdown of the BRB poses a significant problem in eye diseases, on the other hand, the presence of BRB also represents a unique challenge in ocular drug delivery, as it blocks systemic delivery of large molecular therapeutic agents to the eye. Identifying ways to modulate BRB both ways will promote not only better treatment of ocular vascular leakage but also discovery of new methods for improved ocular drug delivery.

1.5 Summary

In summary, studies conducted over the last several decades on retinal vascular development have uncovered important insights into the fundamental cellular and molecular processes that govern blood vessel growth in the eye. These discoveries provided the much needed basis for understanding the pathogenesis of neovascular eye diseases and the development of antiangiogenic therapies. In particular, identification of the role of VEGF in retinal vascular development greatly facilitated the development of the first pharmacological treatment for exudative age-related macular degeneration—anti-VEGF therapy. Currently, there are many active areas of research on retinal vascular development and pathologic ocular angiogenesis, which will continue to expand our knowledge on the roles of cellular interaction within the eye and the signaling pathways and cellular mechanisms involved. Moreover, there is increasing interest towards exploring the impact of cellular energy metabolism, both in endothelial cells (De Bock et al. 2013) and in retinal neurons, as one of the fundamental driving forces of vascular growth. Repercussions of elucidating neurovascular energetics within the eye may have broad implications for a range of neurodegenerative diseases beyond the retina. In addition, valuable biological insights can be gained through studies of rare inherited vascular eye diseases with defective retinal vascular development, which may also generate important implication for other more prevalent vascular eye disorders such as ROP, diabetic retinopathy, and age-related macular degeneration. Together, these ongoing and future studies will provide new directions in the development of novel antiangiogenic or angiomodulatory therapies to prevent or treat pathologic ocular angiogenesis and the breakdown of the blood–retinal barrier that is central to vision loss in children and adults.

Compliance with Ethical Requirements

No human studies were carried out by the authors for this article. For animal studies, all institutional and national guidelines for the care and use of laboratory animals were followed. The authors received research grants from NIH/NEI (R01 EY024963), BrightFocus Foundation, Boston Children's Hospital (BCH) Ophthalmology Foundation, BCH career development award, Mass Lions Eye Research Fund Inc., and Alcon Research Institute (J.C.). The authors declare no conflict of interest.

References

Adams RH, et al. Roles of ephrinB ligands and EphB receptors in cardiovascular development: demarcation of arterial/venous domains, vascular morphogenesis, and sprouting angiogenesis. Genes Dev. 1999;13: 295–306.

Ahmed K, et al. An autocrine lactate loop mediates insulin-dependent inhibition of lipolysis through GPR81. Cell Metab. 2010;11:311–9.

Aiello LP, et al. Suppression of retinal neovascularization in vivo by inhibition of vascular endothelial growth factor (VEGF) using soluble VEGF-receptor chimeric proteins. Proc Natl Acad Sci U S A. 1995;92: 10457–61.

Alon T, et al. Vascular endothelial growth factor acts as a survival factor for newly formed retinal vessels and has implications for retinopathy of prematurity. Nat Med. 1995;1:1024–8.

Argaw AT, Gurfein BT, Zhang Y, Zameer A, John GR. VEGF-mediated disruption of endothelial CLN-5 promotes blood-brain barrier breakdown. Proc Natl Acad Sci U S A. 2009;106:1977–82.

Ash JD, Overbeek PA. Lens-specific VEGF-A expression induces angioblast migration and proliferation and stimulates angiogenic remodeling. Dev Biol. 2000;223:383–98.

Ashton N. Oxygen and the growth and development of retinal vessels. In vivo and in vitro studies The XX Francis I Proctor Lecture. Am J Ophthalmol. 1966; 62:412–35.

Bela Anand-Apte JGH. Developmental anatomy of the retinal and choroidal vasculature. In: Joseph Besharse DB, editor. The retina and its disorders. Oxford: Academic Press; 2011.

Benedito R, et al. The notch ligands Dll4 and Jagged1 have opposing effects on angiogenesis. Cell. 2009; 137:1124–35.

Brunet A, et al. Stress-dependent regulation of FOXO transcription factors by the SIRT1 deacetylase. Science. 2004;303:2011–5.

Buttery RG, Hinrichsen CF, Weller WL, Haight JR. How thick should a retina be? A comparative study of mammalian species with and without intraretinal vasculature. Vision Res. 1991;31:169–87.

Caprara C, Grimm C. From oxygen to erythropoietin: relevance of hypoxia for retinal development, health and disease. Prog Retin Eye Res. 2012;31:89–119.

Caprara C, et al. HIF1A is essential for the development of the intermediate plexus of the retinal vasculature. Invest Ophthalmol Vis Sci. 2011;52:2109–17.

Carmeliet P, Jain RK. Molecular mechanisms and clinical applications of angiogenesis. Nature. 2011;473:298–307.

Carmeliet P, Tessier-Lavigne M. Common mechanisms of nerve and blood vessel wiring. Nature. 2005;436:193–200.

Chan-Ling T, Gock B, Stone J. The effect of oxygen on vasoformative cell division. Evidence that 'physiological hypoxia' is the stimulus for normal retinal vasculogenesis. Invest Ophthalmol Vis Sci. 1995;36:1201–14.

Chase J. The evolution of retinal vascularization in mammals. A comparison of vascular and avascular retinae. Ophthalmology. 1982;89:1518–25.

Checchin D, Sennlaub F, Levavasseur E, Leduc M, Chemtob S. Potential role of microglia in retinal blood vessel formation. Invest Ophthalmol Vis Sci. 2006;47:3595–602.

Chen L, Yang P, Kijlstra A. Distribution, markers, and functions of retinal microglia. Ocul Immunol Inflamm. 2002;10:27–39.

Chen J, Connor KM, Aderman CM, Smith LE. Erythropoietin deficiency decreases vascular stability in mice. J Clin Invest. 2008;118:526–33.

Chen J, et al. Suppression of retinal neovascularization by erythropoietin siRNA in a mouse model of proliferative retinopathy. Invest Ophthalmol Vis Sci. 2009;50:1329–35.

Chen J, et al. Wnt signaling mediates pathological vascular growth in proliferative retinopathy. Circulation. 2011;124:1871–81.

Chen J, et al. Retinal expression of Wnt-pathway mediated genes in low-density lipoprotein receptor-related protein 5 (Lrp5) knockout mice. PLoS One. 2012;7, e30203.

Chen J, et al. Neuronal sirtuin1 mediates retinal vascular regeneration in oxygen-induced ischemic retinopathy. Angiogenesis. 2013.

Choi YK, et al. AKAP12 regulates human blood-retinal barrier formation by downregulation of hypoxia-inducible factor-1alpha. J Neurosci. 2007;27:4472–81.

Chu Y, Hughes S, Chan-Ling T. Differentiation and migration of astrocyte precursor cells and astrocytes in human fetal retina: relevance to optic nerve coloboma. FASEB J. 2001;15:2013–5.

Claxton S, Fruttiger M. Role of arteries in oxygen induced vaso-obliteration. Exp Eye Res. 2003;77:305–11.

Cringle SJ, Yu PK, Su EN, Yu DY. Oxygen distribution and consumption in the developing rat retina. Invest Ophthalmol Vis Sci. 2006;47:4072–6.

Daneman R, et al. Wnt/beta-catenin signaling is required for CNS, but not non-CNS, angiogenesis. Proc Natl Acad Sci U S A. 2009;106:641–6.

De Bock K, Georgiadou M, Carmeliet P. Role of endothelial cell metabolism in vessel sprouting. Cell Metab. 2013;18:634–47.

de Gooyer TE, et al. Retinopathy is reduced during experimental diabetes in a mouse model of outer retinal degeneration. Invest Ophthalmol Vis Sci. 2006;47:5561–8.

De Smet F, Segura I, De Bock K, Hohensinner PJ, Carmeliet P. Mechanisms of vessel branching: filopodia on endothelial tip cells lead the way. Arterioscler Thromb Vasc Biol. 2009;29:639–49.

Dejda A, et al. Neuropilin-1 mediates myeloid cell chemoattraction and influences retinal neuroimmune crosstalk. J Clin Invest. 2014.

Dorrell M, Friedlander M. Mechanisms of endothelial cell guidance and vascular patterning in the developing mouse retina. Prog Retin Eye Res. 2006;25:277–95.

Dorrell MI, Aguilar E, Friedlander M. Retinal vascular development is mediated by endothelial filopodia, a preexisting astrocytic template and specific R-cadherin adhesion. Invest Ophthalmol Vis Sci. 2002;43:3500–10.

Dorrell MI, Otani A, Aguilar E, Moreno SK, Friedlander M. Adult bone marrow-derived stem cells use R-cadherin to target sites of neovascularization in the developing retina. Blood. 2004;103:3420–7.

Dreher B, Robinson SR. Development of the retinofugal pathway in birds and mammals: evidence for a common 'timetable'. Brain Behav Evol. 1988;31:369–90.

Dreher Z, Robinson SR, Distler C. Muller cells in vascular and avascular retinae: a survey of seven mammals. J Comp Neurol. 1992;323:59–80.

Dumont DJ, et al. Dominant-negative and targeted null mutations in the endothelial receptor tyrosine kinase, tek, reveal a critical role in vasculogenesis of the embryo. Genes Dev. 1994;8:1897–909.

Edwards MM, et al. The deletion of Math5 disrupts retinal blood vessel and glial development in mice. Exp Eye Res. 2011.

Epstein AC, et al. C. elegans EGL-9 and mammalian homologs define a family of dioxygenases that regulate HIF by prolyl hydroxylation. Cell. 2001;107:43–54.

Fantin A, et al. Tissue macrophages act as cellular chaperones for vascular anastomosis downstream of VEGF-mediated endothelial tip cell induction. Blood. 2010;116:829–40.

Fruttiger M. Development of the mouse retinal vasculature: angiogenesis versus vasculogenesis. Invest Ophthalmol Vis Sci. 2002;43:522–7.

Fruttiger M. Development of the retinal vasculature. Angiogenesis. 2007;10:77–88.

Fruttiger M, et al. PDGF mediates a neuron-astrocyte interaction in the developing retina. Neuron. 1996;17: 1117–31.

Fukushima Y, et al. Sema3E-PlexinD1 signaling selectively suppresses disoriented angiogenesis in ischemic retinopathy in mice. J Clin Invest. 2011;121:1974–85.

Gariano RF, Gardner TW. Retinal angiogenesis in development and disease. Nature. 2005;438:960–6.

Gariano RF, Sage EH, Kaplan HJ, Hendrickson AE. Development of astrocytes and their relation to blood vessels in fetal monkey retina. Invest Ophthalmol Vis Sci. 1996;37:2367–75.

Gelfand MV, Hong S, Gu C. Guidance from above: common cues direct distinct signaling outcomes in vascular and neural patterning. Trends Cell Biol. 2009;19:99–110.

Gerhardt H, et al. VEGF guides angiogenic sprouting utilizing endothelial tip cell filopodia. J Cell Biol. 2003;161:1163–77.

Gogat K, et al. VEGF and KDR gene expression during human embryonic and fetal eye development. Invest Ophthalmol Vis Sci. 2004;45:7–14.

Grant MB, et al. Adenosine receptor activation induces vascular endothelial growth factor in human retinal endothelial cells. Circ Res. 1999;85:699–706.

Grant MB, et al. Proliferation, migration, and ERK activation in human retinal endothelial cells through A (2B) adenosine receptor stimulation. Invest Ophthalmol Vis Sci. 2001;42:2068–73.

Grant MB, et al. Adult hematopoietic stem cells provide functional hemangioblast activity during retinal neovascularization. Nat Med. 2002;8:607–12.

Gray H. Gray's anatomy. Philadelphia: Elsevier; 2008.

Gutman M, Bonomi F, Pagani S, Cerletti P, Kroneck P. Modulation of the flavin redox potential as mode of regulation of succinate dehydrogenase activity. Biochim Biophys Acta. 1980;591:400–8.

Hackett SF, Wiegand S, Yancopoulos G, Campochiaro PA. Angiopoietin-2 plays an important role in retinal angiogenesis. J Cell Physiol. 2002;192:182–7.

Hartnett ME. Pediatric Retina. Philadelphia, Lippincott Williams & Wilkins. 2013.

Hayreh SS. Orbital vascular anatomy. Eye (Lond). 2006;20:1130–44.

He W, et al. Citric acid cycle intermediates as ligands for orphan G-protein-coupled receptors. Nature. 2004;429:188–93.

Hellstrom A, et al. Low IGF-I suppresses VEGF-survival signaling in retinal endothelial cells: direct correlation with clinical retinopathy of prematurity. Proc Natl Acad Sci U S A. 2001;98:5804–8.

Hellstrom A, et al. IGF-I is critical for normal vascularization of the human retina. J Clin Endocrinol Metab. 2002;87:3413–6.

Hellstrom A, et al. Postnatal serum insulin-like growth factor I deficiency is associated with retinopathy of prematurity and other complications of premature birth. Pediatrics. 2003;112:1016–20.

Hellstrom M, et al. Dll4 signalling through Notch1 regulates formation of tip cells during angiogenesis. Nature. 2007;445:776–80.

Henkind P, Hansen RI, Szalay J, Editors. Ocular circulation. In: Physiology of the human eye and visual system. New York: Harper & Row; 1979, pp. 98–155.

Huber AB, Kolodkin AL, Ginty DD, Cloutier JF. Signaling at the growth cone: ligand-receptor complexes and the control of axon growth and guidance. Annu Rev Neurosci. 2003;26:509–63.

Hughes S, Yang H, Chan-Ling T. Vascularization of the human fetal retina: roles of vasculogenesis and angiogenesis. Invest Ophthalmol Vis Sci. 2000;41:1217–28.

Ishida S, et al. Leukocytes mediate retinal vascular remodeling during development and vaso-obliteration in disease. Nat Med. 2003;9:781–8.

Jaakkola P, et al. Targeting of HIF-alpha to the von Hippel-Lindau ubiquitylation complex by O$_2$-regulated prolyl hydroxylation. Science. 2001;292:468–72.

Janzer RC, Raff MC. Astrocytes induce blood-brain barrier properties in endothelial cells. Nature. 1987; 325:253–7.

Katsura Y, et al. Erythropoietin is highly elevated in vitreous fluid of patients with proliferative diabetic retinopathy. Diabetes Care. 2005;28:2252–4.

Kim J, Oh WJ, Gaiano N, Yoshida Y, Gu C. Semaphorin 3E-Plexin-D1 signaling regulates VEGF function in developmental angiogenesis via a feedback mechanism. Genes Dev. 2011;25:1399–411.

Klagsbrun M, Eichmann A. A role for axon guidance receptors and ligands in blood vessel development and tumor angiogenesis. Cytokine Growth Factor Rev. 2005;16:535–48.

Klinger G, et al. Outcome of early-onset sepsis in a national cohort of very low birth weight infants. Pediatrics. 2010;125:e736–40.

Kubota Y, et al. M-CSF inhibition selectively targets pathological angiogenesis and lymphangiogenesis. J Exp Med. 2009;206:1089–102.

Lahdenranta J, et al. An anti-angiogenic state in mice and humans with retinal photoreceptor cell degeneration. Proc Natl Acad Sci U S A. 2001;98:10368–73.

Larrivee B, Freitas C, Suchting S, Brunet I, Eichmann A. Guidance of vascular development: lessons from the nervous system. Circ Res. 2009;104:428–41.

Lee J, Dammann O. Perinatal infection, inflammation, and retinopathy of prematurity. Semin Fetal Neonatal Med. 2012;17:26–9.

Liebner S, et al. Wnt/beta-catenin signaling controls development of the blood-brain barrier. J Cell Biol. 2008;183:409–17.

Linsenmeier RA, Padnick-Silver L. Metabolic dependence of photoreceptors on the choroid in the normal and detached retina. Invest Ophthalmol Vis Sci. 2000;41:3117–23.

Lobov IB, et al. WNT7b mediates macrophage-induced programmed cell death in patterning of the vasculature. Nature. 2005;437:417–21.

Lofqvist C, et al. Postnatal head growth deficit among premature infants parallels retinopathy of prematurity and insulin-like growth factor-1 deficit. Pediatrics. 2006;117:1930–8.

McLeod DS, Hasegawa T, Prow T, Merges C, Lutty G. The initial fetal human retinal vasculature develops by vasculogenesis. Dev Dyn. 2006;235:3336–47.

Meixner-Monori B, Kubicek CP, Habison A, Kubicek-Pranz EM, Rohr M. Presence and regulation of the alpha-ketoglutarate dehydrogenase multienzyme complex in the filamentous fungus Aspergillus niger. J Bacteriol. 1985;161:265–71.

Michaelson IC. The mode of development of the vascular system of the retina, with some observations on its significance for certain retinal diseases. Trans Ophthalmol Soc UK. 1948;68:137–81.

Michan S. Acetylome regulation by sirtuins in the brain: from normal physiology to aging and pathology. Curr Pharm Des. 2013.

Michan S, et al. SIRT1 is essential for normal cognitive function and synaptic plasticity. J Neurosci. 2010; 30:9695–707.

Mino RP, et al. Adenosine receptor antagonists and retinal neovascularization in vivo. Invest Ophthalmol Vis Sci. 2001;42:3320–4.

Mitchell CA, Risau W, Drexler HC. Regression of vessels in the tunica vasculosa lentis is initiated by coordinated endothelial apoptosis: a role for vascular endothelial growth factor as a survival factor for endothelium. Dev Dyn. 1998;213:322–33.

Mu X, et al. Ganglion cells are required for normal progenitor-cell proliferation but not cell-fate determination or patterning in the developing mouse retina. Curr Biol. 2005;15:525–30.

Nakamura-Ishizu A, et al. The formation of an angiogenic astrocyte template is regulated by the neuroretina in a HIF-1-dependent manner. Dev Biol. 2012;363:106–14.

Netter FH. Atlas of human anatomy. Philadelphia: Elsevier Health Sciences; 2006.

Niehrs C. Norrin and frizzled; a new vein for the eye. Dev Cell. 2004;6:453–4.

Ohh M, et al. Ubiquitination of hypoxia-inducible factor requires direct binding to the beta-domain of the von Hippel-Lindau protein. Nat Cell Biol. 2000;2:423–7.

Ohlmann A, et al. Norrin promotes vascular regrowth after oxygen-induced retinal vessel loss and suppresses retinopathy in mice. J Neurosci. 2010;30: 183–93.

Oshima Y, et al. Angiopoietin-2 enhances retinal vessel sensitivity to vascular endothelial growth factor. J Cell Physiol. 2004;199:412–7.

Paul Riordan-Eva ETC. Vaughan & Asbury's general ophthalmology. New York: McGraw-Hill Professional. 2011.

Pierce EA, Avery RL, Foley ED, Aiello LP, Smith LE. Vascular endothelial growth factor/vascular permeability factor expression in a mouse model of retinal neovascularization. Proc Natl Acad Sci U S A. 1995;92:905–9.

Pierce EA, Foley ED, Smith LE. Regulation of vascular endothelial growth factor by oxygen in a model of retinopathy of prematurity. Arch Ophthalmol. 1996;114: 1219–28.

Provis JM, et al. Development of the human retinal vasculature: cellular relations and VEGF expression. Exp Eye Res. 1997;65:555–68.

Rehm HL, et al. Vascular defects and sensorineural deafness in a mouse model of Norrie disease. J Neurosci. 2002;22:4286–92.

Ross MH, Pawlina W. Histology: a text and atlas with correlated cell and molecular biology. Philadelphia: Lippincott Williams & Wilkins; 2005.

Runkle EA, Antonetti DA. The blood-retinal barrier: structure and functional significance. Methods Mol Biol. 2011;686:133–48.

Rymo SF, et al. A two-way communication between microglial cells and angiogenic sprouts regulates angiogenesis in aortic ring cultures. PLoS One. 2011;6, e15846.

Saint-Geniez M, D'Amore PA. Development and pathology of the hyaloid, choroidal and retinal vasculature. Int J Dev Biol. 2004;48:1045–58.

Santos AM, et al. Embryonic and postnatal development of microglial cells in the mouse retina. J Comp Neurol. 2008;506:224–39.

Sapieha P. Eyeing central neurons in vascular growth and reparative angiogenesis. Blood. 2012;120:2182–94.

Sapieha P, et al. The succinate receptor GPR91 in neurons has a major role in retinal angiogenesis. Nat Med. 2008;14:1067–76.

Sato TN, et al. Distinct roles of the receptor tyrosine kinases Tie-1 and Tie-2 in blood vessel formation. Nature. 1995;376:70–4.

Sato T, Kusaka S, Shimojo H, Fujikado T. Vitreous levels of erythropoietin and vascular endothelial growth factor in eyes with retinopathy of prematurity. Ophthalmology. 2009;116:1599–603.

Scott A, et al. Astrocyte-derived vascular endothelial growth factor stabilizes vessels in the developing retinal vasculature. PLoS One. 2010;5, e11863.

Senger DR, et al. Tumor cells secrete a vascular permeability factor that promotes accumulation of ascites fluid. Science. 1983;219:983–5.

Sengupta N, et al. The role of adult bone marrow-derived stem cells in choroidal neovascularization. Invest Ophthalmol Vis Sci. 2003;44:4908–13.

Shui YB, et al. Vascular endothelial growth factor expression and signaling in the lens. Invest Ophthalmol Vis Sci. 2003;44:3911–9.

Smith LE. IGF-1 and retinopathy of prematurity in the preterm infant. Biol Neonate. 2005;88:237–44.

Smith LE, et al. Essential role of growth hormone in ischemia-induced retinal neovascularization. Science. 1997;276:1706–9.

Smith LE, et al. Regulation of vascular endothelial growth factor-dependent retinal neovascularization by insulin-like growth factor-1 receptor. Nat Med. 1999;5: 1390–5.

Stahl A, et al. The mouse retina as an angiogenesis model. Invest Ophthalmol Vis Sci. 2010a;51:2813–26.

Stahl A, et al. Vitreal levels of erythropoietin are increased in patients with retinal vein occlusion and correlate with vitreal VEGF and the extent of macular edema. Retina. 2010b.

Stefater Iii JA, et al. Regulation of angiogenesis by a noncanonical Wnt-Flt1 pathway in myeloid cells. Nature. 2011;474:511–5.

Sternberg Jr P, Landers 3rd MB, Wolbarsht M. The negative coincidence of retinitis pigmentosa and proliferative diabetic retinopathy. Am J Ophthalmol. 1984; 97:788–9.

Stone J, et al. Development of retinal vasculature is mediated by hypoxia-induced vascular endothelial growth factor (VEGF) expression by neuroglia. J Neurosci. 1995;15:4738–47.

Tolsma KW, et al. Neonatal bacteremia and retinopathy of prematurity: the ELGAN study. Arch Ophthalmol. 2011;129:1555–63.

Torczynski E. Choroid and suprachoroid. Ocular anatomy, embryology and teratology. Philadelphia: Harper & Row; 1982.

Tremblay S, et al. Systemic inflammation perturbs developmental retinal angiogenesis and neuroretinal function. Invest Ophthalmol Vis Sci. 2013;54:8125–39.

Uemura A, Kusuhara S, Wiegand SJ, Yu RT, Nishikawa S. Tlx acts as a proangiogenic switch by regulating extracellular assembly of fibronectin matrices in retinal astrocytes. J Clin Invest. 2006;116:369–77.

Wang GL, Semenza GL. Characterization of hypoxia-inducible factor 1 and regulation of DNA binding activity by hypoxia. J Biol Chem. 1993a;268:21513–8.

Wang GL, Semenza GL. General involvement of hypoxia-inducible factor 1 in transcriptional response to hypoxia. Proc Natl Acad Sci U S A. 1993b;90:4304–8.

Wang GL, Jiang BH, Rue EA, Semenza GL. Hypoxia-inducible factor 1 is a basic-helix-loop-helix-PAS heterodimer regulated by cellular O_2 tension. Proc Natl Acad Sci U S A. 1995;92:5510–4.

Wang Y, et al. Norrin/Frizzled4 signaling in retinal vascular development and blood brain barrier plasticity. Cell. 2012;151:1332–44.

Wangsa-Wirawan ND, Linsenmeier RA. Retinal oxygen: fundamental and clinical aspects. Arch Ophthalmol. 2003;121:547–57.

Watanabe T, Raff MC. Retinal astrocytes are immigrants from the optic nerve. Nature. 1988;332:834–7.

Watanabe D, et al. Erythropoietin as a retinal angiogenic factor in proliferative diabetic retinopathy. N Engl J Med. 2005;353:782–92.

Weidemann A, et al. Astrocyte hypoxic response is essential for pathological but not developmental angiogenesis of the retina. Glia. 2010;58:1177–85.

Wilson BD, et al. Netrins promote developmental and therapeutic angiogenesis. Science. 2006;313:640–4.

Wise GN. Factors influencing retinal new vessel formation. Am J Ophthalmol. 1961;52:637–50.

Xu Q, et al. Vascular development in the retina and inner ear: control by Norrin and Frizzled-4, a high-affinity ligand-receptor pair. Cell. 2004;116:883–95.

Ye X, Smallwood P, Nathans J. Expression of the Norrie disease gene (Ndp) in developing and adult mouse eye, ear, and brain. Gene Expr Patterns. 2011;11:151–5.

Yi X, Mai LC, Uyama M, Yew DT. Time-course expression of vascular endothelial growth factor as related to the development of the retinochoroidal vasculature in rats. Exp Brain Res. 1998;118:155–60.

Zhao S, Overbeek PA. Regulation of choroid development by the retinal pigment epithelium. Mol Vis. 2001;7:277–82.

Zhu M, et al. The human hyaloid system: cell death and vascular regression. Exp Eye Res. 2000;70:767–76.

Retinopathy of Prematurity

2

Andreas Stahl, Ann Hellström, and Lois E.H. Smith

2.1 Natural History and Grading of ROP

In order to understand when and how treatment strategies for ROP can be delivered in a sensible and timely manner, a thorough understanding of ROP disease characteristics and development is essential. ROP develops predominantly in infants born before 32 weeks of gestational age. Among these, most infants will experience only mild forms of ROP that will regress and do not require treatment. Our challenge as ophthalmologists is to identify the few infants that will progress to ROP stages that require treatment. Those most at risk are infants that are either born very prematurely (in developed countries mainly below

A. Stahl (✉)
Eye Center at the Medical Center, University of Freiburg, Freiburg 79106, Germany
e-mail: andreas.stahl@uniklinik-freiburg.de

A. Hellström
Department of Ophthalmology, Institute of Neuroscience and Physiology, The Queen Silvia Children's Hospital, The Sahlgrenska Academy at University of Gothenburg, Gothenburg 416-85, Sweden
e-mail: ann.hellstrom@medfak.gu.se

L.E.H. Smith
Department of Ophthalmology, Harvard Medical School, Boston Children's Hospital, 300 Longwood Avenue, Boston, MA 02465, USA
e-mail: lois.smith@childrens.harvard.edu

25 weeks gestational age) or the ones that are born small for their respective gestational age or show a reduced postnatal growth rate often complicated by accompanying problems like sepsis, anemia, or lung disorders requiring prolonged oxygen supplementation.

The reason that very prematurely born infants in particular may progress to severe ROP stages lies in the nature of physiologic retinal vascularization as it is described in detail in the previous chapter by Chen, Liu, and Sapieha. This physiologic growth of retinal vessels originates from the optic nerve head and proceeds to the ora serrata in a centrifugal pattern. If it is disrupted by premature birth, the peripheral retina remains void of blood vessels in the early postnatal period. The earlier the child is born, the greater the area of avascular retina at birth. Due to the fact that oxygen saturations in the retinal vasculature increase significantly after switching from placental supply to breathing room air, the retinal vessels will sense a *hyper*oxic environment during the first weeks after premature birth, even without additional iatrogenic oxygen supply. This hyperoxic retinal environment leads to slowing or even stalling of physiologic vessel growth. This hyperoxic phase of slowed or stalled vessel growth in the first weeks of life is often referred to as *Phase I* of ROP.

In Phase I ROP, the ophthalmologist finds a vascularized central retina and avascular peripheral retina without a clear demarcation between the two and without signs of pathologic vessel

© Springer International Publishing Switzerland 2016
A. Stahl (ed.), *Anti-Angiogenic Therapy in Ophthalmology*,
Essentials in Ophthalmology, DOI 10.1007/978-3-319-24097-8_2

activation. The retinal vessel growth is stalled but the nonvascularized peripheral retina appears to receive sufficient nutrients and oxygen from the increased oxygen tension after birth. This oversupply of oxygen that is due to switching from placental to pulmonary supply after premature birth is further increased if supplemental oxygen is given (which is often necessary to ensure the development of other organs or even to guarantee survival of the infant (Stenson 2013; Chen et al. 2010)). After usually 6 or more weeks of life, the peripheral avascular retina, which has by that time grown in thickness and has matured to some degree, begins to experience an undersupply of oxygen for its now increased metabolic demand. As a consequence, the retinal microenvironment switches from hyperoxic to hypoxic. This hypoxic phase of ROP is often referred to as *Phase II* and is characterized by a reactivation of vessel growth.

Phase II ROP needs to be monitored closely by strict adherence to the established screening protocols in order to treat if neovascularization progresses to the point of high risk of retinal detachment. During Phase II ROP, the vessels start to resume their centrifugal growth and proceed towards the ora serrata. In most infants, this centrifugal growth progresses without significant disturbance and the ophthalmologist can identify

an increasing area of the retina becoming vascularized from visit to visit. However, in some infants the hypoxic environment in the peripheral retina is so severe that pathologically high levels of the angiogenic growth factor VEGF are produced (Sonmez et al. 2008; Velez-Montoya et al. 2010). This leads to a breakdown of natural growth factor gradients in the retina and to aberrant and uncontrolled growth of retinal vessels.

Several stages of ROP are distinguished during the course of disease development. In *stage 1* of ROP, there is only a non-prominent demarcation line between vascularized and nonvascularized retina. In *stage 2*, the line becomes a prominent demarcation ridge. *Stage 3* is characterized by extraretinal proliferations on the ridge that can be identified on fundoscopy. This is a stage that will develop only in a minority of infants (approximately 5 %), but if it is present, most cases will require treatment, in particular when it is associated with increased tortuosity and dilation of central retinal vessels (referred to as *Plus disease*). An example of ROP stage 3+ is given in Fig. 2.1.

In addition to identifying the correct ROP stages, it is essential for the ophthalmologist to document the zone where the demarcation line or ridge is seen between vascularized and nonvascularized retina. The more central this border lies,

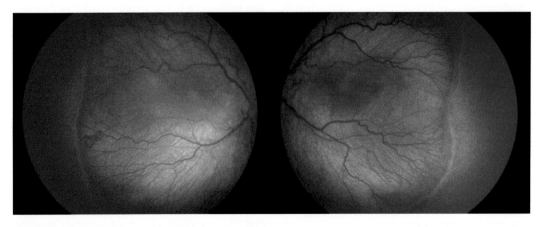

Fig. 2.1 Exemplary images of bilateral ROP stage 3 with plus disease (ROP 3+). The optic nerve head is located on the central margin of each image. Vessel dilation and tortuosity are the defining characteristics of plus disease. The prominent ridge between vascularized and nonvascularized retina with pathologic vessel proliferations defines stage 3 of ROP

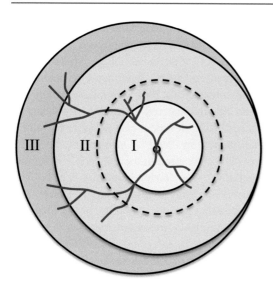

Fig. 2.2 Schematic representation of the three zones of ROP. Zone I is defined as a circle around the optic nerve head (ONH) with a radius of twice the distance ONH-fovea. Central zone II is defined as a *circle* around the ONH with a radius of three times the distance ONH-fovea (*dashed line* in zone II). Peripheral zone II is a circle around the ONH reaching the ora serrata nasally. Zone III is the remaining crescent-shaped temporal retina

the larger the avascular retinal area and the more problematic the potential course of the disease. For the purpose of using standardized descriptions or ROP, the retina is divided into different zones. *Zone I* is defined by a circle around the optic nerve head (ONH) with twice the diameter ONH—fovea. *Central zone II* (or posterior zone II) is defined by a circle around the ONH with three times the diameter ONH—fovea. *Peripheral zone II* (or anterior zone II) is a circle around the ONH reaching the ora serrata nasally. *Zone III* refers to the crescent-shaped remaining retina on the temporal side. The ROP zones are schematically depicted in Fig. 2.2.

Stage 4 and 5 of ROP are characterized by partial or complete retinal detachment and can be avoided in most cases by timely treatment at earlier stages. Stage 4 and 5 of ROP are often associated with poor functional long-term outcomes. However, in some cases ROP can progress so aggressively that even with best-possible screening and treatment protocols in place stage 4 or 5 will develop. This is particularly the case in the

subgroup of aggressive posterior ROP (*AP-ROP*) which is characterized by pronounced angiogenic activation and often very fast progression of pathologic vascular changes that do not in all cases follow the stage-to-stage progression described above but may show variable progression patterns that are challenging to reign in at early stages. AP-ROP is mainly seen in very sick and extremely preterm infants.

2.2 Treatment of ROP

Published in 1990, the CRYO-ROP study defined the underlying principle for ROP treatment for the next decades (Multicenter trial of cryotherapy for retinopathy of prematurity). Three-month outcome. Cryotherapy for Retinopathy of Prematurity Cooperative Group 1990b; Multicenter trial of cryotherapy for retinopathy of prematurity. One-year outcome—structure and function. Cryotherapy for Retinopathy of Prematurity Cooperative Group 1990a). The main finding was that when treated at a point when about 50 % would regress and 50 % would go on to retinal detachment (called "threshold"), those infants treated with cryoablation of avascular peripheral retina had fewer unfavorable structural outcomes compared to non-treated infants. Building on this same principle, laser photocoagulation was introduced in the 1990s providing a treatment alternative to cryotherapy (McNamara et al. 1991; Landers et al. 1992; Fleming et al. 1992). Today, laser photocoagulation of peripheral avascular retina has replaced cryotherapy in most countries in the treatment of ROP (Simpson et al. 2012). Both cryo and laser therapy, however, follow the same principle: avascular retina is destroyed in order to decrease the production of pro-angiogenic growth factors like VEGF from hypoxic retinal cells. The treatment is safe and, when performed properly, will in most cases stop disease progression before stage 4 or 5 of ROP develops. The downside of laser therapy, however, is that potentially viable retinal tissue is replaced by functionless scar tissue and that laser therapy may increase the extent of myopia (Geloneck et al. 2014).

In the recent years, two mutually synergistic medical approaches have been evaluated that have the potential to significantly broaden our range of therapeutic options in ROP. The first of these medical approaches is supplementation of the fetal growth factor insulin-like growth factor 1 (*IGF-1*) during the first weeks of life. This treatment targets Phase I of ROP and has the potential of providing a *preventive* intervention by aiming at normalizing retinal vascular development during the first weeks of life. IGF-1 is essential for the physiologic vascular growth in the retina (Hellstrom et al. 2002; Smith et al. 1999; Hellstrom et al. 2001). In addition, IGF-1 is also an important inducer of overall growth and development of all tissues (Netchine et al. 2011). The role of IGF-1 in ROP may therefore be two-fold: First, IGF-1 may directly promote normal retinal development during Phase I of ROP when vascular growth in the retina is stalled. Augmented retinal vascular growth during Phase I in turn would lead to a reduced size of peripheral avascular retina in later weeks of life and would therefore limit overexpression of angiogenic growth factors, thereby preventing or curtailing Phase II. The second effect of IGF-1 on ROP might be more indirect but nevertheless similarly important. It is known that serum IGF-1 is substantially reduced after preterm birth (Engstrom et al. 2005) and that low IGF-1 levels are associated with poor postnatal weight gain and the development of more severe forms of ROP (Hellstrom et al. 2003; Perez-Munuzuri et al. 2010). Increasing systemic IGF-1 to levels that would be normal during that developmental window could therefore have a beneficial effect on overall postnatal growth and improve the general health and development of a preterm infant—with associated beneficial effects on his or her ROP risk. A phase I study administering IGF-I to preterm infants has been performed (Hellstrom et al. 2003), and a multicenter, international phase II clinical trial is currently ongoing to investigate whether IGF-1 supplementation during Phase I of ROP is safe and well tolerated (clinical trials identifier NCT01096784).

The second medical approach to treat advanced ROP is anti-VEGF treatment. Binding and inhibition of VEGF targets Phase II of ROP when overexpression of angiogenic growth factors and activation of pathologic vessel growth has already occurred. It is therefore potentially complementary to IGF-1 supplementation and could be administered to infants proceeding to Phase II ROP despite a best-possible preventive management in Phase I. Once pathologic vessel growth has occurred in the retina, IGF-1 supplementation is no longer helpful and potentially could even aggravate disease progression by further stimulating vessel growth. During Phase II, an antiangiogenic treatment approach is appealing if found to be safe. And with VEGF being the main angiogenic molecule in the vitreous of ROP infants (Sonmez et al. 2008), it appears sensible to target VEGF for this purpose. The first effect of anti-VEGF therapy is a reduction of plus disease which can often be observed in the first days after treatment (Fig. 2.3).

After several smaller studies were published, the BEAT-ROP study was the first larger trial comparing the effect of standard laser treatment in ROP to the effect of an intravitreal injection of the anti-VEGF antibody bevacizumab (Mintz-Hittner et al. 2011). The primary end point of the BEAT-ROP study was recurrence of active ROP up to 54 weeks postmenstrual age (PMA). The study found that for zone I disease there were fewer recurrences in the bevacizumab group compared to laser and for central zone II disease both treatments were equal with regard to recurrence rates. One caveat when interpreting these results is that the recurrence rate in the zone I laser group of the BEAT-ROP study was relatively high compared to other published studies. Another limitation is the relatively short follow-up window that did not examine if avascular retina persisted long term. Different from laser therapy, recurrences of proliferative disease after bevacizumab therapy may occur later due to the persistence of peripheral avascular retinal tissue. These late recurrences could fall outside the observational window of 54 weeks PMA investigated in the published BEAT-ROP results (Hu et al. 2012; Lee et al. 2012). Systemic effects of anti-VEGF treatment were not evaluated in the BEAT-ROP study.

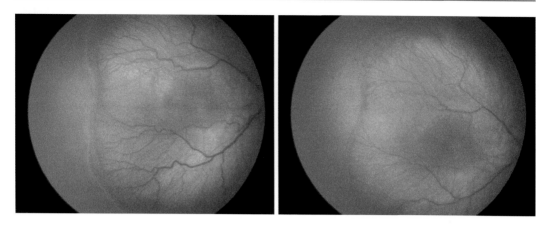

Fig. 2.3 ROP stage 3+ before and three days after treatment with intravitreal anti-VEGF therapy. Note the rapid reduction in plus disease visible by reduced dilatation and reduced tortuosity of the retinal vessels

Despite these caveats, the BEAT-ROP results raised some important points:

(1) Bevacizumab is effective in halting neovascular disease progression in ROP in most cases; (2) unlike laser therapy, the avascular retinal areas are not destroyed but may become (partially) vascularized over time. Whether the vessels and underlying neural retina are fully normal is unknown at this point. Recent data, however, point towards comparable visual acuity results in infants treated with bevacizumab compared to laser-treated infants—with the potential advantage of fewer cases of high myopia in infants with bevacizumab treatment over laser (Harder et al. 2013; Geloneck et al. 2014; Martinez-Castellanos et al. 2013).

Some important questions remain with regard to anti-VEGF treatment in ROP. In particular, only limited data exist on potential systemic effects of intravitreal anti-VEGF treatment. It is known from adult data that after one single bevacizumab injection systemic VEGF levels in the circulation remain suppressed below the detection levels of the most prevalently used ELISA assays over several weeks (Zehetner et al. 2013; Matsuyama et al. 2010). The same appears to be true in infants (Sato et al. 2012) where the currently used dose of bevacizumab (0.625 mg per eye) by far exceeds the standard adult exposure when calculated per body weight or per body surface area. It is currently not known what the ideal dosing for bevacizumab in ROP infants is—nor is it clear whether bevaci-

zumab is the ideal drug in this vulnerable population (Avery 2012). Bevacizumab has a systemic half-life of several days. So even if lower doses of bevacizumab were used intravitreally, bevacizumab would be secreted from the vitreous into the circulation (possibly via active transport through the RPE (Powner et al. 2014)) and would therefore *accumulate* over time in the systemic circulation (Krohne et al. 2014). Whether and how this systemic exposure to an anti-VEGF antibody could affect developmental processes in, for example, brain or lung maturation is currently not known. Ranibizumab, however, is an alternative anti-VEGF agent with comparable efficacy at treating retinal vascular proliferations in adults (Martin et al. 2012; Chakravarthy et al. 2013; Chakravarthy et al. 2012; Martin et al. 2011) and with the possible advantage of much faster systemic clearance rates (Krohne et al. 2014). Ranibizumab is therefore currently being investigated in the CARE-ROP study, a multicenter randomized controlled trial for ROP (clinical trials identifier NCT02134457).

The CARE-ROP study investigates two pertinent questions:

(1) Is ranibizumab with its advantageous systemic clearance rate effective in treating Phase II ROP; and (2) are lower doses than the currently used 50 % adult dose sufficient to treat ROP with the potential benefit of reduced local and systemic drug exposure in a developing infant. In addition to its faster systemic clearance rate,

ranibizumab has been developed explicitly for use in the eye and is approved for intravitreal use in adults for several indications (Rosenfeld et al. 2006; Massin et al. 2010; Brown et al. 2010). The two doses compared in the CARE-ROP study are 24 % vs. 40 % of the standard adult dose. Both these doses are lower than the 50 % adult dose of bevacizumab used in the BEAT-ROP study. The use of lower doses may have an additional beneficial effect. The physiologic vascularization of the peripheral avascular retina may progress better than occurs in infants treated with higher doses. Animal studies found that lower doses of anti-VEGF agents were comparable to high doses in controlling pathologic angiogenic activity but superior in allowing physiologic peripheral vascularization at the same time (Lutty et al. 2011).

It is important to emphasize the significance of sufficient peripheral retinal vascularization after anti-VEGF treatment. Different from laser treatment, the peripheral retina is not rendered a scar tissue by anti-VEGF treatment. If neural retinal development is normal, then these retinal areas retain their potential to contribute to visual function. Further, no scar tissue is induced that might produce traction on the more central retina and macula.

The downside of not using laser is that the peripheral retina may not function properly but will continue to produce VEGF. By not destroying this dysfunctional tissue, there may be a late recurrence of ROP—up to months after an initially successful treatment (Hu et al. 2012; Ittiara et al. 2013). In infants where no or incomplete vascularization can be obtained, a prolonged period of frequent follow-up examinations after anti-VEGF treatment is warranted. In some cases, a sequential approach of first anti-VEGF therapy for central ROP (in zone I or central zone II) followed by laser therapy at a later time point for remaining peripheral avascular retina with signs of recurring ROP activity may be sensible. With lower doses of anti-VEGF agents as they are investigated in the CARE-ROP study, there may be superior peripheral vascularization after anti-VEGF treatment which would reduce the risk for late recurrences while at the same time controlling excessive aberrant vessel growth.

2.3   Summary

ROP therapy is currently at a crucial crossroads: If the currently ongoing clinical trials on IGF-1 supplementation and anti-VEGF treatment provide sufficient evidence for their safety and efficacy, then the current laser therapy for ROP may be supplemented by two potentially complementary medical approaches:

(1) In Phase I, promotion of physiologic retinal vascularization by normalization of IGF-1; and (2) in Phase II inhibition of VEGF with lowest possible anti-VEGF dosing to inhibit pathologic angiogenesis but to allow further peripheral vascularization.

Ideally, ROP management would consist of two steps. In a first step aimed at preventive treatment, all at-risk infants would receive supplemental systemic IGF-1 from birth to normalize their physiologic retinal vascular development. In those infants who despite this preventive treatment proceed to Phase II ROP with aberrant vessel proliferation in relatively central retinal areas (where laser treatment would induce large areas of scarring), anti-VEGF treatment could be applied—in the lowest possible dose and using compounds that are cleared fast from the systemic circulation. After anti-VEGF treatment, all infants would then be followed-up regularly to monitor first the regression of pathologic vessel growth and then (over a longer period of time) the centrifugal progression of physiologic vessel growth in the periphery. If infants develop recurrent ROP, then laser therapy may be warranted to permanently stop the production of angiogenic factors from remaining peripheral avascular areas—ideally at a time when some peripheral vascularization has already occurred due to the prior IGF-1 and anti-VEGF treatments. This sequential approach could in future ROP treatment protocols potentially reduce the number of infants progressing to ROP stages with pathologic vessel proliferation (by IGF-1 supplementation) and for those infants that do progress, reduce the laser-induced scar areas to a minimum (by low-dose anti-VEGF treatment).

Compliance with Ethical Requirements Informed Consent and Animal Studies disclosures are not applicable to this review. The authors received research grants from Deutsche Forschungsgemeinschaft (DFG STA 1102/5-1), Deutsche Ophthalmologische Gesellschaft (DOG), Novartis Pharma (AS), European Commission FP7 project 305485 PREVENT-ROP (AH), NIH/NEI (EY022275, EY017017, P01 HD18655, RPB Sr. Investigator Award, Lowy Medical Foundation, (LEHS). AS is consultant for Novartis Pharma and has received speaker honoraria from Zeiss, Böhringer-Ingelheim, Bausch&Lomb. LEHS and AH are consultants for Shire Pharmaceuticals.

References

Avery RL. Bevacizumab (Avastin) for retinopathy of prematurity: wrong dose, wrong drug, or both? J AAPOS. 2012;16(1):2–4. doi:10.1016/j.jaapos.2011.11.002. S1091-8531(11)00612-4 [pii].

Brown DM, Campochiaro PA, Singh RP, Li Z, Gray S, Saroj N, Rundle AC, Rubio RG, Murahashi WY. Ranibizumab for macular edema following central retinal vein occlusion: six-month primary end point results of a phase III study. Ophthalmology. 2010;117(6):1124–33. doi:10.1016/j.oph-tha.2010.02.022. e1121S0161-6420(10)00186-7 [pii].

Chakravarthy U, Harding SP, Rogers CA, Downes SM, Lotery AJ, Wordsworth S, Reeves BC. Ranibizumab versus bevacizumab to treat neovascular age-related macular degeneration: one-year findings from the IVAN randomized trial. Ophthalmology. 2012;119(7):1399–411. doi:10.1016/j.oph-tha.2012.04.015. S0161-6420(12)00358-2 [pii].

Chakravarthy U, Harding SP, Rogers CA, Downes SM, Lotery AJ, Culliford LA, Reeves BC. Alternative treatments to inhibit VEGF in age-related choroidal neovascularisation: 2-year findings of the IVAN randomised controlled trial. Lancet. 2013;382(9900):1258–67. doi:10.1016/S0140-6736(13)61501-9. S0140-6736(13) 61501-9 [pii].

Chen ML, Guo L, Smith LE, Dammann CE, Dammann O. High or low oxygen saturation and severe retinopathy of prematurity: a meta-analysis. Pediatrics. 2010;125(6):e1483–1492. doi:10.1542/peds.2009-2218. peds.2009-2218 [pii].

Cryotherapy for Retinopathy of Prematurity Cooperative Group. Multicenter trial of cryotherapy for retinopathy of prematurity. Arch Ophthalmol. 1990a; 108(10):1408–16.

Cryotherapy for Retinopathy of Prematurity Cooperative Group. Multicenter trial of cryotherapy for retinopathy of prematurity. Three-month outcome. Arch Ophthalmol. 1990b;108(2):195–204.

Engstrom E, Niklasson A, Wikland KA, Ewald U, Hellstrom A. The role of maternal factors, postnatal nutrition, weight gain, and gender in regulation of serum IGF-I among preterm infants. Pediatr Res. 2005;57(4):605–10. doi:10.1203/01.PDR.0000 155950.67503.BC. 01.PDR.0000155950.67503.BC [pii].

Fleming TN, Runge PE, Charles ST. Diode laser photocoagulation for prethreshold, posterior retinopathy of prematurity. Am J Ophthalmol. 1992;114(5): 589–92.

Geloneck MM, Chuang AZ, Clark WL, Hunt MG, Norman AA, Packwood EA, Tawansy KA, Mintz-Hittner HA. Refractive outcomes following bevacizumab monotherapy compared with conventional laser treatment: a randomized clinical trial. JAMA Ophthalmol. 2014;132(11):1327–33. doi:10.1001/jamaophthalmol.2014.2772. 1893536 [pii].

Harder BC, Schlichtenbrede FC, von Baltz S, Jendritza W, Jendritza B, Jonas JB. Intravitreal bevacizumab for retinopathy of prematurity: refractive error results. Am J Ophthalmol. 2013;155(6):1119–24. doi:10.1016/j. ajo.2013.01.014. e1111S0002-9394(13)00070-6 [pii].

Hellstrom A, Perruzzi C, Ju M, Engstrom E, Hard AL, Liu JL, Albertsson-Wikland K, Carlsson B, Niklasson A, Sjodell L, LeRoith D, Senger DR, Smith LE. Low IGF-I suppresses VEGF-survival signaling in retinal endothelial cells: direct correlation with clinical retinopathy of prematurity. Proc Natl Acad Sci U S A. 2001;98(10):5804–8. doi:10.1073/pnas.101113998. 101113998 [pii].

Hellstrom A, Carlsson B, Niklasson A, Segnestam K, Boguszewski M, de Lacerda L, Savage M, Svensson E, Smith L, Weinberger D, Albertsson Wikland K, Laron Z. IGF-I is critical for normal vascularization of the human retina. J Clin Endocrinol Metab. 2002;87(7):3413–6. doi:10.1210/jcem.87.7.8629.

Hellstrom A, Engstrom E, Hard AL, Albertsson-Wikland K, Carlsson B, Niklasson A, Lofqvist C, Svensson E, Holm S, Ewald U, Holmstrom G, Smith LE. Postnatal serum insulin-like growth factor I deficiency is associated with retinopathy of prematurity and other complications of premature birth. Pediatrics. 2003;112(5):1016–20.

Hu J, Blair MP, Shapiro MJ, Lichtenstein SJ, Galasso JM, Kapur R. Reactivation of retinopathy of prematurity after bevacizumab injection. Arch Ophthalmol.

2012;130(8):1000–6. doi:10.1001/archophthalmol.2012.592. archophthalmol.2012.592 [pii].

Ittiara S, Blair MP, Shapiro MJ, Lichtenstein SJ. Exudative retinopathy and detachment: a late reactivation of retinopathy of prematurity after intravitreal bevacizumab. J AAPOS. 2013;17(3):323–5. doi:10.1016/j.jaapos.2013.01.004. S1091-8531(13)00083-9 [pii].

Krohne TU, Holz FG, Meyer CH. Pharmacokinetics of intravitreally administered VEGF inhibitors. Ophthalmologe. 2014;111(2):113–20. doi:10.1007/s00347-013-2932-9.

Landers 3rd MB, Toth CA, Semple HC, Morse LS. Treatment of retinopathy of prematurity with argon laser photocoagulation. Arch Ophthalmol. 1992;110(1):44–7.

Lee BJ, Kim JH, Heo H, Yu YS. Delayed onset atypical vitreoretinal traction band formation after an intravitreal injection of bevacizumab in stage 3 retinopathy of prematurity. Eye (Lond). 2012;26(7):903–9. doi:10.1038/eye.2012.111. quiz 910eye2012111 [pii].

Lutty GA, McLeod DS, Bhutto I, Wiegand SJ. Effect of VEGF trap on normal retinal vascular development and oxygen-induced retinopathy in the dog. Invest Ophthalmol Vis Sci. 2011;52(7):4039–47. doi:10.1167/iovs.10-6798. iovs.10-6798 [pii].

Martin DF, Maguire MG, Ying GS, Grunwald JE, Fine SL, Jaffe GJ. Ranibizumab and bevacizumab for neovascular age-related macular degeneration. N Engl J Med. 2011;364(20):1897–908. doi:10.1056/NEJMoa1102673.

Martin DF, Maguire MG, Fine SL, Ying GS, Jaffe GJ, Grunwald JE, Toth C, Redford M, Ferris 3rd FL. Ranibizumab and bevacizumab for treatment of neovascular age-related macular degeneration: two-year results. Ophthalmology. 2012;119(7):1388–98. doi:10.1016/j.ophtha.2012.03.053. S0161-6420(12)00321-1 [pii].

Martinez-Castellanos MA, Schwartz S, Hernandez-Rojas ML, Kon-Jara VA, Garcia-Aguirre G, Guerrero-Naranjo JL, Chan RV, Quiroz-Mercado H. Long-term effect of antiangiogenic therapy for retinopathy of prematurity up to 5 years of follow-up. Retina. 2013;33(2):329–38. doi:10.1097/IAE.0b013e318275394a.

Massin P, Bandello F, Garweg JG, Hansen LL, Harding SP, Larsen M, Mitchell P, Sharp D, Wolf-Schnurrbusch UE, Gekkieva M, Weichsberger A, Wolf S. Safety and efficacy of ranibizumab in diabetic macular edema (RESOLVE Study): a 12-month, randomized, controlled, double-masked, multicenter phase II study. Diabetes Care. 2010;33(11):2399–405. doi:10.2337/dc10-0493. dc10-0493 [pii].

Matsuyama K, Ogata N, Matsuoka M, Wada M, Takahashi K, Nishimura T. Plasma levels of vascular endothelial growth factor and pigment epithelium-derived factor before and after intravitreal injection of bevacizumab. Br J Ophthalmol. 2010;94(9):1215–8. doi:10.1136/bjo.2008.156810. bjo.2008.156810 [pii].

McNamara JA, Tasman W, Brown GC, Federman JL. Laser photocoagulation for stage 3+ retinopathy of prematurity. Ophthalmology. 1991;98(5):576–80.

Mintz-Hittner HA, Kennedy KA, Chuang AZ. Efficacy of intravitreal bevacizumab for stage 3+ retinopathy of prematurity. N Engl J Med. 2011;364(7):603–15. doi:10.1056/NEJMoa1007374.

Netchine I, Azzi S, Le Bouc Y, Savage MO. IGF1 molecular anomalies demonstrate its critical role in fetal, postnatal growth and brain development. Best Pract Res Clin Endocrinol Metab. 2011;25(1):181–90. doi:10.1016/j.beem.2010.08.005. S1521-690X(10)00090-4 [pii].

Perez-Munuzuri A, Fernandez-Lorenzo JR, Couce-Pico ML, Blanco-Teijeiro MJ, Fraga-Bermudez JM. Serum levels of IGF1 are a useful predictor of retinopathy of prematurity. Acta Paediatr. 2010;99(4):519–25. doi:10.1111/j.1651-2227.2009.01677.x. APA1677 [pii].

Powner MB, McKenzie JA, Christianson GJ, Roopenian DC, Fruttiger M. Expression of neonatal Fc receptor in the eye. Invest Ophthalmol Vis Sci. 2014;55(3):1607–15. doi:10.1167/iovs.13-12574. iovs.13-12574 [pii].

Rosenfeld PJ, Brown DM, Heier JS, Boyer DS, Kaiser PK, Chung CY, Kim RY. Ranibizumab for neovascular age-related macular degeneration. N Engl J Med. 2006;355(14):1419–31.

Sato T, Wada K, Arahori H, Kuno N, Imoto K, Iwahashi-Shima C, Kusaka S. Serum concentrations of bevacizumab (avastin) and vascular endothelial growth factor in infants with retinopathy of prematurity. Am J Ophthalmol. 2012;153(2):327–33. doi:10.1016/j.ajo.2011.07.005. e321S0002-9394(11)00582-4 [pii].

Simpson JL, Melia M, Yang MB, Buffenn AN, Chiang MF, Lambert SR. Current role of cryotherapy in retinopathy of prematurity: a report by the American Academy of Ophthalmology. Ophthalmology. 2012;119(4):873–7. doi:10.1016/j.ophtha.2012.01.003. S0161-6420(12)00005-X [pii].

Smith LE, Shen W, Perruzzi C, Soker S, Kinose F, Xu X, Robinson G, Driver S, Bischoff J, Zhang B, Schaeffer JM, Senger DR. Regulation of vascular endothelial growth factor-dependent retinal neovascularization by insulin-like growth factor-1 receptor. Nat Med. 1999;5(12):1390–5. doi:10.1038/70963.

Sonmez K, Drenser KA, Capone Jr A, Trese MT. Vitreous levels of stromal cell-derived factor 1 and vascular endothelial growth factor in patients with retinopathy of prematurity. Ophthalmology. 2008;115(6):1065–70. doi:10.1016/j.ophtha.2007.08.050. e1061S0161-6420(07)00976-1 [pii].

Stenson BJ. Oxygen targets for preterm infants. Neonatology. 2013;103(4):341–5. doi:10.1159/000349936. 000349936 [pii].

Terry TL. Retrolental fibroplasia in the premature infant: V. Further studies on fibroblastic overgrowth of the persistent tunica vasculosa lentis. Trans Am Ophthalmol Soc. 1944;42:383–96.

Velez-Montoya R, Clapp C, Rivera JC, Garcia-Aguirre G, Morales-Canton V, Fromow-Guerra J, Guerrero-Naranjo JL, Quiroz-Mercado H. Intraocular and systemic levels of vascular endothelial growth factor in advanced cases of retinopathy of prematurity. Clin Ophthalmol. 2010;4:947–53.

Zehetner C, Kirchmair R, Huber S, Kralinger MT, Kieselbach GF. Plasma levels of vascular endothelial growth factor before and after intravitreal injection of bevacizumab, ranibizumab and pegaptanib in patients with age-related macular degeneration, and in patients with diabetic macular oedema. Br J Ophthalmol. 2013;97(4):454–9. doi:10.1136/bjophthalmol-2012-302451. bjophthalmol-2012-302451 [pii].

Anti-vascular Endothelial Growth Factor (VEGF) Treatment in Neovascular Age-Related Macular Degeneration: Outcomes and Outcome Predictors

3

Dujon Fuzzard, Robyn H. Guymer, and Robert P. Finger

Abbreviations

ABC	Aflibercept (Eylea®)
ABC-Trial	Bevacizumab for neovascular age-related macular degeneration—multicenter randomized double-masked study
AMD	Age-related macular degeneration
ANCHOR	Anti-VEGF antibody for the treatment of predominantly classic choroidal neovascularization in AMD—phase III clinical trial
APOE	Apolipoprotein E
AREDS	Age-Related Eye Disease study
ARMS2	Age-related maculopathy susceptibility 2 gene
BCVA	Best corrected visual acuity
BMES	Blue Mountains Eye Study
BVZ	Bevacizumab (Avastin®)
C2	Complement factor 2
C3	Complement factor 3
C5	Complement factor 5
CATT	Comparisons of Age-Related Macular Degeneration Treatments Trial
CFB	Complement factor B
CFT	Central foveal thickness
CFH	Complement factor H
CFHR	Complement factor H receptor
CI	Confidence interval
CMT	Central macular thickness
CNV	Choroidal neovascularization
CRT	Central retinal thickness
CSMT	Central subfield macular thickness
ETDRS	Early Treatment Diabetic Retinopathy Study
EXCITE	Efficacy and safety of monthly versus quarterly ranibizumab treatment in neovascular age-related macular degeneration—phase IIIb clinical trial
EXTEND-I	Long-term efficacy and safety of ranibizumab administered pro re nata in Japanese patients with neovascular age-related macular degeneration—open label phase I/II study

D. Fuzzard (✉) • R.H. Guymer • R.P. Finger
Department of Ophthalmology, Centre for Eye Research Australia, Royal Victorian Eye and Ear Hospital, University of Melbourne, East Melbourne, VIC 3002, Australia
e-mail: dujonfuzzard@gmail.com; robyn.guymer@unimelb.edu.au; robert.finger@unimelb.edu.au

© Springer International Publishing Switzerland 2016
A. Stahl (ed.), *Anti-Angiogenic Therapy in Ophthalmology*, Essentials in Ophthalmology, DOI 10.1007/978-3-319-24097-8_3

FA	Fluorescein angiography		Ranibizumab—phase III clinical trial
FLT1	fms-related tyrosine kinase 1 (vascular endothelial growth factor/vascular permeability factor receptor)	MedDRA SOC	Medical Dictionary for Regulatory Activities System Organ Classes
FOCUS	Ranibizumab combined with verteporfin photodynamic therapy in neovascular age-related macular degeneration—phase I/II randomized-controlled trial	MT	Macular thickness. In the context of this chapter, this encompasses a variety of anatomical measures, including CFT, CMT, CRT, CSMT, and FT
FT	Foveal thickness	NR	Not reported
GEFAL	Ranibizumab versus bevacizumab for neovascular age-related macular degeneration—a non-inferiority randomized trial	nv	Neovascular
		OCT	Optical coherence tomography
		PCV	Polypoidal choroidal vasculopathy
HELIOS	Real-world variability in ranibizumab treatment and associated clinical quality of life and safety outcomes over 24 months—prospective, observation open-label study with arms based in Belgium and the Netherlands	PDT	Photodynamic therapy
		PED	Pigment epithelial detachment
		PIER	Randomized double-masked, sham-controlled trial of ranibizumab for neovascular age-related macular degeneration
HORIZON	Open label extension trial of ranibizumab for choroidal neovascularization secondary to age-related macular degeneration	PLA2G12A	Group 12 secretory phospholipase A2 gene
		PRN	Pro re nata, i.e., as required
		PrONTO	Prospective OCT Study with Lucentis for Neovascular AMD
HTRA1	High-temperature requirement A-1	RAP	Retinal angiomatous proliferations
IL	Interleukin	RBZ	Ranibizumab (Lucentis®)
IQR	Inter-quartile range	RCT	Randomized-controlled trial
IVAN	Randomized-Controlled Trial of Alternative Treatments to Inhibit VEGF in Age-related Choroidal Neovascularization	RPE	Retinal pigment epithelium
		SD	Standard deviation
LogMAR	Logarithm of the minimum angle of resolution	SAILOR	A phase IIb study to evaluate the safety of ranibizumab in subjects with neovascular age-related macular degeneration
LUMINOUS	Safety of ranibizumab in routine clinical practice: 1-year retrospective pooled analysis of four European neovascular AMD registries.	SE	Standard error
		SECURE	Long-term safety of ranibizumab 0.5 mg in neovascular age-related macular degeneration—24-month phase IV extension study
MANTA	A randomized double-masked trial comparing the visual outcome after treatment with ranibizumab or bevacizumab in patients with neovascular age-related macular degeneration	SEVEN-UP	Seven-year outcome in ranibizumab-treated patients in ANCHOR MARINA and HORIZON—a multicenter cohort study
MARINA	Minimally Classic/Occult Trial of Anti-VEGF antibody	SNP	Single nucleotide polymorphisms

SUSTAIN	Safety and efficacy of a flexible dosing regimen of ranibizumab in neovascular age-related macular degeneration—12-month phase III single arm study
UK	United Kingdom
US	United States
VA	Visual acuity
VEGF	Vascular endothelial growth factor
VIEW	VEGF Trap-Eye: Investigation of efficacy and safety in wet AMD—non-inferiority trial comparing aflibercept with ranibizumab
WAVE	Lucentis in wet AMD: Evaluation of visual acuity and quality of life—German non-interventional clinical practice study

3.1 Introduction

The late-stage neovascular form of age-related macular degeneration (nvAMD) is the largest single cause of irreversible, severe vision loss in all developed countries (Lim et al. 2012b). Current treatment options that preserve sight and lead to a considerable improvement in some patients are based on the inhibition of vascular endothelial growth factor (anti-VEGF) and are delivered as regular intravitreal injections (Brown et al. 2006; Rosenfeld et al. 2006). As anti-VEGF treatment does not cure nvAMD but only controls it, treatment is for the long term and is often required until either the eye worsens to levels, where treatment is no longer indicated or the patient dies. To date, however, data on treatment outcomes and their predictors beyond 2 years are sparse (Rasmussen and Sander 2014). In just 1 year in the USA, an estimated 151,340 non-Hispanic whites develop nvAMD in one eye, of whom one third have preexisting nvAMD in the other eye (Bressler et al. 2011). Out of these, 103,582 new cases are in need of anti-VEGF treatment. Without treatment, it is estimated that 16 %

would be legally blind due to their nvAMD within 2 years (Bressler et al. 2011). This highlights not only the devastating natural history of the disease, but also the importance of data on long-term outcomes and the predictors of outcomes for this potentially lifelong treatment.

Several anti-VEGF agents are available, including aflibercept (ABC; Eylea®, Regeneron, Tarrytown, New York, approved use), ranibizumab (RBZ, Lucentis®, Genetech, San Francisco, approved use), and bevacizumab (BVZ, Avastin®, Roche, Basel, Switzerland, off-label) (Wickremasinghe et al. 2011). BVZ is approved for intravenous use in treatment of some cancers; however, due to its similar pharmacological profile to RBZ (Braithwaite et al. 2014), it is used off-label as a less-expensive alternative agent (Miller et al. 2013). Also available, but less commonly used due to its lower clinical effectiveness compared with RBZ, ABC, and BVZ is pegaptanib (Macugen®, Pfizer, New York), the first anti-VEGF treatment registered for treatment in the eye (Takeda et al. 2007). Currently, available data on treatment outcomes and their predictors for RBZ, BVZ, and ABC are summarized in this chapter.

3.2 Overview of Anti-VEGF Treatment Outcomes

Establishment of optimized treatment regimes in terms of agent choice and frequency of injections, based on patient factors at presentation, remains an important focus of current research, to achieve optimally effective and safe anti-VEGF treatment outcomes (Finger et al. 2014). In this chapter, treatment outcomes will be presented by visual acuity (VA) outcomes, anatomical outcomes as assessed by optical coherence tomography (OCT), the incidence of legal blindness and safety.

3.2.1 Visual Acuity Outcomes

There are considerable differences between the patient populations and treatment outcomes of phase III clinical trials published to date and those encountered in routine clinical practice (Table 3.1) (Finger et al. 2014). To illustrate this point, available information from each setting is discussed separately. Whilst it exists as a treatment option, pegaptanib has not been included in this work, due to the cessation of its use in clinical practice. The volume of high-level evidence available varies considerably between agents.

3.2.1.1 Phase III Clinical Trials

Ranibizumab

The efficacy of RBZ in treatment of AMD was demonstrated to be superior to no treatment or photodynamic therapy (PDT) over a 2-year period in the ANCHOR and MARINA phase III clinical trials (Brown et al. 2009; Rosenfeld et al. 2006). Where different doses of RBZ have been studied, 0.5 mg has appeared superior to 0.3 mg in terms of the mean numbers of letters gained (Mitchell 2011). Outcomes in terms of VA and central retinal thickness (CRT) have been best with regular 4-weekly treatment regimes compared to regular 3-monthly or as required (pro re nata (PRN)) treatment strategies (Lanzetta et al. 2013). Quarterly RBZ dosing has been demonstrated not to maintain initial treatment gains at 12 months after an initial loading phase or monthly injections for 3 months in the EXCITE and PIER studies (Schmidt-Erfurth et al. 2011; Regillo et al. 2008). A similar pattern has been observed with PRN treatment regimes in the SUSTAIN and SAILOR trials, where the full extent of treatment gains after a loading phase is not maintained to the 12-month mark (Holz et al. 2011; Boyer et al. 2009). Where PRN regimes are more aggressive (i.e., averaging greater than six injections in 12 months as in the CATT and HARBOR studies) initial gains are maintained to the 12-month mark (Martin et al. 2011; Busbee et al. 2013), although regular 4-weekly treatment regimes yielded overall better results (Martin et al. 2012; Busbee et al. 2013). The mean gain in VA reported with regular 4-weekly regimes across phase III clinical trials has varied between 7 and 11 Early Treatment Diabetic Retinopathy Study (EDTRS) letters (Lanzetta et al. 2013).

Long-term follow-up of patients treated with RBZ was reported in the SEVEN-UP study (Rofagha et al. 2013), a multicenter cohort study which reviewed 65 study eyes, which had successfully completed ANCHOR or MARINA protocols within the RBZ arms (which received 4-weekly RBZ for 2 years) followed by completion of the HORIZON study protocol (Singer et al. 2012), which administered RBZ to participants on a PRN basis for a further 2 years. On average, SEVEN-UP participants were followed up 7.3 years (range 6.33–8.49 years) after entering either the ANCHOR or MARINA trials (Rofagha et al. 2013). Vision outcomes varied widely; whilst 37 % of eyes had VA of 20/70 or better and 43 % of eyes had a stable VA compared with baseline, 37 % of eyes were legally blind, with a VA of 20/200 or worse in the study eye. This corresponded to a mean decrease in VA of 8.6 ETDRS letters when compared with baseline measures. Despite being the longest period of follow-up available in a cohort of patients treated for nvAMD with anti-VEGF agents, this study had multiple limitations. The low enrollment rate of eligible participants (42 %) that were not randomly sampled may have resulted in selection bias. Furthermore, the absence of a treatment protocol during the 3–4-year period following completion of the HORIZON trial resulted in wide differences in the number of injections given to different patients, with 41 % receiving no further anti-VEGF therapy at all. Like the PIER study (Regillo et al. 2008), SEVEN-UP demonstrated that under-treatment of nvAMD with anti-VEGF agents would lead to worsening of visual outcomes (Rofagha et al. 2013).

Aflibercept

The efficacy of ABC 2.0 mg administered 8-weekly was compared to that of RBZ 0.5 mg administered 4-weekly in the VIEW studies (Heier et al. 2012; Schmidt-Erfurth et al. 2014). These comprised two multinational, double-blinded randomized-controlled trials (RCTs). VIEW-1 was conducted in the USA and Canada with 1217 patients, whilst VIEW-2 was performed in Europe with 1240 patients across Europe, Asia Pacific, and Latin America (Heier

Table 3.1 Visual acuity (VA) outcomes of anti-VEGF treatment reported in clinical trials and clinical practice settings

Study	Setting (clinical practice or clinical trial)	Drug and dose (if reported)	Treatment regime (n per regime at baseline)	Mean age at baseline	Mean VA at baseline	VA at 3 months (n at 3 months)	Injections at 3 months	VA at 1 year (n at 1 year)	Injections at 1 year	VA at 2 years (n at 2 years)	Injections at 2 years	VA at >2 years (Time point) (n at given time point)	Injections at specified time point
CATT (Martin et al. 2011, 2012)	Clinical trial	RBZ 0.5 mg	Monthly (n=146)	79.5 (SD 7.4)	59.9 (SD 12.2)	65.0 (SD 12.7) (n=273)	NR	68.8 (SD 17.7) (n=284)	11.7 (SD 1.5)	68.5 (SD 18.9) (n=134)	22.4 (SD 3.9)	NR	NR
			Monthly (1 year) then PRN (n=138)	78.8 (SD 7.5)	60.9 (SD 14.3)					67.7 (SD 18.5) (n=130)	NR (5.0 in second year)		
			PRN (n=298)	78.3 (SD 7.8)	61.6 (SD 13.1)	67.2 (SD 13.8) (n=277)		68.4 (SD 16.4) (n=285)	6.9 (SD 3.0)	68.5 (SD 15.3) (n=264)	12.6 (SD 6.6)		
		BVZ 1.25 mg	Monthly (n=135)	79.7 (SD 7.5)	60.2 (SD 13.6)	66.3 (SD 14.3) (n=260)		68.4 (SD 18.2) (n=265)	11.9 (SD 1.2)	68.2 (SD 16.1) (n=129)	23.4 (SD 2.8)		
			Monthly (1 year) then PRN (n=131)	80.4 (SD 7.1)	60.4 (SD 12.4)				7.7 (SD 3.5)	65.0 (SD 21.8) (n=122)	NR (5.8 in second year)		
			PRN (n=300)	78.9 (SD 7.4)	60.6 (SD 13.0)	66.2 (SD 13.7) (n=275)		66.5 (SD 19.0) (n=271)		66.0 (SD 19.9) (n=251)	14.1 (SD 7.0)		
IVAN[a] (Chakravarthy et al. 2012, 2013)	Clinical trial	RBZ 0.5 mg	Monthly (n=157)	77.8 (SD 7.6)	61.8 (SD 15.0)	NR	NR	69.0 (SD 16.0) (n=287)	NR	67.8 (SD 17.0) (n=271)	NR	NR	NR
			3-dose loading phase, then PRN (n=155)										
		BVZ 1.25 mg	Monthly (n=149)	77.8 (SD 8.0)	61.1 (SD 15.6)			66.1 (SD 17.4) (n=274)		66.1 (SD 18.4) (n=254)			
			3-dose loading phase, then PRN (n=145)										
		Analysis combining agents	Monthly (agents combined) (n=308)	77.8 (SD 8.0)	60.0 (SD 15.5)			66.8 (SD 17.4) (n=277)		66.6 (SD 17.9) (n=261)			
			3-dose loading phase, then PRN (agents combined) (n=302)	77.6 (SD 6.8)	62.9 (SD 15.0)			68.4 (SD 16.1) (n=284)		67.3 (SD 17.5) (n=264)			
GEFAL (Kodjikian et al. 2013)	Clinical trial	RBZ 0.5 mg	3-dose loading phase, then PRN (n=183)	78.68 (SD 7.27)	55.78 (SD 13.99)	59.9 (SD 11.9) (n=176)	NR	59.4 (SD 14.2) (n=176)	6.5 (SD 2.4)	NR	NR	NR	NR
Data for cohort which completed study protocol		BVZ 1.25 mg	3-dose loading phase, then PRN (n=191)	79.62 (SD 6.90)	54.62 (SD 14.07)	59.9 (SD 10.6) (n=187)		60.0 (SD 14.4) (n=187)	6.8 (SD 2.7)				
MANTA (Krebs et al. 2013)	Clinical trial	BVZ 1.25 mg	3-dose loading phase, then PRN (n=154)	76.7 (SD 7.8)	57.0 (SD 13.0)	NR	NR	62.2 (CI 60.1–64.3) (n=121)	9.1 (SD 2.8)	NR	NR	NR	NR
		RBZ 0.5 mg	3-dose loading phase, then PRN (n=163)	77.6 (SD 8.1)	56.4 (SD 13.5)			60.7 (CI 58.7–62.8) (n=127)	8.8 (SD 2.7)				

(continued)

Table 3.1 (continued)

Study	Setting (clinical practice or clinical trial)	Drug and dose (if reported)	Treatment regime (n per regime at baseline)	Mean age at baseline	Mean VA at baseline	VA at 3 months (n at 3 months)	Injections at 3 months	VA at 1 year (n at 1 year)	Injections at 1 year	VA at 2 years (n at 2 years)	Injections at 2 years	VA at >2 years (Time point) (n at given time point)	Injections at specified time point
VIEW 1 (Heier et al. 2012)	Clinical trial	RBZ 0.5 mg	4-weekly (n=304)	78.2 (SD 7.6)	54.0 (SD 13.4)	NR	NR	62.1 (SD 15.3) (n=269)	12.1–12.5 for all monthly treatment arms (SD NR)	NR	NR	NR	NR
		ABC 0.5 mg	4-weekly (n=301)	78.4 (SD 8.1)	55.6 (SD 13.1)			62.5 (SD 13.4) (n=270)					
		ABC 2 mg	4-weekly (n=304)	77.7 (SD 7.9)	55.2 (SD 13.2)			66.1 (SD 13.8) (n=285)					
			3-month loading phase, then 8-weekly (n=301)	77.9 (SD 8.4)	55.7 (SD 12.8)			63.6 (SD 15.0) (n=265)	7.5 (SD NR)				
VIEW 2 (Heier et al. 2012)	Clinical trial	RBZ 0.5 mg	4-weekly (n=291)	73.0 (SD 9.0)	53.8 (SD 13.5)	NR	NR	63.4 (SD 13.5) (n=269)	12.2–12.4 for all monthly treatment arms (SD NR)	NR	NR	NR	NR
		ABC 0.5 mg	4-weekly (n=296)	74.7 (SD 8.6)	51.6 (SD 14.2)			61.3 (SD 14.1) (n=268)					
		ABC 2 mg	4-weekly (n=309)	74.1 (SD 8.5)	52.8 (SD 13.9)			60.4 (SD 12.6) (n=274)					
			3-month loading phase, then 8-weekly (n=306)	73.8 (SD 8.6)	51.6 (SD 13.9)			60.5 (SD 14.4) (n=270)	7.5 (SD NR)				
VIEW studies combined (Heier et al. 2012; Schmidt-Erfurth et al. 2014)	Clinical trial	RBZ 0.5 mg	4-weekly (n=595)	75.6 (SD 8.7)	53.9 (SD 13.4)	NR	NR	62.6 (SD NR) (n=560)	12.1–12.5 for all monthly treatment arms (SD NR)	61.8 (n=519)	16.5 (SD 3.7)	NR	NR
		ABC 0.5 mg	4-weekly (n=597)	76.5 (SD 8.5)	53.6 (13.8)			61.9 (n=551)		60.2 (n=502)	16.2 (SD 4.0)		
		ABC 2 mg	4-weekly (n=613)	75.9 (SD 8.4)	54.0 (13.6)			63.3 (n=574)		61.6 (n=529)	16.0 (SD 3.2)		
			3-month loading phase, then 8-weekly (n=607)	75.8 (SD 8.8)	53.6 (13.5)			62 (n=560)	7.5 (SD NR)	61.2 (n=513)	11.2 (SD 2.9)		
PIER (Regillo et al. 2008; Abraham et al. 2010)	Clinical trial	RBZ 0.3 mg	3-month loading phase, then quarterly. Switched to monthly at month19 (n=60)	78.7 (SD 6.3)	55.8 (SD 12.2)	NR	NR	54.2 (SD 15.1) (n=59)	NR	53.6 (SD 15.6) (n=53)	NR	NR	NR
		RBZ 0.5 mg	3-month loading phase, then quarterly. Switched to monthly at month19 (n=61)	78.8 (SD 7.9)	53.7 (SD 15.5)			53.5 (SD 13.1) (n=58)		51.4 (SD 14.4) (n=54)			

Study	Type	Drug	Regimen (n)										
EXCITE (Schmidt-Erfurth et al. 2011)	Clinical trial	RBZ 0.3 mg	Monthly (0.3 mg) (n=115)	75 (SD 8.26)	56.5 (SD 12.19)	64.0 (SD NR) (n=NR)	NR	64.5 (SD 16.27) (n=101)	11.4 (SD 1.69)	NR	NR	NR	NR
			3-dose loading phase, then quarterly (0.3 mg) (n=120)	75.1 (SD 7.45)	55.8 (SD 11.81)	62.6 (SD NR) (n=NR)		60.2 (SD 16.01) (n=104)	5.7 (SD 0.80)				
		RBZ 0.5 mg	3-dose loading phase, then quarterly (0.5 mg) (n=118)	75.8 (SD 6.96)	57.7 (SD 13.06)	64.3 (SD NR) (n=NR)		61.3 (SD 16.32) (n=88)	5.5 (SD 1.05)				
SUSTAIN (Holz et al. 2011)	Clinical trial	RBZ 0.3 mg/0.5 mg	3-dose loading phase, then PRN (n=513)	75.1 (SD 8.06)	56.1 (SD 12.19)	61.9 (SD 11.12) (n=509)	2.9 (SD 0.35)	59.7 (SD 13.89) (n=509)	5.6 (SD 2.37)	NR	NR	NR	NR
SECURE (Silva et al. 2013)	Clinical trial	RBZ 0.3 mg/0.5 mg	Completion of EXCITE or SUSTAIN protocol (1 year), then PRN (n=234)	74.5 (SD 7.62)	NR	NR	NR	60.7 (SD 16.14) (n=231)	NR	58.7 (SD 10.44) (n=230)	NR	56.4 (SD 13.04) (n=230)	6.1 (SD 5.67) Number of injections from end of Year 1 to 36 months
SAILOR (Boyer et al. 2009) (Note: only treatment naïve cohorts are included)	Clinical trial	RBZ 0.3 mg	3-dose loading phase, then PRN (n=462)	79.9 (SD 7.9)	55.0 (SD 12.5)	60.8 (SD NR) (n=NR)	96 % of cohort received 3 doses in first 3 months	55.5 (SD NR)	4.6 (combined figure for both groups) (SD NR) (81.7 % follow-up reported)	NR	NR	NR	NR
		RBZ 0.5 mg	3-dose loading phase, then PRN (n=490)	75.8 (SD 8.0)	48.9 (SD 13.8)	55.9 (SD NR)		51.3 (SD NR)					
ANCHOR (Brown et al. 2006, 2009)	Clinical trial	RBZ 0.3 mg	Monthly (n=140)	77.4 (SD 7.5)	47.0 (SD 13.1)	53.8 (SD NR) (n=NR)	NR	55.5 (SD 14.6) (n>126)	11.0 (SD NR)	55.1 (SD 16.2) (n=117)	21.5 (SD NR)	NR	NR
		RBZ 0.5 mg	Monthly (n=139)	76.0 (SD 8.6)	47.1 (SD 13.2)	57.1 (SD NR) (n=NR)		58.4 (SD 14.6) (n>126)	11.2 (SD NR)	57.8 (SD 16.5) (n=116)	21.3 (SD NR)		
MARINA (Rosenfeld et al. 2006)	Clinical trial	RBZ 0.3 mg	Monthly (n=238)	77 (SD 8)	53.1 (SD 12.9)	58.2 (SD NR) (n=NR)	NR	59.6 (SD) (n=226)	NR	58.5 (SD) (n=210)	NR	NR	NR
		RBZ 0.5 mg	Monthly (n=240)	77 (SD 8)	53.7 (SD 12.8)	59.6 (SD NR) (n=NR)		60.9 (SD) (n=226)		60.3 (SD) (n=215)			
HORIZON (Singer et al. 2012)	Clinical trial	RBZ 0.5 mg	Monthly for 2 years (in ANCHOR, MARINA or FOCUS), then PRN (n=600)	76.1 (SD 7.6)	51.6 (SD 13.0)	NR	NR	NR	NR	60.5 (SD 17.9) (n=600)	NR	55.7 (SD NR) (n=481) 36 months; 53.6 (SD NR) (n=388) 48 months; 51.5 (SD NR) (n=73) 60 months	NR

(continued)

Table 3.1 (continued)

Study	Setting (clinical practice or clinical trial)	Drug and dose (if reported)	Treatment regime (n per regime at baseline)	Mean age at baseline	Mean VA at baseline	VA at 3 months (n at 3 months)	Injections at 3 months	VA at 1 year (n at 1 year)	Injections at 1 year	VA at 2 years (n at 2 years)	Injections at 2 years	VA at >2 years (Time point) (n at given time point)	Injections at specified time point
SEVEN-UP (Rofagha et al. 2013)	Clinical practice follow-up of a Clinical trial sample	RBZ 0.5 mg (n=36) and 0.3 mg (n=29). Data pooled	Monthly for 2 years (in ANCHOR or MARINA), then PRN for 2 years in HORIZON, then PRN (n=65)	74.9 (SD 7.7)	54.3 (SD 12.4)	NR	NR	NR	NR	NR	NR	45.7 (SE 2.8) (n=65) 7 year follow-up	6.8 (Range 0–46) Since exit from HORIZON (from 4 years onwards)
EXTEND-I (Tano and Ohji 2010, 2011)	Clinical trial	RBZ 0.3 mg	Monthly (n=35)	70.7 (SD NR)	46.7 (SD 11.8)	NR	NR	57.2 (SD NR) (n=31)	11.2 (Range 3–12)	NR	NR	55.4 (SD 17.14) (n=28) 2.7 years (SD 0.35)	4.1 (SD 4.12) No. of injections/year after 12 months
		RBZ 0.5 mg	Monthly (n=41)	71.6 (SD NR)	48.1 (SD 10.8)			57.6 (SD NR) (n=37)	11.1 (Range 3–12)			57.6 (SD 15.36) (n=33) 2.93 years (SD 0.09)	3.9 (SD 4.63) No. of injections/year after 12 months
PrONTO (Fung et al. 2007; Lalwani et al. 2009)	Clinical trial	RBZ 0.5 mg	3-dose loading phase, then PRN (n=40)	83.5 (SD 7.2)	56.2 (SD NR)	67.0 (SD NR) (n=40)	3 (SD NR)	65.5 (SD NR) (n=40)	5.6 (SD 2.3)	67.0 (SD 12.2) (n=37)	9.9 (SD 5.3)	NR	NR
ABC-Trial (Tufail et al. 2010)	Clinical trial	BVZ 1.25 mg	3-dose loading phase (6-weekly intervals) then PRN (n=65)	79 (SD NR)	50 (IQR 43–61)	56.7 (SD NR) (n=NR)	NR	57 (SD NR) (n=64)	7.1 (Range 3–9)	NR	NR	NR	NR
Sacu et al. (2009)	Clinical trial	BVZ 1 mg	3-dose loading phase, then PRN (n=14)	78 (SD 8)	50 (SD NR) (n=14)	62 (SD NR) (n=14)	NR	58 (SD NR) (n=14)	6.8 (SD NR)	NR	NR	NR	NR
Kruger Falk et al. (2013)	Clinical Practice	RBZ	3-month loading phase, then variable regimes (n=855)	77.3 (Range 54–98)	53.2 (Range 1–85)	NR	NR	NR		NR	NR	50.5 (Variable follow-up time. Mean 23.3 months, range 4–48 months) (n=855)	8.7 (Range 1–35)
Rasmussen et al. (2013)	Clinical Practice	RBZ	3-dose loading phase, then PRN (n=600)	79.9 (SD 9.9)	0.24 (SD NR)	0.26 (SD NR)	NR	NR	NR	NR	NR 10.2 (SD NR)	0.18 (SD NR) 4 years – last visit carried forward (n=600)	NR
			Subgroup who completed 4 years of screening and re-treatment (n=192)	78.0 (SD 11.5)	0.30 (95%CI 0.28–0.33) (n=192)	0.38 (95%CI 0.35–0.42) (n=192)		0.35 (95%CI NR)	5.2 (SD NR)			0.32 (95%CI 0.29–0.35) (n=192)	22.1 (SD NR)

Note: Visual acuity recorded as Snellen equivalent

Study	Setting	Drug	Regimen										
Muniraju et al. (Muniraju et al. 2013)	Clinical Practice	RBZ	3-dose loading phase, then PRN (n=292)	82.7 (Range 55–97)	48.2 (SD 16.9)	NR	NR	51.2 (SD 18.7) (n=NR)	4.8 (SD 2.2)	50.4 (SD 20.8) (n=NR)	7.8 (SD 4.2)	49.1 (SD 21.7) (n=192) 36 months	10.2 (SD 6.2)
Marques et al. (Marques et al. 2013)	Clinical Practice	RBZ	PRN (n=84)	77.39 (Range 61–94)	49.3 (SD 15.2)	52.6 (SD 15.3) (n=67)	1.53 (SD 0.53)	50.7 (SD 15.9) (n=84)	3.75 (SD 1.20)	48.8 (SD 18.8) (n=77)	6.35 (SD 2.3)	47.7 (SD 18.7) (n=52) 34.3 months (SD 6.9)	8.67 (SD 3.3)
Rung and Lovestam-Adrian (Rung and Lovestam-Adrian 2013)	Clinical Practice	RBZ	3-dose loading phase, then PRN (n=66)	76 (SD 7)	53 (SD 14)	61 (SD 14)	NR	NR	NR	NR	NR	44 (SD 24) (n=51) 37-month follow-up	7.8 (SD 5.0)
WAVE Germany (Finger et al. 2013; Holz et al. 2013) Note: Visual acuity at 3 months recorded using LogMAR scale	Clinical Practice	RBZ	3-month loading phase, then PRN (n=3470)	77.6 (SD 7.8)	48.8 (SD 18.7)	0.64 (SE 0.01) (n=3124)	2.95 (SE 0.01)	48.0 (SD 11.7) (n=2587)	4.34 (SD 1.9)	NR	NR	NR	NR
HELIOS Netherlands (Holz et al. 2013)	Clinical Practice	RBZ	3-dose loading phase, then PRN (n=243)	77.9 (SD 8.0)	45.1 (SD 21.5)	NR	NR	50.7 (SD 24.0) (n=208)	5.1 (SD 2.4)	NR	NR	NR	NR
HELIOS Belgium (Rakic et al. 2013)	Clinical Practice	RBZ	3-dose loading phase, then PRN (n=267)	78.5 (SD 7.3)	56.3 (SD 14.3)	61.7 (SD 14.9) (n=NR) (2.5-month follow-up)	2.5 (SD 0.7)	58.5 (SD 17.8) (n=206)	5.0 (SD 2.1)	53.3 (SD 19.3) (n=184)	7.6 (SD 4.1)	NR	NR
Sweden ranibizumab registry (Hjelmqvist et al. 2011) Data reported for patients who remained in treatment for 12 months (370/471)	Clinical Practice	RBZ	3-dose loading phase, then PRN (n=370)	77.7 (SD 8.0)	58.3 (SD 12.2)	63.3 (SD 12.5)	95 % of patients had 3 injections at 3 months	59.3 (SD 16.2) (n=370)	4.7 (SD 1.6)	NR	NR	NR	NR

(continued)

Table 3.1 (continued)

Study	Setting (clinical practice or clinical trial)	Drug and dose (if reported)	Treatment regime (n per regime at baseline)	Mean age at baseline	Mean VA at baseline	VA at 3 months (n at 3 months)	Injections at 3 months	VA at 1 year (n at 1 year)	Injections at 1 year	VA at 2 years (n at 2 years)	Injections at 2 years	VA at >2 years (Time point) (n at given time point)	Injections at specified time point
NvAMD database, UK (The neovascular age-related macular degeneration database: multicenter study of 92 976 ranibizumab injections: report 1: visual acuity 2014)	Clinical Practice	RBZ	3-month loading phase, then PRN (n=12,951)	79.1 (IQR 75–85)	55	NR	NR	57 (n=8598)	5.7 (Range 1–13)	55 (n=4990)	9.4 (mean 3.7 in second year, range 0–13)	53 (n=2470) (3 years)	13.1 (mean 3.7 in third year, range 0–12)

Only studies reporting outcomes to 1 year or greater have been included. All VA measurements were reported using the Early Treatment Diabetic Retinopathy Study (ETDRS) measurement unless otherwise stated. Loading doses were spaced in 4-weekly intervals unless otherwise stated

NR not reported, *IQR* inter-quartile range, *SD* standard deviation, *SE* standard error

[a]IVAN trial reported findings according to drug allocation and regime allocation, but did not report findings for individual subgroups.

et al. 2012). This work demonstrated 8-weekly ABC 2.0 mg to be non-inferior to 4-weekly RBZ 0.5 mg in terms of vision and anatomical outcomes over 52 weeks (Heier et al. 2012). Both cohorts were subsequently followed up to 96 weeks (Schmidt-Erfurth et al. 2014). For weeks 52–96, patients were treated on a PRN basis, with ongoing monthly monitoring and a 12-weekly minimum injection frequency. Small losses from gains achieved at 52 weeks were noted in both cohorts; however, equal efficacy between 4-weekly RBZ 0.5 mg and 8-weekly ABC 2.0 mg was demonstrated (Schmidt-Erfurth et al. 2014).

Bevacizumab

Due to its off-label use, highly standardized clinical trials testing BVZ for nvAMD have only recently been completed. A review published in 2011 (Mitchell 2011) identified only one study constituting Level I evidence (Tufail et al. 2010), which demonstrated a positive effect of BVZ compared to pegaptanib, PDT, and sham injections. In 2009, a small study compared the efficacy of BVZ with RBZ over a 6-month period for the first time (Subramanian et al. 2009). Since then, four large comparative studies have reported results (Martin et al. 2011; 2012; Chakravarthy et al. 2012, 2013; Krebs et al. 2013; Kodjikian et al. 2013). In 2012, 2-year results were published for the CATT study, which compared RBZ 0.5 mg and BVZ 1.25 mg across regular 4-weekly and PRN injection regimes, which did not include a loading phase (Martin et al. 2012). Of the 1185 patients enrolled in the study, 1107 (93.4 %) were followed up during the second year. This trial found similar efficacy of the two agents on VA over a 2-year period, despite a significant difference in the proportion of participants without the presence of fluid on OCT in favor of RBZ (Martin et al. 2012). Groups receiving regular 4-weekly injections with either agent achieved higher visual gains than those receiving PRN regimes. In the case of BVZ, the mean reported gains after 2 years were 7.8 letters for 4-weekly dosing and 5.0 letters for PRN regimes. A second multicenter, non-inferiority factorial trial (IVAN) studied 610 patients with nvAMD over 2 years, comparing regular and PRN treatment regimes of

BVZ and RBZ. Like the CATT study, this work demonstrated a similar efficacy of the two agents; however, a difference in efficacy between regular and PRN treatment regimes was not found (Chakravarthy et al. 2013). The MANTA (Krebs et al. 2013) and GEFAL (Kodjikian et al. 2013) studies have contributed further comparative data between BVZ and RBZ over a 1-year treatment duration, utilizing a protocol of three initial treatments spaced monthly followed by further treatment as required. Participants in the MANTA study received more treatments across both treatment arms than the GEFAL cohorts; however, VA outcomes were comparable. Both studies found BVZ to be non-inferior to RBZ for VA outcomes after 1 year (Krebs et al. 2013; Kodjikian et al. 2013). A subsequent meta-analysis, including all above-mentioned comparison studies performed by the research group who conducted the GEFAL study, concluded that the BVZ and RBZ treatments achieved similar VA outcomes (Kodjikian et al. 2014).

3.2.1.2 Outcomes Achieved in Routine Medical Practice

Treatment outcomes of nvAMD using anti-VEGF agents appear to be worse in routine medical practice, when compared with data generated from phase III clinical trials (Finger et al. 2014; Rasmussen and Sander 2014; the neovascular age-related macular degeneration database: multicenter study of 92,976 ranibizumab injections: report 1: visual acuity 2014). In much of the published work from the clinical trial setting, a stable VA was defined as a loss of less than 15 EDTRS letters (Martin et al. 2011; Brown et al. 2009; Rosenfeld et al. 2006; Krebs et al. 2013; Tufail et al. 2010). In the trial setting, approximately 90 % of participants achieved stable VA after 2 years of treatment according to this definition (Martin et al. 2011; Brown et al. 2009; Rosenfeld et al. 2006; Krebs et al. 2013; Tufail et al. 2010). In comparison, research in clinical practice has tended to find 70–80 % of patients maintained stable vision with treatment (Rasmussen and Sander 2014). Clinical practice studies have focused almost exclusively on RBZ, with a regime consisting of three initial monthly doses followed by monthly reviews and treatment on a PRN basis. Fewer studies have reported outcomes for a Treat & Extend regimen, in which intravitreal injections are given monthly until disease inactivity has been achieved, defined as stable VA, absence of fluid on OCT, and no new hemorrhage. Following this, patient visits are extended by a 2-week interval from 4 to 6 to 8, etc., weeks with an intravitreal injection given at each visit as long as there is no sign of disease activity (no loss of VA, a dry OCT, and no new hemorrhage). In case of a reactivation (loss of VA or increase/presence of fluid on OCT, or fresh hemorrhage), intervals are reduced again.

Several studies have reported treatment outcomes of Treat & Extend regimes for nvAMD, which achieved improvements in VA ranging from an 11 letter gain at 1 year to a 15 letter gain at 2 years with a very similar mean number of injections (7–8 in year 1 and 5–6 in year 2) (Oubraham et al. 2011; Abedi et al. 2014). The OCT-guided Treat & Extend treatment protocol has been shown to lead to treatment outcomes comparable to outcomes in phase III clinical trials with fewer injections over the first 2 years (Lalwani et al. 2009; Gupta et al. 2010; Abedi et al. 2014).

Populations that received fewer injections have not fared as well. A large study produced in Demark followed a cohort of 855 patients undergoing PRN treatment with RBZ for AMD over a 4-year period, with a mean follow-up time of 23.3 months (Kruger Falk et al. 2013). A mean VA loss of 3 ETDRS letters was recorded, with a mean of 8.7 injections over the time frame studied. During the study period, 399 patients (46.7 %) discontinued treatment for several different reasons. Chiefly, this was due to the absence of further disease activity in 181 cases, treatment being deemed futile in 113 cases and 36 cases where patients declined further injections (Kruger Falk et al. 2013). Three clinical practice studies have documented VA outcomes after approximately 3 years (34–37 months) from commencing treatment (Muniraju et al. 2013; Marques et al. 2013; Rung and Lovestam-Adrian 2013). Whilst patients in the largest of these studies maintained a modest gain from baseline (0.9 ETDRS letters)

with 10.2 (SD 6.2) injections (Muniraju et al. 2013), the other studies recorded losses of 1.6 and 7 ETDRS letters with 8.67 (SD 3.3) and 7.8 (SD 5.0) injections, respectively (Marques et al. 2013; Rung and Lovestam-Adrian 2013). A very large study utilized the United Kingdom national nvAMD database to examine VA outcomes of 12,951 eyes of 11,135 individuals over a treatment period of up to 3 years (The neovascular age-related macular degeneration database: multicenter study of 92,976 ranibizumab injections: report 1: visual acuity 2014). The 2470 eyes that completed 3 years of follow-up had a loss of 2 ETDRS letters on average, with a mean of 13.1 injections over this time period. Whilst longer term follow-up has demonstrated a further decline in vision over time, the relatively low number of injections administered to patients in clinical practice studies may indicate under-treatment in this setting (Rasmussen and Sander 2014).

The need for ongoing follow-up of patients with nvAMD was highlighted in a Danish longitudinal study over 4 years, where 192 of 600 eyes (32 %) followed were still receiving active treatment (Rasmussen et al. 2013). Vision had been maintained over 4 years compared with baseline readings with a mean of 22.1 injections over this period and was significantly better than those who had discontinued treatment. Furthermore, of 120 eyes (20 %) that had ceased treatment as a result of apparent disease inactivity, 25 were subsequently referred for further treatment (Rasmussen et al. 2013).

Patient registries have been examined in Germany, the Netherlands, Belgium, and Sweden through the LUMINOUS program to assess the efficacy of RBZ for nvAMD in clinical practice over a 1-year treatment period (Holz et al. 2013). Patient age was similar across the four registries, between 77.6 (SD 7.8) in Germany and 78.7 (SD 6.8) in Belgium; however, the mean baseline VAs were higher in the Belgian (56.3, SD 14.2) and Swedish (58.3, SD 12.2) registries compared with those of the Netherlands (45.1, SD 21.5) and Germany (48.8, SD 18.7). Over 1 year of treatment, three populations gained between 1.0 and 5.6 letters with between 4.7 and 5.7 injections, however the German cohort lost 0.73 letters during the same time period with a mean of 4.3 injections in patients who completed a year of follow-up (Holz et al. 2013; Finger et al. 2013). These results further demonstrate that VA outcomes in clinical practice are inferior to those in phase III clinical trials, with under-treatment of patients in the clinical practice setting being a likely contributing factor.

3.2.2 Anatomical Outcomes Based on Optical Coherence Tomography

The response of macular tissue to anti-VEGF therapy has been examined with OCT in a number of studies. Changes in macular thickness (MT) viewed with OCT have been the most commonly reported outcome (see Table 3.2) (Finger et al. 2014). Extensive variation of thickness measurements exists between studies, due to differences in methods of measurement as well as different OCT machines being used. Terminology is similarly variable between papers, with foveal thickness (FT), CRT, central macular thickness (CMT), central subfield macular thickness (CSMT), and central foveal thickness (CFT) all used in various clinical trials (Mitchell 2011). Of these, CRT is the most often reported, however variation in reported measurements exists even within this subgroup. Despite this high level of variance, trends observed in macular thickness changes with anti-VEGF therapy are apparent when comparing agents and treatment regimes (see Table 3.2).

3.2.2.1 Ranibizumab

RBZ has been extensively demonstrated to reduce the thickness of macular tissue in the treatment of nvAMD (Martin et al. 2011, 2012; Chakravarthy et al. 2012, 2013; Kodjikian et al. 2013; Krebs et al. 2013; Heier et al. 2012; Schmidt-Erfurth et al. 2011; Holz et al. 2011; Boyer et al. 2009; Lalwani et al. 2009; Fung et al. 2007; Marques et al. 2013; Finger et al. 2013). This reduction in thickness is mostly due to resolution of edema and is evident in most patients followed up 4 weeks after their first injection

(Subramanian et al. 2009; Martin et al. 2011; Heier et al. 2012; Schmidt-Erfurth et al. 2011; Holz et al. 2011; Boyer et al. 2009; Fung et al. 2007). Reductions in mean MT at 3 months are often not maintained to the 12-month mark (Kodjikian et al. 2013; Holz et al. 2011; Boyer et al. 2009; Fung et al. 2007; Finger et al. 2013); however, as most studies reporting 3-month figures involve a loading phase of three 4-weekly injections, followed by PRN treatment, this may reflect under-treatment post-loading phase. Reductions in mean MT seen after 1 year are maintained at 2 years (Martin et al. 2012; Chakravarthy et al. 2013; Lalwani et al. 2009; Marques et al. 2013), regardless of treatment regime (4-weekly or PRN). However, the CATT study found regular 4-weekly treatment to be more effective than PRN therapy for reducing foveal thickness, and a switch from 4-weekly therapy to PRN after 1 year resulted in an increase in MT to the level of participants that received PRN treatment from the commencement of therapy (Martin et al. 2012).

Minimal evidence is available on long-term changes in MT from anti-VEGF therapy for nvAMD. However a clinical practice-based 36-month follow-up of 52 patients in Portugal found reductions in CMT to be maintained, despite a relatively low injection-rate throughout the study (Marques et al. 2013). The SEVEN-UP study performed retinal imaging to assess the anatomical status of previous participants in the ANCHOR or MARINA trials (Brown et al. 2006; Rosenfeld et al. 2006), followed by the HORIZON study (Singer et al. 2012). As baseline measurements of MT were not published in these trials, figures published in SEVEN-UP cannot shed light on long-term changes in MT with RBZ therapy. However, no association was found between OCT findings (including measures of retinal thickness) in SEVEN-UP and the visual acuity outcomes of its participants. The authors discussed the complexity of the relationship between anatomical outcomes within the macula and VA (Rofagha et al. 2013), implying that MT may be an overly simplistic outcome measure. Almost all of the participants followed up at this late time point (7 years post entering ANCHOR or

Table 3.2 Anatomical outcomes in terms of macular thickness (MT) changes from anti-VEGF therapy reported in clinical trials and clinical practice settings. Only studies reporting outcomes to 1 year or greater have been included

Study	Setting (clinical practice or clinical trial) and measure used	Drug and dose (if reported)	Treatment regime (n or per regime at baseline)	Mean age at baseline	Mean MT (in μm) at baseline	MT at 3 months (n at 3 months)	Injections at 3 months	MT (in μm) at 1 year (n at 1 year)	Injections at 1 year	MT (in μm) at 2 years (n at 2 years)	Injections at 2 years	MT at >2 years (in μm) (Time point) (n at given time point)	Injections at specified time point
CATT (Martin et al. 2011, 2012)	Clinical trial	RBZ 0.5 mg	Monthly (n=146)	79.5 (SD 7.4)	460 (SD 194)	NR	NR	266 (SD 125) (n=280)	11.7 (SD 1.5)	267 (SD 143) (n=134)	22.4 (SD 3.9)	NR	NR
	FT		Monthly (1 year) then PRN (n=138)	78.8 (SD 7.5)	462 (SD 184)					295 (SD 135) (n=130)	NR (5.0 in second year)		
			PRN (n=298)	78.3 (SD 7.8)	462 (SD 195)			294 (SD 139) (n=281)	6.9 (SD 3.0)	293 (SD 129) (n=264)	12.6 (SD 6.6)		
		BVZ 1.25 mg	Monthly (n=135)	79.7 (SD 7.5)	462 (SD 205)			300 (SD 149) (n=261)	11.9 (SD 1.2)	274 (SD 137) (n=129)	23.4 (SD 2.8)		
			Monthly (1 year) then PRN (n=131)	80.4 (SD 7.1)	471 (SD 185)					334 (SD 190) (n=122)	NR (5.8 in second year)		
			PRN (n=300)	78.9 (SD 7.4)	459 (SD 173)			308 (SD 127) (n=266)	7.7 (SD 3.5)	306 (SD 134) (n=251)	14.1 (SD 7.0)		
IVAN[a] (Chakravarthy et al. 2012, 2013)	Clinical trial	RBZ 0.5 mg	Monthly (n=157)	77.8 (SD 7.6)	468 (SD 187) (n=302)	NR	NR	322 (SD 139) (n=287)	NR	322.4 (SD 137.3) (n=271)	NR	NR	NR
	FT		3-dose loading phase, then PRN (n=155)										
		BVZ 1.25 mg	Monthly (n=149)	77.8 (SD 8.0)	465 (SD 184) (n=279)			325 (SD 134) (n=274)		331.0 (SD 144.2) (n=254)			
			3-dose loading phase, then PRN (n=145)										
		Analysis combining agents	Monthly (agents combined) (n=308)	77.8 (SD 8.0)	474 (SD 188) (n=293)			311 (SD 126) (n=277)		314.7 (SD 137.1) (n=261) (n=261)			
			3-dose loading phase, then PRN (agents combined) (n=302)	77.6 (SD 6.8)	459 (SD 182) (n=289)			459 (SD 182) (n=289)		338.5 (SD 143.3) (n=264)			
GEFAL (Kodjikian et al. 2013)	Clinical trial	RBZ 0.5 mg	3-dose loading phase, then PRN (n=183)	78.68 (SD 7.27)	354.75 (SD 109.90)	239 (SD NR) (n=183)	NR	248 (SD 103) (n=183)	6.5 (SD 2.4)	NR	NR	NR	NR
Data for cohort which completed study protocol	CSMT	BVZ 1.25 mg	3-dose loading phase, then PRN (n=187)	79.62 (SD 6.90)	359.21 (SD 120.72)	258 (SD NR) (n=187)		264 (SD 133) (n=187)	6.8 (SD 2.7)				

MANTA (Krebs et al. 2013)	Clinical trial	BVZ 1.25 mg	3-dose loading phase, then PRN (n=154)	76.7 (SD 7.8)	374.6 (SD 8.4)	NR	288.3 (SD 8.0) (n=121)	9.1 (SD 2.8)	NR	NR	NR	NR
	CRT	RBZ 0.5 mg	3-dose loading phase, then PRN (n=163)	77.6 (SD 8.1)	365.0 (SD 8.1)		275.1 (SD 6.8) (n=127)	8.8 (SD 2.7)				
VIEW 1 (Heier et al. 2012)	Clinical trial	RBZ 0.5 mg	4-weekly (n=304)	78.2 (SD 7.6)	315.3 (SD 108.3)	NR	198.5 (SD 109.0) (n=269)	12.1–12.5 for all monthly treatment arms (SD NR)	NR	NR	NR	NR
	CRT	ABC 0.5 mg	4-weekly (n=301)	78.4 (SD 8.1)	313.2 (SD 106.0)		197.6 (SD 104.1) (n=270)					
		ABC 2 mg	4-weekly (n=304)	77.7 (SD 7.9)	313.6 (SD 103.4)		197.1 (SD 98.4) (n=285)					
			3-month loading phase, then 8-weekly (n=301)	77.9 (SD 8.4)	324.4 (SD 111.2)		195.9 (SD 108.5) (n=265)	7.5 (SD NR)				
VIEW 2 (Heier et al. 2012)	Clinical trial	RBZ 0.5 mg	4-weekly (n=291)	73.0 (SD 9.0)	325.9 (SD 110.9)	NR	187.4 (SD 122.2) (n=269)	12.2–12.4 for all monthly treatment arms (SD NR)	NR	NR	NR	NR
	CRT	ABC 0.5 mg	4-weekly (n=296)	74.7 (SD 8.6)	326.5 (SD 116.5)		196.7 (SD 114.8) (n=268)					
		ABC 2 mg	4-weekly (n=309)	74.1 (SD 8.5)	334.6 (SD 119.8)		177.8 (SD 122.8) (n=274)					
			3-month loading phase, then 8-weekly (n=306)	73.8 (SD 8.6)	342.6 (SD 124.0)		193.4 (SD 119.7) (n=270)	7.5 (SD NR)				
VIEW studies combined (Heier et al. 2012; Schmidt-Erfurth et al. 2014)	Clinical trial	RBZ 0.5 mg	4-weekly (n=594)	75.6 (SD 8.7)	296 (SD 123)	NR	NR	12.1–12.5 for all monthly treatment arms (SD NR)	+10 µm from 1 year	NR	16.5 (SD 3.7)	NR
	CRT	ABC 0.5 mg	4-weekly (n=594)	76.5 (SD 8.5)	296 (SD 132)				+10 µm from 1 year		16.2 (SD 4.0)	
		ABC 2 mg	4-weekly (n=611)	75.9 (SD 8.4)	299 (SD 126)				+10 µm from 1 year		16.0 (SD 3.2)	
			3-month loading phase, then 8-weekly (n=603)	75.8 (SD 8.8)	306 (SD 134)			7.5 (SD NR)	+6 µm from 1 year		11.2 (SD 2.9)	

(continued)

Table 3.2 (continued)

Study	Setting (clinical practice or clinical trial) and measure used	Drug and dose (if reported)	Treatment regime (n per regime at baseline)	Mean age at baseline	Mean MT (in µm) at baseline	MT at 3 months (n at 3 months)	Injections at 3 months	MT (in µm) at 1 year (SD (n at 1 year)	Injections at 1 year	MT (in µm) at 2 years (n at 2 years)	Injections at 2 years	MT at >2 years (in µm) (Time point) (n at given time point)	Injections at specified time point
EXCITE (Schmidt-Erfurth et al. 2011)	Clinical trial / CRT	RBZ 0.3 mg	Monthly (0.3 mg) (n=95)	75 (SD=8.26)	320.6 (SD=118.55)	NR	NR	215.3 (SD NR) (n NR)	11.4 (SD=1.69)	NR	NR	NR	NR
			3-dose loading phase, then quarterly (0.3 mg) (n=100)	75.1 (SD=7.45)	313.6 (SD=85.05)			217.6	5.7 (SD=0.80)				
		RBZ 0.5 mg	3-loading phase, then quarterly (0.5 mg) (n=100)	75.8 (SD=6.96)	324.5 (SD=115.94)			218.9	5.5 (SD=1.05)				
SUSTAIN (Holz et al. 2011)	Clinical trial / CRT	RBZ 0.3 mg/0.5 mg	3-dose loading phase, then PRN (n=512)	75.1 (SD=8.06)	340.5 (SD 113.19)	239.4 (SD NR) (n=509)	2.9 (SD 0.35)	249.0 (SD NR) (n=509)	5.6 (SD 2.37)	NR	NR	NR	NR
SAILOR (Boyer et al. 2009) (Note: only treatment naïve cohorts are included)	Clinical trial	RBZ 0.3 mg	3-dose loading phase, then PRN (n=462)	79.9 (SD 7.9)	312 (SD 104)	205 (SD NR) (n=NR)	96 % of total cohort received 3 doses in first 3 months	240 (SD NR) (n=NR)	4.6 (combined figure for both groups) (SD NR) (81.7 % follow-up reported)	NR	NR	NR	NR
	CFT	RBZ 0.5 mg	3-dose loading phase, then PRN (n=490)	75.8 (SD 8.0)	322 (SD 116)	200 (SD NR) (n=NR)		230 (SD NR) (n=NR)					
PrONTO (Fung et al. 2007; Lalwani et al. 2009)	Clinical trial / CRT	RBZ 0.5 mg	3-dose loading phase, then PRN (n=40)	83.5 (SD 7.2)	393.9 (SD NR)	204.3 (SD NR)	3 (SD NR)	216.1 (SD NR)	5.6 (SD 2.3)	179.3 (SD NR) (n=37)	9.9 (SD 5.3)	NR	NR
ABC-Trial (Tufail et al. 2010)	Clinical trial / CMT	BVZ 1.25 mg	3-dose loading phase (6-weekly intervals) then PRN (n=65)	79 (SD NR)	328 (IQR 271–376)	NR	NR	239 (IQR 127–350) (n=64)	7.1 (Range 3–9)	NR	NR	NR	NR
Sacu et al. (2009)	Clinical trial / CRT	BVZ 1 mg	3-dose loading phase, then PRN (n=14)	78 (SD 8)	357 (SD NR) (n=14)	230 (SD NR) (n=14)	NR	244 (SD NR) (n=14)	6.8 (SD NR)	NR	NR	NR	NR
Marques et al. (Marques et al. 2013)	Clinical Practice / CMT	RBZ	PRN (n=84)	77.39 (Range 61–94)	373.3 (SD 102.7)	314.2 (SD 102.7) (n=67)	1.53 (SD 0.53)	296.3 (SD 68.6) (n=84)	3.75 (SD 1.20)	259.4 (SD 67.9) (n=77)	6.35 (SD 2.3)	264.3 (SD 67.7) (n=52) 36 months	8.67 (SD 3.3)
WAVE Germany (Finger et al. 2013)	Clinical Practice / CRT	RBZ	3-month loading phase, then PRN (n=871)	NR	349.4 (SE 4.31)	250.8 (SE 5.42) (n=679)	2.95 (SE 0.01)	270.5 (SE 7.31) (n=545)	4.34 (SE 0.05)	NR	NR	NR	NR

NR Not reported, *IQR* inter-quartile range, *SD* standard deviation, *SE* standard error, *FT* foveal thickness, *CRT* central retinal thickness, *CFT* central foveal thickness, *CMT* central macular thickness, *CSMT* central subfield macular thickness

[a]IVAN trial reported findings according to drug allocation and regime allocation, but did not report findings for individual sub-groups

MARINA) showed some degree of macular atrophy (Rofagha et al. 2013). Indeed, the interplay between the variable and concurrent effects of nvAMD, atrophic AMD, and intravitreal RBZ may limit the value of MT as a predictor of long-term treatment outcome.

3.2.2.2 Aflibercept

The VIEW studies compared 8-weekly ABC 2.0 mg to 4-weekly RBZ 0.5 mg over 96 weeks (Heier et al. 2012; Schmidt-Erfurth et al. 2014). In those receiving 8-weekly ABC treatment, a small degree of retinal thickening was regularly observed 8-week post injection (Heier et al. 2012). However, overall comparable reductions in CRT were recorded in all treatment groups at all time points to 96 weeks. It is noteworthy that the reported baseline CRT values in the 96-week follow-up paper (Schmidt-Erfurth et al. 2014) were different to those reported in the 52-week paper (Heier et al. 2012) (see Table 3.2). No reason for this difference was cited in the 96-week paper; however, given that this subsequent paper had baseline CRT values consistently 20–30 μm thinner, it is plausible that a different anatomical landmark was used for measurement in the second analysis. This discrepancy highlights the difficulty of comparing MT measurements between different studies, or even amongst subsamples of the same study. However, although far less evidence exists for ABC than for RBZ, available data suggests they are similarly efficacious in reducing MT.

3.2.2.3 Bevacizumab

BVZ therapy reduces MT in nvAMD compared with PDT (Tufail et al. 2010). Results beyond 2 years of treatment are yet to be reported. As with RBZ, continuous 4-weekly treatment has a greater magnitude of effect than PRN treatment, and reductions seen after a year of continuous treatment were not maintained with a second year of PRN treatment (Martin et al. 2012). Most available evidence is from head-to-head comparisons with RBZ 0.5 mg under highly standardized clinical trial conditions (Martin et al. 2012; Chakravarthy et al. 2013; Kodjikian et al. 2013; Krebs et al. 2013). These results have consistently found the magnitude of MT reduction to be greater with RBZ 0.5 mg than BVZ 1.25 mg, when continuous and PRN regimes are compared.

3.2.3 Incidence of Legal Blindness

The impact of RBZ on the incidence of legal blindness has been modeled in the United States (Bressler et al. 2011) and Australia (Mitchell et al. 2014). The US model (applied to the non-Hispanic white population only) combined national population data with the incidence of nvAMD found in the Beaver Dam Eye Study (Klein et al. 2007) to derive an estimate of disease incidence and progression across the country (Bressler et al. 2011). The effectiveness of RBZ was based on treatment outcomes in the Age-related Eye Disease Study (ARED) (Bressler et al. 2003), ANCHOR, and MARINA phase III clinical trials (Brown et al. 2009; Rosenfeld et al. 2006). This model found that regular 4-weekly treatment with RBZ over 2 years would reduce the incidence of legal blindness (defined as BCVA ≤ 20/200 in both eyes) by 72 % (95%CI: 70–74 %) from 16,268 to 4484 individuals, of the 103,582 modeled to develop nvAMD. The same model estimated this treatment regime would reduce development of visual impairment (BCVA ≤ 20/40 in both eyes) by 37 % (95%CI: 35–39 %) from 34,702 to 21,919 cases (Bressler et al. 2011). The Australian model used the same treatment outcome data (Brown et al. 2009; Rosenfeld et al. 2006; Bressler et al. 2003), combined with population data from 2010 and the 10-year cumulative incidence of AMD in the Blue Mountains Eye Study (BMES) (Wang et al. 2007). In addition to studying the effect of 4-weekly RBZ, this model estimated the effectiveness of PRN treatment, based on results of the CATT study (Martin et al. 2012). Using the same criteria to define legal blindness and visual impairment, the estimated effect of 4-weekly RBZ over 2 years was most similar to that of the US model, estimating a 72 % (95%CI: 70–74 %) reduced incidence of legal blindness and a 37 % (95%CI: 34–39 %)

decrease in the development of visual impairment (Mitchell et al. 2014). The modeled effectiveness of PRN RBZ was relatively poorer, estimating a 68 % (95%CI: 64–71 %) reduction in incidence of legal blindness and a 28 % (95%CI: 23–33 %) decrease in visual impairment development (Mitchell et al. 2014).

Decreases in the incidence of blindness from AMD have been observed in population studies based on national registers of blind persons since the introduction of anti-VEGF therapy. In Denmark, a nation with a similar population incidence of AMD to Australia and the United States (Buch et al. 2005; Wang et al. 2007; Klein et al. 2007), a dramatic decrease in the incidence of registered blindness (defined in terms of visual acuity as BCVA $\leq$ 20/200 in both eyes) from AMD was observed over a decade, from 52.2 per 100,000 people in 2000 to 25.7 per 100,000 people in 2010 (Bloch et al. 2012). The rate of decline was greatest in the years following the introduction of anti-VEGF therapy in 2006 (Bloch et al. 2012). Another population register study from Israel also reported a declining incidence of blindness from AMD (Skaat et al. 2012). Blindness was defined differently in terms of visual acuity in this study, as BCVA < 1/60 in both eyes; however, from 1999 to 2008 the incidence decreased from 511 cases out of a population of 6.13 million (8.34 per 100,000) to 440 out of a population of 7.31 million (6.02 per 100,000) (Skaat et al. 2012). Anti-VEGF agents were introduced into Israeli clinical practice in 2004 (Skaat et al. 2012). Neither population study was able to separate AMD patients into wet and dry subgroups, nor did they find the same magnitude effect as models based on phase III clinical trials. However, these results point to a significant benefit of anti-VEGF therapy for prevention of legal blindness in the clinical practice setting.

3.2.4 Safety

Variable degrees of evidence exist for the safety of the available anti-VEGF agents used for treatment of nvAMD. Due to differences between agents at the molecular level (Chen et al. 1999),

their target profiles and binding affinity for VEGF, available data for the safety of one agent should not be extrapolated to others (Mitchell 2011). Some of the available data are summarized in Table 3.3.

3.2.4.1 Ranibizumab

The safety of intravitreal RBZ is supported by extensive, robust evidence generated by large prospective clinical studies (Mitchell 2011; Holz et al. 2013). Evidence has been collected from over 12,500 patients enrolled in RCTs for multiple treatment indications, including nvAMD (Brown et al. 2009; Rosenfeld et al. 2006; Abraham et al. 2010; Boyer et al. 2009; Holz et al. 2011), diabetic macular edema (Mitchell et al. 2011) as well as macular edema following branch (Brown et al. 2011) and central retinal vein occlusions (Campochiaro et al. 2011). Following the conclusion of phase III clinical trials involving RBZ, long-term safety outcomes have been recorded in extension studies. The SECURE study followed 234 patients that had been treated with RBZ for 12 months in the EXCITE and SUSTAIN studies for an additional 2 years (Silva et al. 2013). The HORIZON study followed 600 patients who had received RBZ for 2 years in the ANCHOR, MARINA, and FOCUS studies for an additional 2 years (Singer et al. 2012). These two extension studies reported similar rates of adverse ocular and systemic events. In SECURE, the most commonly reported adverse ocular events were retinal hemorrhage (12.8 %), cataract formation (11.5 %), and increased intra-ocular pressure (6.4 %) (Silva et al. 2013). In HORIZON, the most common adverse ocular events were cataract (12.5 %) and post-dose IOP rises to $\geq$ 30 mmHg (9.2 %) (Singer et al. 2012). The incidence of endophthalmitis was low; 0.2 % in HORIZON and 0.9 % in SECURE. The most common nonocular events in both studies were nasopharyngitis (9.5 % in HORIZON and 9.0 % in SECURE) and hypertension, affecting 8.7 % and 9.0 % of the HORIZON and SECURE populations, respectively (Singer et al. 2012; Silva et al. 2013). The incidence of arterial thromboembolic events (including hemorrhagic and ischemic cerebrovascular conditions, myocardial infarction as well as

Table 3.3 RCTs comparing the systemic safety of BVZ and RBZ, included in a Cochrane meta-analysis, 2014 (Moja et al. 2014)

Study name	Total number of participants	Length of follow-up	BVZ			RBZ			Risk ratio for death, 95%CI[a]	Risk ratio for all serious adverse events, 95%CI
			Deaths	All serious systemic adverse events	Total number	Deaths	All serious systemic adverse events	Total number		
Biswas 2011 (Biswas et al. 2011)	120	18 months	0	0	60	0	0	60	Not estimable	Not estimable
BRAMD (unpublished) (Schauwvlieghe et al. 2014)	327	1 year	Not available	34	161	Not available	37	166	Not estimable	0.95 [0.63–1.43]
CATT (Martin et al. 2012)	1185	2 years	36	234	586	32	190	599	1.15 [0.72–1.83]	1.26 [1.08–1.47]
GEFAL (Kodjikian et al. 2013)	485	1 year	2	30	246	3	24	239	0.65 [0.11–3.84]	1.21 [0.73–2.02]
IVAN (Chakravarthy et al. 2013)	610	2 years	15	80	296	15	81	314	1.06 [0.53–2.13]	1.05 [0.80–1.37]
LUCAS (unpublished) (Berg 2013)	432	2 years	3	33	214	3	51	218	1.02 [0.21–4.99]	0.66 [0.44–0.98]
MANTA (Krebs et al. 2013)	317	1 year	3	18	154	2	15	163	1.59 [0.27–9.37]	1.27 [0.66–2.43]
Subramanian et al. (2010)	28	1 year	2	2	20	0	0	8	2.14 [0.11–40.30]	2.14 [0.11–40.30]
VIBERA (unpublished) (NCT00559715 2007)	161	1 year	1	22	107	1	6	54	0.50 [0.03–7.91]	1.85 [0.80–4.29]
Total	3665		62	453	1844	56	404	1821	1.10 [0.78–1.57]	1.08 [0.90–1.31]

Data reproduced from Moja L, Lucenteforte E, Kwag KH, Bertele V, Campomori A, Chakravarthy U, D'Amico R, Dickersin K, Kodjikian L, Lindsley K, Loke Y, Maguire M, Martin DF, Mugelli A, Muhlbauer B, Puntmann I, Reeves B, Rogers C, Schmucker C, Subramanian ML, Virgili G (2014) Systemic safety of bevacizumab versus ranibizumab for neovascular age-related macular degeneration. The Cochrane Database of Systematic Reviews 9:Cd011230. doi:10.1002/14651858.CD011230.pub2, with permission of Wiley

[a]Risk ratio above one favors events in the BVZ group, risk ratio below one favors events in the RBZ group

other embolic and thrombotic events) was 5.6 % in SECURE and 5.3 % in HORIZON (Singer et al. 2012; Silva et al. 2013). In the PIER study, a similar incidence of death, arterial thromboembolic events, and other adverse events was found in the RBZ 0.5 mg and sham injection groups (Abraham et al. 2010).

Safety data for RBZ has also been collected in the clinical practice setting. The LUMINOUS program combined data from treatment registries in Germany, Sweden, Belgium, and the Netherlands to study the "real-world safety" of 1 year of treatment with RBZ (Holz et al. 2013). Adverse events of interest to the reviewers were those thoughts that pertain to the mechanism of action of RBZ and the intravitreal injection procedure. Of the 4444 patients included in the analysis, 73 (1.64 %) experienced ocular complications of particular interest, the most common of these being retinal pigment epithelial tear (27, 0.61 %), intraocular pressure-related events (12, 0.27 %), and traumatic cataract (10, 0.23 %). 55 (1.24 %) suffered non-ocular adverse events during data collection, the most common of which comprised stroke (19, 0.43 %), hypersensitivity (8, 0.18 %; the specifics of such hypersensitivity were not specified), and hypertension (7, 0.16 %). The reviewers concluded that RBZ was associated with a low rate of adverse events (Holz et al. 2013). However, potential undertreatment of patients, particularly in the German WAVE study data (Finger et al. 2013), may explain the low number of adverse events (Holz et al. 2013). Similarly, treatment registers tend to not follow patients up who are lost to follow-up; thus, information on particular severe adverse events which will stop patients attending treating ophthalmologists' practices are likely to be considerably under-reported.

3.2.4.2 Aflibercept

The VIEW studies have compared the safety of ABC 2 mg with RBZ 0.5 mg over 96 weeks (Schmidt-Erfurth et al. 2014). No significant difference in rates of death, adverse ocular, thromboembolic, or other systemic events were found (Schmidt-Erfurth et al. 2014), although the trial was insufficiently powered to identify differences in rare but serious intraocular or systemic complications (Heier et al. 2012). Nevertheless, a reduction in the number of injections required with regular 8-weekly treatment with ABC compared with monthly RBZ is likely to cause a substantial reduction in cumulative risk of adverse events related to intraocular injections. Whether ABC can be extended further using an Inject & Extend regime compared to RBZ or BVZ in clinical routine practice is yet to be established. If not, side effects related to the intraocular injection procedure are likely to be similar between all agents.

3.2.4.3 Bevacizumab

Sufficient safety data for the intravitreal use of BVZ for nvAMD has been much slower to emerge compared to RBZ. This is due to the fact that BVZ was initially developed and approved by drug regulatory authorities for treatment of cancers via systemic intravenous administration (Moja et al. 2014), whereas RBZ was bespoke designed for intravitreal administration and has been approved for use accordingly (Moja et al. 2014). Publication of the CATT study provided important data on the safety of BVZ compared to RBZ (Martin et al. 2012). Prior to this, only one study (the ABC-trial) had provided high-level evidence for use of BVZ in nvAMD (Tufail et al. 2010), with its relatively small size ($n = 131$) limiting its findings with regard to safety. CATT study findings raised concerns about the systemic safety of BVZ, with a significantly increased incidence of participants in this group developing one or more serious systemic adverse events (adjusted risk ratio 1.30; 95%CI: 1.07–1.57) (Martin et al. 2012). Both agents have been shown to reach the systemic circulation post intravitreal injections; however, BVZ has a longer systemic half-life, due to its larger molecular structure (Avery et al. 2014). This has been discussed as a possible mechanism for potential differences in the risk profiles of the two agents, should a difference exist.

In the subsequent 2 years following publication of the CATT study findings, a number of other RCTs were conducted comparing BVZ with RBZ whilst recording adverse events. In September 2014, the Cochrane Collaboration published a review directly comparing the systemic safety of the two agents (Moja et al. 2014). Results were obtained from a random-effects meta-analysis involving nine nonindustry sponsored RCTs (see Table 3.3), which included 3665 participants, who were followed up for up to 2 years after commencing treatment. All studies directly compared the two agents; however, variable treatment regimes were included. Three of the nine trials were unpublished at this time, comprising 482 individuals who received BVZ and 438 that were treated with RBZ, which limited assessment of the quality of evidence in this subgroup. However, for the two primary outcomes of all-cause deaths and all serious systemic adverse events, the review did not find a significant difference between the two agents on either outcome (Moja et al. 2014). A number of secondary outcomes were also assessed, including myocardial infarction, stroke, arteriothrombotic events, serious hemorrhage, serious neutropenia, gastrointestinal perforation, serious infection, treatment related drug discontinuation, serious systemic adverse events classified as per the Medical Dictionary for Regulatory Activities System Organ Classes (MedDRA SOC) (ICH 2014), and serious adverse events previously associated with drugs affecting the VEGF pathway (Moja et al. 2014). Variable levels of evidence existed for various secondary outcomes, however only one positive association was found across these. A higher incidence of MedDRA classified gastrointestinal disorders was identified in study participants who had received BVZ, at a rate of 2.9 % compared to 1.6 % in the RBZ cohorts (risk ratio 1.82, 95%CI: 1.04–3.19) (Moja et al. 2014). Gastrointestinal disorders included abdominal pain, vomiting, dyspepsia, duodenal ulcer, pancreatitis, intestinal obstruction, intestinal perforation, faecaloma, colitis, and Crohn's disease (ICH 2014). In summary, this review drew on nine nonindustry sponsored head-to-head RCTs and was comprehensive in its acquisition and analysis of available data. Its authors concluded that systemic safety data does not provide significant evidence to support preferential use of either RBZ or BVZ for nvAMD (Moja et al. 2014). The release of yet to be published data from three RCTs will provide additional useful evidence on the subject. The authors also proposed that the safety of both drugs might vary between patients and recommended an individual patient data meta-analysis to explore the impact of predisposing risk factors and the effect of different treatment regimes.

3.3　Predictors of Outcomes

The response to anti-VEGF therapy in nvAMD varies greatly amongst patients. Whilst patients treated monthly for 2 years in phase III clinical trials showed an average gain of 7–15 ETDRS letters, a subgroup 10–15 % continued to lose vision despite treatment. In contrast, a second subgroup of approximately 30 % shows significant visual improvement (Brown et al. 2009; Rosenfeld et al. 2006, 2011; Martin et al. 2012). Most studies have used a change in vision threshold of 15 ETDRS letters (Rosenfeld et al. 2011). In the clinical practice setting, where treatment tends to involve fewer injections, the rate of poor response to treatment has been reported to be as high as 20–30 % (Rasmussen and Sander 2014). To date, the wide variance in treatment outcomes is not well understood; however, a number of genetic and clinical factors have been suggested as potential predictors for treatment outcomes, with variable levels of proposed effect (Finger et al. 2014). Whilst evidence for single nucleotide polymorphisms (SNPs) in the complement factor H (CFH) and VEGF-A genes has been found to be somewhat associated with treatment outcomes, clinical factors recorded at baseline, including age, visual acuity, choroidal neovascularization (CNV) lesion size, and a delay in treatment of more than 3 weeks from symptom onset appear to be of greater importance in determining anti-VEGF treatment outcomes (Finger et al. 2014).

3.3.1　Genetic Factors

A number of genes have been linked to an elevated risk of developing AMD, including CFH, age-related maculopathy susceptibility 2 (ARMS2)/

high-temperature requirement A-1 (HTRA1), complement factor 3 (C3), complement factor B (CFB)/complement factor 2 (C2), and apolipoprotein E (APOE) genes (Chamberlain et al. 2006). However, the role these genetic polymorphisms may play in the response of nvAMD to anti-VEGF therapy remains to be well understood, with inconsistencies in the nature and extent of their associations in the literature published to date (Finger et al. 2014). The most evidence currently available is for the CFH gene, where almost half of all SNPs assessed have been found to be associated with visual outcomes and the number of injections required. Approximately, 15 % of SNPs assessed in the VEGF gene have also been linked to treatment outcomes (Finger et al. 2014).

3.3.1.1 Complement Factor H (CFH) Gene

The CFH gene complex has been investigated with mixed results. Several studies have identified associations pertaining to VA (Imai et al. 2010; Tian et al. 2012; McKibbin et al. 2012; Nischler et al. 2011; Brantley et al. 2007; Lee et al. 2009; Francis 2011; Kloeckener-Gruissem et al. 2011), for as long as 12 months after commencing treatment (Francis 2011; Kloeckener-Gruissem et al. 2011). Others, however, did not find any association with treatment (Inglehearn et al. 2012; Orlin et al. 2012; Teper et al. 2010; Wickremasinghe et al. 2011), including the largest study to date ($n=834$) which was based on the CATT study cohort (Hagstrom et al. 2013). This study also returned negative findings for associations with lesion size, leakage seen on fluorescein angiography (FA), OCT findings of mean foveal thickness changes and the presence of fluid and also the mean of number of injections required in the first 12 months of treatment (Hagstrom et al. 2013). Where associations have been identified with CFH and treatment outcomes, the CC risk genotype of SNP rs1061170 (Y402 H) has been linked to poorer treatment outcomes including reduced VA improvement (Brantley et al. 2007; Kloeckener-Gruissem et al. 2011) and a greater number of injections required (Lee et al. 2009). Congruently, the CT genotype has been identified as predictive of favorable visual outcomes up to 24 months after

initiation of treatment (Menghini et al. 2012). However, in complete contrast, a different paper previously found the CT genotype of this SNP to be linked to the worst outcomes (Imai et al. 2010). A greater number of injections in the first 12 months of therapy were found for the AG genotypes of SNP rs194918455 when compared to the AA genotype (Francis 2011). Whilst evidence has accrued over time for an effect of the CFH gene on nvAMD treatment outcomes, the picture painted by research to-date is far from clear. A number of factors affect visual acuity measured by commonly used ETDRS or Snellen distance visual acuity letter charts, and thus determining the effect of genetic factors on visual anti-VEGF treatment outcomes is per se very challenging.

3.3.1.2 Age-Related Maculopathy Susceptibility 2 (ARMS2)/ High-Temperature Requirement A-1 (HTRA1) Genes

Papers examining ARMS2/HTRA1 for associations with treatment outcomes have reported variable results. Homozygous carriers of the SNP rs10490924 (A69 S) TT genotype of the ARMS2 gene have an increased risk of not improving or continuing to lose vision (Teper et al. 2010). The presence of the TT genotype (independent of homozygosity) has also been associated with a lack of treatment response (Kitchens et al. 2013; Tian et al. 2012). Congruently, the CC genotype is associated with a better response to treatment (Abedi et al. 2013a). A higher risk of AMD development has been shown, where the T-allele at SNP rs10490924 is present (Rivera et al. 2005). In the HTRA1 gene, homozygous carriers of the AA genotype at SNP rs11200638 are at an increased risk of developing AMD and (confusingly) have been associated with improved (Abedi et al. 2013a) and worsened (Tian et al. 2012) vision outcomes. Despite the presence of several papers that identify associations between ARMS2/HTRA1 and treatment outcomes, a number of negative studies have also been published (Hagstrom et al. 2013; Inglehearn et al. 2012; Kloeckener-Gruissem et al. 2011, 2012; Yamashiro et al. 2012).

3.3.1.3 Vascular Endothelial Growth Factor (VEGF) Gene

The VEGF gene has been examined at length for an effect on treatment outcomes with anti-VEGF therapy for nvAMD. Approximately, 15 % of the SNPs studied within this gene have been linked to treatment outcomes (Finger et al. 2014). A small proportion of studies have identified associations of VEGF-A SNPs rs699946 and rs699947 with VA outcomes (Imai et al. 2010; Nakata et al. 2011; Park et al. 2014) whilst another found the SNP rs3025000 to be associated with improved visual outcome 6 months after initiation of treatment (Abedi et al. 2013b). In addition, the VEGF-A gene has been linked to fewer injections over a 12-month period (Francis 2011). The SNP rs833069 of VEGF-A has been associated with reductions in CSMT over 6 months of treatment (Chang et al. 2013), whilst SNP rs943080 has also been associated with anatomical outcomes over 12 months (Zhao et al. 2013). Positive associations have been identified in studies that comprised different ethnic groups, further complicating analysis of these results (Finger et al. 2014). The majority of research into the effect of the VEGF gene has not found an association with treatment outcomes (Inglehearn et al. 2012; Kitchens et al. 2013; Kloeckener-Gruissem et al. 2011; McKibbin et al. 2012; Tian et al. 2012; Wang et al. 2012), or only found an association that did not remain when factors such as age and baseline BCVA had been controlled for (Boltz et al. 2012).

3.3.1.4 Apolipoprotein E (APOE) Gene

Available evidence suggests that variants of the APOE gene can affect both the risk of development of AMD, as well the response to anti-VEGF treatment. The ε2 variant appears to increase the risk of AMD development compared to ε3 and ε4 alleles (Wickremasinghe et al. 2011). Furthermore, a comparison between the ε2 and ε4 polymorphisms found ε4 to be associated with superior treatment outcomes (Wickremasinghe et al. 2011).

3.3.1.5 Complement System-Related Genes

Genes comprising the complement system, including complement factors two (C2), three (C3), five (C5), B (CFB), and complement factor H receptor (CFHR) genes, have been examined for associations with treatment outcomes. One study linked C3 to reduced CRT on OCT, as well as reduced leakage on FA (Francis 2011). However, the bulk of published work did not find links between these genes and treatment outcomes (Abedi et al. 2013a; Hagstrom et al. 2013; Kloeckener-Gruissem et al. 2011; Tian et al. 2012; Kloeckener-Gruissem et al. 2012).

3.3.1.6 Other Genes

The influence of other genes on nvAMD treatment outcomes with anti-VEGF agents has been assessed in variable degrees of detail. One study has suggested that various polymorphisms within the C-reactive protein gene might be associated with poorer vision outcomes after treatment (Brantley et al. 2007). An interesting association was reported for patients heterozygous for two SNPs; rs1061170 within the CFH gene and rs10896563 in the frizzled family receptor 4 gene. These patients had an improved response to treatment after 12 months (Kloeckener-Gruissem et al. 2011); however, the same association was not found at 24 months (Kloeckener-Gruissem et al. 2012). A study focused primarily on the interleukin (IL) 23 R gene identified an association between the Group 12 secretory phospholipase A2 (PLA2G12A) gene; however, after adjustment for multiple testing by the false discovery rate had been made the association was no longer present (Wang et al. 2012). The study did not find any association between the 11 tested SNPs of the IL-23 R gene and treatment outcomes (Wang et al. 2012). Several genes known to increase patient risk of developing AMD have not been associated with treatment outcomes from anti-VEGF agents, including complement factor I gene, the tissue inhibitor of metalloproteinase 3 gene as well as genes involved in cholesterol metabolism in addition to APOE (Finger et al. 2014).

3.3.1.7 Genome Wide Association Studies

A genome-wide association study comprising 65 patients identified a number of genetic associations relating to various treatment outcomes. Within the CFH gene, the AA genotype in the SNP rs1065489 was associated with less improvement, whilst comparison of the AG and AA genotypes of the SNP rs3766404 found the former to be associated with a higher number of required injections over the first 12 months of treatment (Francis 2011). Two genotypes within the VEGF-A gene also impacted the number of required injections. The AG genotypes within SNPs rs833068 and rs833069 both predicted the need for more intensive treatment than the AA and GG genotypes, respectively (Francis 2011). With regard to the C3 gene, the SNP rs6660704 contained a genotype (AA) that was associated with reduced CRT on OCT examination after 1 year of anti-VEGF treatment (Francis 2011). This work yielded the discovery of the fms-related tyrosine kinase 1 (FLT1) gene's involvement in treatment outcomes. It was associated with the persistence of leakage on FA as well as the number of required injections over 1 year (Francis 2011).

In 2012 a large pharmacogenetic study examined a number of risk alleles within the CFH, ARMS2/HTRA1, and VEGF-A genes and their cumulative impact on treatment outcomes with RBZ (Smailhodzic et al. 2012). This work found that patients with higher numbers of risk alleles required treatment earlier; with a mean increase of up to 10 years earlier when those with four high-risk alleles in the VEGF gene were compared to those with zero (Smailhodzic et al. 2012). In addition, an increased number of high-risk alleles corresponded to poorer treatment outcomes (Smailhodzic et al. 2012).

3.3.2 Clinical Factors

Clinical factors predictive of treatment outcomes have been searched for and examined within the cohorts of several large phase III clinical trials (Boyer et al. 2007; Kaiser et al. 2007; Rosenfeld et al. 2011; Ying et al. 2013). Much of this work has focused on functional outcomes, identifying predictive factors for improvements in BCVA (Finger et al. 2014). However, other outcome measures such as anatomical changes, adverse events, and the number of injections required by patients have also been studied.

3.3.2.1 Vision Outcomes

Factors at presentation that predispose individuals to poorer vision outcomes include reduced VA, increasing age and a larger CNV lesion, whilst a higher baseline VA places at increased risk of losing vision (Boyer et al. 2007; Kaiser et al. 2007; Rosenfeld et al. 2011; Ying et al. 2013). These findings are supported by studies performed in the clinical practice setting (Kang and Roh 2009; Lim et al. 2012a; Wickremasinghe et al. 2011; Yamashiro et al. 2012).

A past history of other treatments for AMD has been implicated in predicting future treatment outcomes with anti-VEGF therapy. Previous intravitreal triamcinolone or PDT has been reported to limit achievable visual outcomes (Jyothi et al. 2010; Levy et al. 2009; Lux et al. 2007). An elevated intraocular pressure has also been associated with reduced visual gains (Ying et al. 2013).

Different types of CNV lesion have been linked to vision outcomes with a variety of conflicting results. Classical CNV lesions (both minimally and predominantly classic) have been linked with reduced visual improvement (Ying et al. 2013) and a greater number of recurrences requiring further injections (Horster et al. 2011). Other studies have not replicated these findings (Lalwani et al. 2009; Lux et al. 2007) whilst some research have found minimally and predominantly classical CNVs to gain more vision (Heimes et al. 2011; Jyothi et al. 2010). Eyes with retinal angiomatous proliferations (RAP) made favorable vision gains compared with other lesions in the CATT study cohort (Ying et al. 2013).

Various OCT findings have been linked to vision outcomes. Atrophic changes in the outer retina at baseline are predictive of poor VA outcomes after 12 months of treatment (Ristau et al. 2014). An intact external limiting membrane and ellipsoid zone have been independently associated with good prognosis for VA after three consecutive injections (Kwon et al. 2014) to as long as 12 months after commencement of treatment (Mathew et al. 2013). The anatomical integrity of the retina viewed on OCT, looking at features including the continuity of the external limiting membrane and inner/outer segment band were linked to superior visual acuity outcomes following more than 6 months of anti-VEGF therapy (Oishi et al. 2013). Despite this, the same study identified baseline VA to be of stronger predictive value for long-term vision outcomes (Oishi et al. 2013). Although such results are encouraging that OCT characteristics may hold predictive value for vision outcomes, other research has been unable to link OCT baseline features to 12-month visual outcomes (Kolb et al. 2012).

Features of retinal pigment epithelium (RPE) dysfunction have been linked to vision loss after 2 years of treatment. A pooled analysis of individuals with a gain or loss of ≥15 EDTRS letters in the ANCHOR and MARINA trials found a greater number of signs including pigmentary abnormalities and atrophic scars (Rosenfeld et al. 2011). Conversely, two smaller studies found RPE abnormalities viewed on fundus autofluorescence to be the only factors linked to better treatment outcomes (Heimes et al. 2008, 2011). However, the strength of these findings was diminished by not controlling for confounders in multivariate testing (Finger et al. 2014). The presence of a pigment epithelial detachment (PED) seen at baseline might suggest a higher probability of secondary vision loss after three initial monthly injections of RBZ (Mariani et al. 2011).

The interval between symptom onset and treatment has been identified as an important predictive factor for treatment outcomes. A delay of over 21 days between first symptoms and administration of treatment was shown to predict an increased risk for vision loss or lack of improvement after 12 months (Lim et al. 2012a).

3.3.2.2 Anatomical Outcomes

The type of macular edema viewed on OCT has been studied for its predictive value. Cystoid edema (intraretinal cystic spaces visible on OCT) has been linked to the largest reductions in CRT, when compared with a PED, subretinal fluid, or other types of macular edema (Guber et al. 2014). Other work, however, reported cystoid macular edema to have a higher risk of nonresponse after 12 months of treatment and follow-up (Byun et al. 2010). CRT reductions have been found to occur during the initial six injections, but not beyond this volume of treatment (Guber et al. 2014). Age and baseline BCVA have not been shown to be predictive for CRT response to treatment (Guber et al. 2014).

Utilization of indocyanine green angiography has found persistent lesion activity to be associated with the presence of an arteriolarized vascular complex or a polypoidal choroidal vasculopathy (PCV) in serous PEDs (Mettu et al. 2012). The capillary subtype in classic membranes has indicated a greater chance of resolution of activity after 3–5 monthly injections (Lad et al. 2012).

3.3.2.3 Adverse Events

Minimal research has been published on baseline factors that might predict adverse events (Finger et al. 2014). One study found that individuals with a higher baseline BCVA and the presence of a CNV lesion, instead of an RAP lesion, predicted a higher risk of developing an RPE tear (Introini et al. 2012). However, possible confounders were not adjusted for in this work (Finger et al. 2014). There is a paucity of evidence for predictors of adverse outcomes such as retinal atrophy or hemorrhage (Finger et al. 2014).

3.3.2.4 Predictors of Required Injections

Both predominantly and minimally classic CNV lesions have been linked to a greater number of required injections (Horster et al. 2011). Baseline subretinal fluid on OCT has been associated with a greater likelihood of ongoing treatment requirement over 20 months (Tannan et al. 2010); however, other research has not identified any link between OCT characteristics and the number of required injections in the first 12 months of therapy (Jeng and Sadda 2010). Studies commonly report the number of injections administered to participants, but seldom report the intervals between injections in PRN treatment regimes. Consequently, predictive factors to assess the possibility of extending an individual's retreatment interval have not been assessed (Finger et al. 2014).

3.3.3 Behavioral Factors

Little research has been published on the effect of behavioral and lifestyle risk factors on the treatment outcomes with anti-VEGF therapy (Finger et al. 2014). Conflicting evidence exists for the impact of smoking. A Korean study of 125 eyes found current smoking to be independently associated with poor visual acuity outcomes after 3 months of treatment (Lee et al. 2013). Another study found that an increasing number of pack years correlated with less gain in vision after 2 years of follow-up in both current and former smokers (Menger et al. 2012). Other research found the opposite, where current and former smokers gained vision (Inglehearn et al. 2012), whilst no relationship either way has also been reported (Naj et al. 2013). Individuals receiving antihypertensive therapy gained less vision in one study (Menger et al. 2012). The use of anticoagulants may predispose those with nvAMD to intraocular hemorrhage more so than patient age and disease duration (Kiernan et al. 2010); however, anticoagulant use has not been assessed as a potential predictive factor in larger studies (Finger et al. 2014).

3.3.4 Summary of Evidence

To date, clinical factors have been implicated to a much greater degree in predicting treatment outcomes than genetic factors. Those baseline clinical features that are chiefly involved are age, VA, the size of the CNV lesion, and the delay to initiation of treatment. A higher risk of vision loss or reduced vision gains has been associated with increased age, a better baseline VA, a larger CNV at presentation, and delay of greater than 21 days from symptom onset to commencement of treatment. Patients with better baseline VA are more likely to have good vision outcomes; however, they are less likely to gain vision than their counterparts with relatively poorer vision at baseline. This is the result of a ceiling effect (Finger et al. 2014). Available evidence pertaining to baseline CNV characteristics observed using FA and OCT remains unclear, with variable evidence for and against predictive usefulness for VA outcomes or the frequency of injections required. Evidence for an effect from smoking is equally conflicted, with different studies pointing to both better and worse treatment outcomes in smokers, whilst another paper reported no association (Finger et al. 2014).

A large number of studies have assessed a range of SNPs and their association with treatment outcomes, with the highest yield of evidence being for the CFH and VEGF genes. The outcomes that these have most often been associated with are VA or the number of injections required by an individual during follow-up. Assessment of genetic factors has varied between studies in terms of the length of follow-up, time points, and racial characteristics of samples (Finger et al. 2014). Despite the large number of papers on this topic, most of these are uncontrolled, prospective or retrospective case series. Data is available from only one large randomized-controlled trial (the CATT study) for assessment of pharmacogenetic associations in treatment of nvAMD with anti-VEGF drugs (Hagstrom et al. 2013). The presence of an increasing number of known risk alleles in higher risk genes (namely, CFH, ARMS2/HTRA1, and polymorphisms in the VEGF gene) has been associated with a younger age of nvAMD onset and poorer treatment outcomes (Smailhodzic et al. 2012). Overall, genetic factors appear to have an association with treatment outcomes that is weak at best (Gorin 2012).

3.4   Need for Further Research

Despite the unrivalled dominance of anti-VEGF as the most effective available treatment option for nvAMD, a number of questions regarding its use remain to be answered. Given the absence of a comparably effective alternative treatment, studies must remain uncontrolled for now, as it is not ethical to leave nvAMD untreated. This creates challenges when attempting to determine useful prognostic factors of treatment outcomes. A greater uniformity of study design between projects would allow results to be synthesized, which may provide an improved understanding of the predictive value of baseline factors (Finger et al. 2014). Studies produced to date often fail to separate AMD into its various subtypes. Separation of subtypes (i.e., PCV and RAP) will produce data of greater comparative value with other work (Finger et al. 2014). Improved consistency of treatment regimes and follow-up time points between studies would improve the comparability of studies further (Finger et al. 2014).

Variable amounts of data exist for the different anti-VEGF agents available. There is robust evidence from multiple randomized clinical trials for the efficacy and safety of RBZ (Mitchell 2011). Extensive data has been produced comparing BVZ with RBZ, with further trials yet to be published (Moja et al. 2014), which has found the two agents to be comparable in terms of efficacy and systemic safety. Similarly, ABC has been compared to RBZ and found to be non-inferior (Heier et al. 2012; Schmidt-Erfurth et al. 2014). Despite the number of clinical trials produced on treatment outcomes, only one of these (the CATT study) produced data relating outcomes to AMD susceptibility genes (Hagstrom et al. 2013). As new anti-VEGF treatment options become available (through development of new agents and/or drug combinations) pharmacogenetics may aid in identifying certain subgroups likely to respond better to particular drugs (Finger et al. 2014).

Knowledge of reliable predictors of treatment outcomes serves patient care in numerous ways.

Informing patients of their individual prognosis and allowing treatment to be planned in the most cost-effective way are certainly valuable; however, predictors of treatment outcome can also guide selection of the most appropriate therapy and treatment protocol (Finger et al. 2014). Whilst a comparative alternative therapy does not exist (Gorin 2012), the relevance of this point is diminished. However, whilst currently available anti-VEGF options produce comparable outcomes, subgroups may respond better to different treatment selections. One US study explored the effect of switching patients refractory to or relapsing with BVZ or RBZ (with a mean of 20.4 previous RBZ/BVZ injections) to ABC in 94 patients (Yonekawa et al. 2013). After a mean follow-up of 18 weeks and 3.4 ABC injections, vision had stabilized, and CMT had improved significantly. This study has several limitations, including the pooling of eyes that had relapsed whilst not on treatment with refractory cases and also the grouping together of patients treated with RBZ and BVZ. However, it raises the possibility that some subgroups may be better suited to particular anti-VEGF agents. An improved understanding of predictive factors (genetic, clinical, behavioral, or otherwise) might aid in selection of the best appropriate agent selection and treatment protocol for a given individual.

In the current climate of nvAMD management, clinicians can control several factors, including the frequency of injections and follow-up interval. Furthermore, the standard recommended dose of RBZ (0.5 mg) may be increased to 2 mg in poor responders (Brown et al. 2013). Whilst this does not appear to have benefit in treatment naive patients (Busbee et al. 2013), one small study found improved functional and anatomical outcomes in cases refractory to ongoing conventional 0.5 mg RBZ with an increased RBZ dose (Brown et al. 2013). Such treatment decisions might be guided by further knowledge of predictive factors for treatment outcomes.

A current discussion as to whether long-term anti-VEGF treatment leads to chorioretinal atrophy and/or the development of GA in a dose–response manner, i.e., the probability of atrophy increases with the number of injections, will need to be answered with more longer term follow-up data of large cohorts of patients with detailed imaging, in particular OCTs. Most studies today cannot control for small areas of atrophy present at the initiation of anti-VEGF treatment, or preclinical areas of atrophy, with only loss of certain bands on OCT, which needs to be incorporated in future studies to accurately assess the effect of anti-VEGF on the development of atrophy. Furthermore, clinicians need to be more specific and potentially develop new language to assess changes on OCT, as not every small "black" spot (or "white" spot, depending on standard image settings) indicates fluid in the sense of CNV activity. Some may be chronic cystic changes, others preceding atrophy, and yet others a "looseness" in the tissue following retinal cell death. All this will aid in more accurately determining not only the need for ongoing anti-VEGF, but also the risk of atrophy development associated with long-term anti-VEGF treatment.

3.5   Conclusions

Anti-VEGF treatment maintains vision in most and improves vision in a considerable proportion of patients with nvAMD. Several clinical factors can predict anti-VEGF treatment outcomes. Those who present at a younger age, with better baseline vision and smaller CNV lesions are more likely to have a better final vision outcome, although individuals with a better visual acuity at baseline stand to gain fewer letters due to a ceiling effect. Genetic factors implicated in the development of nvAMD, predominantly related to CFH and VEGF-A gene polymorphisms, may also be associated with anti-VEGF treatment outcomes. However, the overall effect of genetic factors implicated to date appears to be small. Clinical factors at presentation as well as intensity of treatment largely determine current anti-VEGF treatment outcomes.

Compliance with Ethical Requirements

Conflict of Interest: No authors have any conflicts of interests related to this book chapter.

Informed Consent: No human or animal studies were carried out by the authors for this book chapter.

References

Abedi F, Wickremasinghe S, Richardson AJ, Islam AF, Guymer RH, Baird PN. Genetic influences on the outcome of anti-vascular endothelial growth factor treatment in neovascular age-related macular degeneration. Ophthalmology. 2013a;120(8):1641–8. doi:10.1016/j.ophtha.2013.01.014.

Abedi F, Wickremasinghe S, Richardson AJ, Makalic E, Schmidt DF, Sandhu SS, Baird PN, Guymer RH. Variants in the VEGFA gene and treatment outcome after anti-VEGF treatment for neovascular age-related macular degeneration. Ophthalmology. 2013b;120(1):115–21. doi:10.1016/j.ophtha.2012.10.006.

Abedi F, Wickremasinghe S, Islam AF, Inglis KM, Guymer RH. Anti-VEGF treatment in neovascular age-related macular degeneration: a treat-and-extend protocol over 2 years. Retina. 2014;34(8):1531–8. doi:10.1097/iae.0000000000000134.

Abraham P, Yue H, Wilson L. Randomized, double-masked, sham-controlled trial of ranibizumab for neovascular age-related macular degeneration: PIER study year 2. Am J Ophthalmol. 2010;150(3):315–24. doi:10.1016/j.ajo.2010.04.011. e311S0002-9394(10)00267-9 [pii].

Avery RL, Castellarin AA, Steinle NC, Dhoot DS, Pieramici DJ, See R, Couvillion S, Nasir MA, Rabena MD, Le K, Maia M, Visich JE. Systemic pharmacokinetics following intravitreal injections of ranibizumab, bevacizumab or aflibercept in patients with neovascular AMD. Br J Ophthalmol. 2014. doi:10.1136/bjophthalmol-2014-305252.

Berg K. Lucentis Compared to Avastin Study (LUCAS). AAO annual meeting, 2013 subspecialty day. 2013.

Biswas P, Sengupta S, Choudhary R, Home S, Paul A, Sinha S. Comparative role of intravitreal ranibizumab versus bevacizumab in choroidal neovascular membrane in age-related macular degeneration. Indian J Ophthalmol. 2011;59(3):191–6. doi:10.4103/0301-4738.81023. IndianJOphthalmol_2011_59_3_191_81023 [pii].

Bloch SB, Larsen M, Munch IC. Incidence of legal blindness from age-related macular degeneration in Denmark:

year 2000 to 2010. Am J Ophthalmol. 2012;153(2):209–13. doi:10.1016/j.ajo.2011.10.016. e202.

Boltz A, Ruiss M, Jonas JB, Tao Y, Rensch F, Weger M, Garhofer G, Frantal S, El-Shabrawi Y, Schmetterer L. Role of vascular endothelial growth factor polymorphisms in the treatment success in patients with wet age-related macular degeneration. Ophthalmology. 2012;119(8):1615–20. doi:10.1016/j.ophtha.2012.02.001.

Boyer DS, Antoszyk AN, Awh CC, Bhisitkul RB, Shapiro H, Acharya NR. Subgroup analysis of the MARINA study of ranibizumab in neovascular age-related macular degeneration. Ophthalmology. 2007;114(2):246–52. doi:10.1016/j.ophtha.2006.10.045. S0161-6420(06) 01484-9 [pii].

Boyer DS, Heier JS, Brown DM, Francom SF, Ianchulev T, Rubio RG. A Phase IIIb study to evaluate the safety of ranibizumab in subjects with neovascular age-related macular degeneration. Ophthalmology. 2009;116(9):1731–9.doi:10.1016/j.ophtha.2009.05.024. S0161-6420(09)00543-0 [pii].

Braithwaite T, Nanji AA, Lindsley K, Greenberg PB. Anti-vascular endothelial growth factor for macular oedema secondary to central retinal vein occlusion. Cochrane Database Syst Rev. 2014;5:Cd007325. doi:10.1002/14651858.CD007325.pub3.

Brantley Jr MA, Fang AM, King JM, Tewari A, Kymes SM, Shiels A. Association of complement factor H and LOC387715 genotypes with response of exudative age-related macular degeneration to intravitreal bevacizumab. Ophthalmology. 2007;114(12):2168–73. doi:10.1016/j.ophtha.2007.09.008. S0161-6420(07) 01026-3 [pii].

Bressler NM, Bressler SB, Congdon NG, Ferris 3rd FL, Friedman DS, Klein R, Lindblad AS, Milton RC, Seddon JM. Potential public health impact of Age-Related Eye Disease Study results: AREDS report no. 11. Arch Ophthalmol. 2003;121(11):1621–4. doi:10.1001/archopht.121.11.1621.

Bressler NM, Doan QV, Varma R, Lee PP, Suner IJ, Dolan C, Danese MD, Yu E, Tran I, Colman S. Estimated cases of legal blindness and visual impairment avoided using ranibizumab for choroidal neovascularization: non-Hispanic white population in the United States with age-related macular degeneration. Arch Ophthalmol. 2011;129(6):709–17. doi:10.1001/archophthalmol.2011.140. 129/6/709 [pii].

Brown DM, Kaiser PK, Michels M, Soubrane G, Heier JS, Kim RY, Sy JP, Schneider S. Ranibizumab versus verteporfin for neovascular age-related macular degeneration. N Engl J Med. 2006;355(14):1432–44. doi:10.1056/NEJMoa062655. 355/14/1432 [pii].

Brown DM, Michels M, Kaiser PK, Heier JS, Sy JP, Ianchulev T. Ranibizumab versus verteporfin photodynamic therapy for neovascular age-related macular degeneration: two-year results of the ANCHOR study. Ophthalmology. 2009;116(1):57–65. doi:10.1016/j.ophtha.2008.10.018. e55S0161-6420(08)01075-0 [pii].

Brown DM, Campochiaro PA, Bhisitkul RB, Ho AC, Gray S, Saroj N, Adamis AP, Rubio RG, Murahashi WY. Sustained benefits from ranibizumab for macular edema following branch retinal vein occlusion: 12-month outcomes of a phase III study. Ophthalmology. 2011;118(8):1594–602. doi:10.1016/j.ophtha.2011.02.022.

Brown DM, Chen E, Mariani A, Major Jr JC. Super-dose anti-VEGF (SAVE) trial: 2.0 mg intravitreal ranibizumab for recalcitrant neovascular macular degeneration-primary end point. Ophthalmology. 2013;120(2):349–54. doi:10.1016/j.ophtha.2012.08.008.

Buch H, Nielsen NV, Vinding T, Jensen GB, Prause JU, la Cour M. 14-Year incidence, progression, and visual morbidity of age-related maculopathy: the Copenhagen City Eye Study. Ophthalmology. 2005;112(5):787–98. doi:10.1016/j.ophtha.2004.11.040.

Busbee BG, Ho AC, Brown DM, Heier JS, Suner IJ, Li Z, Rubio RG, Lai P. Twelve-month efficacy and safety of 0.5 mg or 2.0 mg ranibizumab in patients with subfoveal neovascular age-related macular degeneration. Ophthalmology. 2013;120(5):1046–56. doi:10.1016/j.ophtha.2012.10.014.

Byun YJ, Lee SJ, Koh HJ. Predictors of response after intravitreal bevacizumab injection for neovascular age-related macular degeneration. Jpn J Ophthalmol. 2010;54(6):571–7. doi:10.1007/s10384-010-0866-1.

Campochiaro PA, Brown DM, Awh CC, Lee SY, Gray S, Saroj N, Murahashi WY, Rubio RG. Sustained benefits from ranibizumab for macular edema following central retinal vein occlusion: twelve-month outcomes of a phase III study. Ophthalmology. 2011;118(10):2041–9. doi:10.1016/j.ophtha.2011.02.038.

Chakravarthy U, Harding SP, Rogers CA, Downes SM, Lotery AJ, Wordsworth S, Reeves BC. Ranibizumab versus bevacizumab to treat neovascular age-related macular degeneration: one-year findings from the IVAN randomized trial. Ophthalmology. 2012;119(7):1399–411. doi:10.1016/j.ophtha.2012.04.015.

Chakravarthy U, Harding SP, Rogers CA, Downes SM, Lotery AJ, Culliford LA, Reeves BC. Alternative treatments to inhibit VEGF in age-related choroidal neovascularisation: 2-year findings of the IVAN randomised controlled trial. Lancet. 2013;382(9900):1258–67. doi:10.1016/s0140-6736(13)61501-9.

Chamberlain M, Baird P, Dirani M, Guymer R. Unraveling a complex genetic disease: age-related macular degeneration. Surv Ophthalmol. 2006;51(6):576–86. doi:10.1016/j.survophthal.2006.08.003.

Chang W, Noh DH, Sagong M, Kim IT. Pharmacogenetic association with early response to intravitreal ranibizumab for age-related macular degeneration in a Korean population. Mol Vis. 2013;19:702–9.

Chen Y, Wiesmann C, Fuh G, Li B, Christinger HW, McKay P, de Vos AM, Lowman HB. Selection and analysis of an optimized anti-VEGF antibody: crystal structure of an affinity-matured Fab in complex with antigen. J Mol Biol. 1999;293(4):865–81. doi:10.1006/jmbi.1999.3192.

Finger RP, Wiedemann P, Blumhagen F, Pohl K, Holz FG. Treatment patterns, visual acuity and quality-of-life outcomes of the WAVE study—a noninterventional study of ranibizumab treatment for neovascular age-related macular degeneration in Germany. Acta Ophthalmol.2013;91(6):540–6.doi:10.1111/j.1755-3768.2012.02493.x.

Finger RP, Wickremasinghe SS, Baird PN, Guymer RH. Predictors of anti-VEGF treatment response in neovascular age-related macular degeneration. Surv Ophthalmol. 2014;59(1):1–18. doi:10.1016/j.survophthal.2013.03.009.

Francis PJ. The influence of genetics on response to treatment with ranibizumab (Lucentis) for age-related macular degeneration: the Lucentis Genotype Study (an American Ophthalmological Society thesis). Trans Am Ophthalmol Soc. 2011;109:115–56.

Fung AE, Lalwani GA, Rosenfeld PJ, Dubovy SR, Michels S, Feuer WJ, Puliafito CA, Davis JL, Flynn Jr HW, Esquiabro M. An optical coherence tomography-guided, variable dosing regimen with intravitreal ranibizumab (Lucentis) for neovascular age-related macular degeneration. Am J Ophthalmol. 2007;143(4):566–83. doi:10.1016/j.ajo.2007.01.028. S0002-9394(07)00068-2 [pii].

Gorin MB. Genetic insights into age-related macular degeneration: controversies addressing risk, causality, and therapeutics. Mol Aspects Med. 2012;33(4):467–86. doi:10.1016/j.mam.2012.04.004.

Guber J, Josifova T, Henrich PB, Guber I. Clinical risk factors for poor anatomic response to ranibizumab in neovascular age-related macular degeneration. Open Ophthalmol J. 2014;8:3–6. doi:10.2174/1874364101408010003.

Gupta OP, Shienbaum G, Patel AH, Fecarotta C, Kaiser RS, Regillo CD. A treat and extend regimen using ranibizumab for neovascular age-related macular degeneration clinical and economic impact. Ophthalmology. 2010;117(11):2134–40. doi:10.1016/j.ophtha.2010.02.032. S0161-6420(10)00244-7 [pii].

Hagstrom SA, Ying GS, Pauer GJ, Sturgill-Short GM, Huang J, Callanan DG, Kim IK, Klein ML, Maguire MG, Martin DF. Pharmacogenetics for genes associated with age-related macular degeneration in the Comparison of AMD Treatments Trials (CATT). Ophthalmology. 2013;120(3):593–9. doi:10.1016/j.ophtha.2012.11.037.

Heier JS, Brown DM, Chong V, Korobelnik JF, Kaiser PK, Nguyen QD, Kirchhof B, Ho A, Ogura Y, Yancopoulos GD, Stahl N, Vitti R, Berliner AJ, Soo Y, Anderesi M, Groetzbach G, Sommerauer B, Sandbrink R, Simader C, Schmidt-Erfurth U. Intravitreal afliber-cept (VEGF trap-eye) in wet age-related macular degeneration. Ophthalmology. 2012;119(12):2537–48. doi:10.1016/j.ophtha.2012.09.006.

Heimes B, Lommatzsch A, Zeimer M, Gutfleisch M, Spital G, Bird AC, Pauleikhoff D. Foveal RPE auto-fluorescence as a prognostic factor for anti-VEGF therapy in exudative AMD. Graefes Arch Clin Exp Ophthalmol. 2008;246(9):1229–34. doi:10.1007/s00417-008-0854-z.

Heimes B, Lommatzsch A, Zeimer M, Gutfleisch M, Spital G, Pauleikhoff D. Anti-VEGF therapy of exudative AMD: Prognostic factors for therapy success. Ophthalmologe. 2011;108(2):124–31. doi:10.1007/s00347-010-2210-z.

Hjelmqvist L, Lindberg C, Kanulf P, Dahlgren H, Johansson I, Siewert A. One-year outcomes using ranibizumab for neovascular age-related macular degeneration: results of a prospective and retrospective observational multicentre study. J Ophthalmol. 2011;2011:405724. doi:10.1155/2011/405724.

Holz FG, Amoaku W, Donate J, Guymer RH, Kellner U, Schlingemann RO, Weichselberger A, Staurenghi G. Safety and efficacy of a flexible dosing regimen of ranibizumab in neovascular age-related macular degeneration: the SUSTAIN study. Ophthalmology. 2011;118(4):663–71. doi:10.1016/j.ophtha.2010.12.019. S0161-6420(10)01372-2 [pii].

Holz FG, Bandello F, Gillies M, Mitchell P, Osborne A, Sheidow T, Souied E, Figueroa MS. Safety of ranibizumab in routine clinical practice: 1-year retrospective pooled analysis of four European neovascular AMD registries within the LUMINOUS programme. Br J Ophthalmol. 2013;97(9):1161–7. doi:10.1136/bjophthalmol-2013-303232.

Horster R, Ristau T, Sadda SR, Liakopoulos S. Individual recurrence intervals after anti-VEGF therapy for age-related macular degeneration. Graefes Arch Clin Exp Ophthalmol. 2011;249(5):645–52. doi:10.1007/s00417-010-1588-2.

ICH (2014) International conference on harmonisation of technical requirements for registration of pharmaceuticals for human use (ICH). Introductory guide MedDRA version 17.0. http://www.meddra.org/sites/default/files/guidance/file/intguide_17_0_english.pdf. Accessed 21 September 2014.

Imai D, Mori K, Horie-Inoue K, Gehlbach PL, Awata T, Inoue S, Yoneya S. CFH, VEGF, and PEDF genotypes and the response to intravitreous injection of bevacizumab for the treatment of age-related macular degeneration. J Ocul Biol Dis Infor. 2010;3(2):53–9. doi:10.1007/s12177-010-9055-1.

Inglehearn CF, Ali M, Gale R, Cassidy F, Varma D, Downey LM, Baxter PD, McKibbin M. Improved response to ranibizumab in ex and current smokers with Age-related Macular Degeneration (AMD), but no evidence that CFH, ARMS2/HTRA1 or VEGF Genotypes Predict Treatment Outcome. Invest Ophthalmol Vis Sci. 2012;53(6):3325.

Introini U, Torres Gimeno A, Scotti F, Setaccioli M, Giatsidis S, Bandello F. Vascularized retinal pigment epithelial detachment in age-related macular degeneration: treatment and RPE tear incidence. Graefes Arch Clin Exp Ophthalmol. 2012;250(9):1283–92. doi:10.1007/s00417-012-1955-2.

Jeng DJ, Sadda SR. Commonly evaluated optical coherence tomography features are not predictive of number of anti-VEGF injections in neovascular age-related macular degeneration. Invest Ophthalmol Vis Sci. 2010;51.

Jyothi S, Chowdhury H, Elagouz M, Sivaprasad S. Intravitreal bevacizumab (Avastin) for age-related macular degeneration: a critical analysis of literature. Eye (Lond). 2010;24(5):816–24. doi:10.1038/eye.2009.219.

Kaiser PK, Brown DM, Zhang K, Hudson HL, Holz FG, Shapiro H, Schneider S, Acharya NR. Ranibizumab for predominantly classic neovascular age-related macular degeneration: subgroup analysis of first-year ANCHOR results. Am J Ophthalmol. 2007;144(6):850–7. doi:10.1016/j.ajo.2007.08.012. S0002-9394(07)00718-0 [pii].

Kang S, Roh YJ. One-year results of intravitreal ranibizumab for neovascular age-related macular degeneration and clinical responses of various subgroups. Jpn J Ophthalmol. 2009;53(4):389–95. doi:10.1007/s10384-009-0670-y.

Kiernan DF, Hariprasad SM, Rusu IM, Mehta SV, Mieler WF, Jager RD. Epidemiology of the association between anticoagulants and intraocular hemorrhage in patients with neovascular age-related macular degeneration. Retina. 2010;30(10):1573–8. doi:10.1097/IAE.0b013e3181e2266d.

Kitchens JW, Kassem N, Wood W, Stone TW, Isernhagen R, Wood E, Hancock BA, Radovich M, Waymire J, Li L, Schneider BP. A pharmacogenetics study to predict outcome in patients receiving anti-VEGF therapy in age related macular degeneration. Clin Ophthalmol. 2013;7:1987–93. doi:10.2147/opth.s39635.

Klein R, Klein BE, Knudtson MD, Meuer SM, Swift M, Gangnon RE. Fifteen-year cumulative incidence of age-related macular degeneration: the Beaver Dam Eye Study. Ophthalmology. 2007;114(2):253–62. doi:10.1016/j.ophtha.2006.10.040.

Kloeckener-Gruissem B, Barthelmes D, Labs S, Schindler C, Kurz-Levin M, Michels S, Fleischhauer J, Berger W, Sutter F, Menghini M. Genetic association with response to intravitreal ranibizumab in patients with neovascular AMD. Invest Ophthalmol Vis Sci. 2011;52(7):4694–702. doi:10.1167/iovs.10-6080. iovs.10-6080 [pii].

Kloeckener-Gruissem B, Menghini M, Sutter F, Fleischhauer J, Kurz-Levin MM, Berger W, Barthelmes D. Long-term studies on the anti-VEGF treatment success in age-related macular degeneration (AMD). Invest Ophthalmol Vis Sci. 2012;53:5168.

Kodjikian L, Souied EH, Mimoun G, Mauget-Faÿsse M, Behar-Cohen F, Decullier E, Huot L, Aulagner G. Ranibizumab versus bevacizumab for neovascular age-related macular degeneration: results from the GEFAL Noninferiority Randomized Trial. Ophthalmology. 2013;120(11):2300–9. doi:10.1016/j.ophtha.2013.06.020.

Kodjikian L, Decullier E, Souied EH, Girmens JF, Durand EE, Chapuis FR, Huot L. Bevacizumab and ranibizumab for neovascular age-related macular degenera-

tion: an updated meta-analysis of randomised clinical trials. Graefes Arch Clin Exp Ophthalmol. 2014;252(10):1529–37. doi:10.1007/s00417-014-2764-6.

Kolb S, Menghini M, Barthelmes D, Sutter F, Kurz-Levin M. The predictive value of OCT characteristics for the visual outcome in neovascular AMD. Klin Monbl Augenheilkd. 2012;229(4):343–7. doi:10.1055/s-0031-1299250.

Krebs I, Schmetterer L, Boltz A, Told R, Vecsei-Marlovits V, Egger S, Schonherr U, Haas A, Ansari-Shahrezaei S, Binder S. A randomised double-masked trial comparing the visual outcome after treatment with ranibizumab or bevacizumab in patients with neovascular age-related macular degeneration. Br J Ophthalmol. 2013;97(3):266–71. doi:10.1136/bjophthalmol-2012-302391.

Kruger Falk M, Kemp H, Sorensen TL. Four-year treatment results of neovascular age-related macular degeneration with ranibizumab and causes for discontinuation of treatment. Am J Ophthalmol. 2013;155(1):89–95. doi:10.1016/j.ajo.2012.06.031. e83.

Kwon YH, Lee DK, Kim HE, Kwon OW. Predictive findings of visual outcome in spectral domain optical coherence tomography after ranibizumab treatment in age-related macular degeneration. Korean J Ophthalmol. 2014;28(5):386–92. doi:10.3341/kjo.2014.28.5.386.

Lad EM, Grunwald L, Mettu PS, Serrano NP, Crowell S, Cousins SW. Lesion morphology on indocyanine green angiography in age-related macular degeneration with classic choroidal neovascular membrane: implications for response to anti-VEGF treatment. Invest Ophthalmol Vis Sci. 2012;53: 5161.

Lalwani GA, Rosenfeld PJ, Fung AE, Dubovy SR, Michels S, Feuer W, Davis JL, Flynn Jr HW, Esquiabro M. A variable-dosing regimen with intravitreal ranibizumab for neovascular age-related macular degeneration: year 2 of the PrONTO Study. Am J Ophthalmol. 2009;148(1):43–58. doi:10.1016/j.ajo.2009.01.024. e41S0002-9394(09)00102-0 [pii].

Lanzetta P, Mitchell P, Wolf S, Veritti D. Different anti-vascular endothelial growth factor treatments and regimens and their outcomes in neovascular age-related macular degeneration: a literature review. Br J Ophthalmol. 2013;97(12):1497–507. doi:10.1136/bjophthalmol-2013-303394.

Lee AY, Raya AK, Kymes SM, Shiels A, Brantley Jr MA. Pharmacogenetics of complement factor H (Y402H) and treatment of exudative age-related macular degeneration with ranibizumab. Br J Ophthalmol. 2009;93(5):610–3. doi:10.1136/bjo.2008.150995. bjo.2008.150995 [pii].

Lee S, Song SJ, Yu HG. Current smoking is associated with a poor visual acuity improvement after intravitreal ranibizumab therapy in patients with exudative age-related macular degeneration. J Korean Med Sci. 2013;28(5):769–74. doi:10.3346/jkms.2013.28.5.769.

Levy J, Shneck M, Rosen S, Klemperer I, Rand D, Weinstein O, Pitchkhadze A, Belfair N, Lifshitz T. Intravitreal bevacizumab (Avastin) for subfoveal neovascular age-related macular degeneration. Int Ophthalmol. 2009;29(5):349–57. doi:10.1007/s10792-008-9243-1.

Lim JH, Wickremasinghe SS, Xie J, Chauhan DS, Baird PN, Robman LD, Hageman G, Guymer RH (2012a) Delay to treatment and visual outcomes in patients treated with anti-vascular endothelial growth factor for age-related macular degeneration. Am J Ophthalmol. 153(4):678–686, 686.e671-672;2012a. doi:10.1016/j.ajo.2011.09.013

Lim LS, Mitchell P, Seddon JM, Holz FG, Wong TY. Age-related macular degeneration. Lancet. 2012b;379(9827):1728–38. doi:10.1016/S0140-6736(12)60282-7.

Lux A, Llacer H, Heussen FM, Joussen AM. Non-responders to bevacizumab (Avastin) therapy of choroidal neovascular lesions. Br J Ophthalmol. 2007;91(10):1318–22. doi:10.1136/bjo.2006.113902.

Mariani A, Deli A, Ambresin A, Mantel I. Characteristics of eyes with secondary loss of visual acuity receiving variable dosing ranibizumab for neovascular age-related macular degeneration. Graefes Arch Clin Exp Ophthalmol. 2011;249(11):1635–42. doi:10.1007/s00417-011-1734-5.

Marques IP, Fonseca P, Luz Cachulo M, Pires I, Figueira J, Faria de Abreu JR, Silva R. Treatment of exudative age-related macular degeneration with intravitreal ranibizumab in clinical practice: a 3-year follow-up. Ophthalmologica. 2013;229(3):158–67. doi:10.1159/000343709.

Martin DF, Maguire MG, Ying GS, Grunwald JE, Fine SL, Jaffe GJ. Ranibizumab and bevacizumab for neovascular age-related macular degeneration. N Engl J Med. 2011;364(20):1897–908. doi:10.1056/NEJMoa1102673.

Martin DF, Maguire MG, Fine SL, Ying GS, Jaffe GJ, Grunwald JE, Toth C, Redford M, Ferris 3rd FL. Ranibizumab and bevacizumab for treatment of neovascular age-related macular degeneration: two-year results. Ophthalmology. 2012;119(7):1388–98. doi:10.1016/j.ophtha.2012.03.053.

Mathew R, Richardson M, Sivaprasad S (2013) Predictive value of spectral-domain optical coherence tomography features in assessment of visual prognosis in eyes with neovascular age-related macular degeneration treated with ranibizumab. Am J Ophthalmol. 155(4):720–726, 726.e721. doi:10.1016/j.ajo.2012.11.003

McKibbin M, Ali M, Bansal S, Baxter PD, West K, Williams G, Cassidy F, Inglehearn CF. CFH, VEGF and HTRA1 promoter genotype may influence the response to intravitreal ranibizumab therapy for neovascular age-related macular degeneration. Br J Ophthalmol. 2012;96(2):208–12. doi:10.1136/bjo.2010.193680.

Menger JF, Haubitz I, Keilhauer-Strachwitz CN. Influence Of AMD-risk factors on the effectiveness of anti-VEGF therapy in neovascular age-related macular degeneration. Invest Ophthalmol Vis Sci. 2012; 53(6):857.

Menghini M, Kloeckener-Gruissem B, Fleischhauer J, Kurz-Levin MM, Sutter FK, Berger W, Barthelmes D. Impact of loading phase, initial response and CFH genotype on the long-term outcome of treatment for neovascular age-related macular degeneration. PLoS One. 2012;7(7), e42014. doi:10.1371/journal.pone.0042014.

Mettu PS, Crowell S, Shaw J, Grunwald L, Lad EM, Serrano N, Cousins SW. Neovascular morphology on ICG angiography predicts response to anti-VEGF therapy in eyes with serous pigment epithelial detachments and age related macular degeneration. Invest Ophtholmol Vis Sci. 2012;53:2654.

Miller JW, Le Couter J, Strauss EC, Ferrara N. Vascular endothelial growth factor a in intraocular vascular disease. Ophthalmology. 2013;120(1):106–14. doi:10.1016/j.ophtha.2012.07.038.

Mitchell P. A systematic review of the efficacy and safety outcomes of anti-VEGF agents used for treating neovascular age-related macular degeneration: comparison of ranibizumab and bevacizumab. Curr Med Res Opin. 2011;27(7):1465–75. doi:10.1185/03007995.2011.585394.

Mitchell P, Bandello F, Schmidt-Erfurth U, Lang GE, Massin P, Schlingemann RO, Sutter F, Simader C, Burian G, Gerstner O, Weichselberger A. The RESTORE study: ranibizumab monotherapy or combined with laser versus laser monotherapy for diabetic macular edema. Ophthalmology. 2011;118(4):615–25. doi:10.1016/j.ophtha.2011.01.031.

Mitchell P, Bressler N, Doan QV, Dolan C, Ferreira A, Osborne A, Rochtchina E, Danese M, Colman S, Wong TY. Estimated cases of blindness and visual impairment from neovascular age-related macular degeneration avoided in Australia by ranibizumab treatment. PLoS One. 2014;9(6), e101072. doi:10.1371/journal.pone.0101072.

Moja L, Lucenteforte E, Kwag KH, Bertele V, Campomori A, Chakravarthy U, D'Amico R, Dickersin K, Kodjikian L, Lindsley K, Loke Y, Maguire M, Martin DF, Mugelli A, Muhlbauer B, Puntmann I, Reeves B, Rogers C, Schmucker C, Subramanian ML, Virgili G. Systemic safety of bevacizumab versus ranibizumab for neovascular age-related macular degeneration. Cochrane Database Syst Rev. 2014;9:Cd011230. doi:10.1002/14651858.CD011230.pub2.

Muniraju R, Ramu J, Sivaprasad S. Three-year visual outcome and injection frequency of intravitreal ranibizumab therapy for neovascular age-related macular degeneration. Ophthalmologica. 2013;230(1):27–33. doi:10.1159/000350238.

Naj AC, Scott WK, Courtenay MD, Cade WH, Schwartz SG, Kovach JL, Agarwal A, Wang G, Haines JL, Pericak-Vance MA. Genetic factors in nonsmokers with age-related macular degeneration revealed through genome-wide gene-environment interaction analysis. Ann Hum Genet. 2013;77(3):215–31. doi:10.1111/ahg.12011.

Nakata I, Yamashiro K, Nakanishi H, Tsujikawa A, Otani A, Yoshimura N. VEGF gene polymorphism and response to intravitreal bevacizumab and triple therapy in age-related macular degeneration. Jpn J Ophthalmol. 2011;55(5):435–43. doi:10.1007/s10384-011-0061-z.

NCT00559715 (2007) Prevention of Vision Loss in Patients With Age-Related Macular Degeneration (AMD) by Intravitreal Injection of Bevacizumab and Ranibizumab (VIBERA). http://clinicaltrials.gov/show/NCT00559715.

Nischler C, Oberkofler H, Ortner C, Paikl D, Riha W, Lang N, Patsch W, Egger SF. Complement factor H Y402H gene polymorphism and response to intravitreal bevacizumab in exudative age-related macular degeneration. Acta Ophthalmol. 2011;89(4):e344–9. doi:10.1111/j.1755-3768.2010.02080.x.

Oishi A, Shimozono M, Mandai M, Hata M, Nishida A, Kurimoto Y. Recovery of photoreceptor outer segments after anti-VEGF therapy for age-related macular degeneration. Graefes Arch Clin Exp Ophthalmol. 2013;251(2):435–40. doi:10.1007/s00417-012-2034-4.

Orlin A, Hadley D, Chang W, Ho AC, Brown G, Kaiser RS, Regillo CD, Godshalk AN, Lier A, Kaderli B, Stambolian D. Association between high-risk disease loci and response to anti-vascular endothelial growth factor treatment for wet age-related macular degeneration. Retina. 2012;32(1):4–9. doi:10.1097/IAE.0b013e31822a2c7c.

Oubraham H, Cohen SY, Samimi S, Marotte D, Bouzaher I, Bonicel P, Fajnkuchen F, Tadayoni R. Inject and extend dosing versus dosing as needed: a comparative retrospective study of ranibizumab in exudative age-related macular degeneration. Retina. 2011;31(1):26–30. doi:10.1097/IAE.0b013e3181de5609.

Park UC, Shin JY, Kim SJ, Shin ES, Lee JE, McCarthy LC, Newcombe PJ, Xu CF, Chung H, Yu HG. Genetic factors associated with response to intravitreal ranibizumab in Korean patients with neovascular age-related macular degeneration. Retina. 2014;34(2):288–97. doi:10.1097/IAE.0b013e3182979e1e.

Rakic JM, Leys A, Brie H, Denhaerynck K, Pacheco C, Vancayzeele S, Hermans C, Macdonald K, Abraham I. Real-world variability in ranibizumab treatment and associated clinical, quality of life, and safety outcomes over 24 months in patients with neovascular age-related macular degeneration: the HELIOS study. Clin Ophthalmo. 2013;7:1849–58. doi:10.2147/opth.s49385.

Rasmussen A, Sander B. Long-term longitudinal study of patients treated with ranibizumab for neovascular age-related macular degeneration. Curr Opin Ophthalmol. 2014. doi:10.1097/ICU.0000000000000050.

Rasmussen A, Bloch SB, Fuchs J, Hansen LH, Larsen M, Lacour M, Lund-Andersen H, Sander B. A 4-year longitudinal study of 555 patients treated with ranibizumab for neovascular age-related macular degeneration. Ophthalmology. 2013;120(12):2630–6. doi:10.1016/j.ophtha.2013.05.018.

Regillo CD, Brown DM, Abraham P, Yue H, Ianchulev T, Schneider S, Shams N. Randomized, double-masked, sham-controlled trial of ranibizumab for neovascular age-related macular degeneration: PIER Study year 1. Am J Ophthalmol. 2008;145(2):239–48. doi:10.1016/j.ajo.2007.10.004. S0002-9394(07)00881-1 [pii].

Ristau T, Keane PA, Walsh AC, Engin A, Mokwa N, Kirchhof B, Sadda SR, Liakopoulos S. Relationship between visual acuity and spectral domain optical coherence tomography retinal parameters in neovascular age-related macular degeneration. Ophthalmologica. 2014;231(1):37–44. doi:10.1159/000354551.

Rivera A, Fisher SA, Fritsche LG, Keilhauer CN, Lichtner P, Meitinger T, Weber BH. Hypothetical LOC387715 is a second major susceptibility gene for age-related macular degeneration, contributing independently of complement factor H to disease risk. Hum Mol Genet. 2005;14(21):3227–36. doi:10.1093/hmg/ddi353.

Rofagha S, Bhisitkul RB, Boyer DS, Sadda SR, Zhang K. Seven-year outcomes in ranibizumab-treated patients in ANCHOR, MARINA, and HORIZON: a multicenter cohort study (SEVEN-UP). Ophthalmology. 2013;120(11):2292–9. doi:10.1016/j.ophtha.2013.03.046.

Rosenfeld PJ, Brown DM, Heier JS, Boyer DS, Kaiser PK, Chung CY, Kim RY. Ranibizumab for neovascular age-related macular degeneration. N Engl J Med. 2006;355(14):1419–31. doi:10.1056/NEJMoa054481. 355/14/1419 [pii].

Rosenfeld PJ, Shapiro H, Tuomi L, Webster M, Elledge J, Blodi B. Characteristics of patients losing vision after 2 years of monthly dosing in the phase III ranibizumab clinical trials. Ophthalmology. 2011;118(3):523–30. doi:10.1016/j.ophtha.2010.07.011. S0161-6420(10)00747-5 [pii].

Rung L, Lovestam-Adrian M. Three-year follow-up of visual outcome and quality of life in patients with age-related macular degeneration. Clin Ophthalmol. 2013;7:395–401. doi:10.2147/opth.s41585.

Sacu S, Michels S, Prager F, Weigert G, Dunavoelgyi R, Geitzenauer W, Pruente C, Schmidt-Erfurth U. Randomised clinical trial of intravitreal Avastin vs photodynamic therapy and intravitreal triamcinolone: long-term results. Eye (Lond). 2009;23(12):2223–7. doi:10.1038/eye.2008.423.

Schauwvlieghe A-SM, Dijkman G, Hooymans JM, Verbraak FD, Dijkgraaf MG, Peto T, Vingerling JR, Hoyng C, Schlingemann RO (2014) Comparing the effectiveness of bevacizumab to ranibizumab in patients with exudative age-related macular degeneration. BRAMD. Invest Ophthalmol Vis Sci 55 (ARVO E-Abstract 870).

Schmidt-Erfurth U, Eldem B, Guymer R, Korobelnik JF, Schlingemann RO, Axer-Siegel R, Wiedemann P, Simader C, Gekkieva M, Weichselberger A. Efficacy and safety of monthly versus quarterly ranibizumab treatment in neovascular age-related macular degeneration: the EXCITE study. Ophthalmology. 2011;118(5):831–9. doi:10.1016/j.ophtha.2010.09.004. S0161-6420(10)00972-3 [pii].

Schmidt-Erfurth U, Kaiser PK, Korobelnik JF, Brown DM, Chong V, Nguyen QD, Ho AC, Ogura Y, Simader C, Jaffe GJ, Slakter JS, Yancopoulos GD, Stahl N, Vitti R, Berliner AJ, Soo Y, Anderesi M, Sowade O, Zeitz O, Norenberg C, Sandbrink R, Heier JS. Intravitreal aflibercept injection for neovascular age-related macular degeneration: ninety-six-week results of the VIEW studies. Ophthalmology. 2014;121(1):193–201. doi:10.1016/j.ophtha.2013.08.011.

Silva R, Axer-Siegel R, Eldem B, Guymer R, Kirchhof B, Papp A, Seres A, Gekkieva M, Nieweg A, Pilz S. The SECURE study: long-term safety of ranibizumab 0.5 mg in neovascular age-related macular degeneration. Ophthalmology. 2013;120(1):130–9. doi:10.1016/j.ophtha.2012.07.026.

Singer MA, Awh CC, Sadda S, Freeman WR, Antoszyk AN, Wong P, Tuomi L. HORIZON: an open-label extension trial of ranibizumab for choroidal neovascularization secondary to age-related macular degeneration. Ophthalmology. 2012;119(6):1175–83. doi:10.1016/j.ophtha.2011.12.016.

Skaat A, Chetrit A, Belkin M, Kinori M, Kalter-Leibovici O. Time trends in the incidence and causes of blindness in Israel. Am J Ophthalmol. 2012;153(2):214–21. doi:10.1016/j.ajo.2011.08.035. e211.

Smailhodzic D, Muether PS, Chen J, Kwestro A, Zhang AY, Omar A, Van de Ven JP, Keunen JE, Kirchhof B, Hoyng CB, Klevering BJ, Koenekoop RK, Fauser S, den Hollander AI. Cumulative effect of risk alleles in CFH, ARMS2, and VEGFA on the response to ranibizumab treatment in age-related macular degeneration. Ophthalmology. 2012;119(11):2304–11. doi:10.1016/j.ophtha.2012.05.040.

Subramanian ML, Ness S, Abedi G, Ahmed E, Daly M, Feinberg E, Bhatia S, Patel P, Nguyen M, Houranieh A. Bevacizumab vs ranibizumab for age-related macular degeneration: early results of a prospective double-masked, randomized clinical trial. Am J Ophthalmol. 2009;148(6):875–82. doi:10.1016/j.ajo.2009.07.009. e871S0002-9394(09)00505-4 [pii].

Subramanian ML, Abedi G, Ness S, Ahmed E, Fenberg M, Daly MK, Houranieh A, Feinberg EB. Bevacizumab vs ranibizumab for age-related macular degeneration: 1-year outcomes of a prospective, double-masked randomised clinical trial. Eye (Lond). 2010;24(11):1708–15. doi:10.1038/eye.2010.147. eye2010147 [pii].

Takeda AL, Colquitt J, Clegg AJ, Jones J. Pegaptanib and ranibizumab for neovascular age-related macular degeneration: a systematic review. Br J Ophthalmol. 2007;91(9):1177–82. doi:10.1136/bjo.2007.118562. bjo.2007.118562 [pii].

Tannan A, Li C, Stevens TS. Predicting treatment outcomes in patients with newly diagnosed exudative age-related macular degeneration based on initial presentation. Invest Ophtholmol Vis Sci. 2010;51.

Tano Y, Ohji M. EXTEND-I: safety and efficacy of ranibizumab in Japanese patients with subfoveal choroidal neovascularization secondary to age-related macular degeneration. Acta Ophthalmol. 2010;88(3):309–16. doi:10.1111/j.1755-3768.2009.01843.x. AOS1843 [pii].

Tano Y, Ohji M. Long-term efficacy and safety of ranibizumab administered pro re nata in Japanese patients with neovascular age-related macular degeneration in the EXTEND-I study. Acta Ophthalmol. 2011;89(3):208–17. doi:10.1111/j.1755-3768.2010.02065.x.

Teper SJ, Nowinska A, Pilat J, Palucha A, Wylegala E. Involvement of genetic factors in the response to a variable-dosing ranibizumab treatment regimen for age-related macular degeneration. Mol Vis. 2010;16:2598–604.

The Neovascular Age-Related Macular Degeneration Database. Multicenter study of 92 976 ranibizumab injections: report 1: visual acuity. Ophthalmology. 2014;121(5):1092–101. doi:10.1016/j.ophtha.2013.11.031.

Tian J, Qin X, Fang K, Chen Q, Hou J, Li J, Yu W, Chen D, Hu Y, Li X. Association of genetic polymorphisms with response to bevacizumab for neovascular age-related macular degeneration in the Chinese population. Pharmacogenomics. 2012;13(7):779–87. doi:10.2217/pgs.12.53.

Tufail A, Patel PJ, Egan C, Hykin P, da Cruz L, Gregor Z, Dowler J, Majid MA, Bailey C, Mohamed Q, Johnston R, Bunce C, Xing W. Bevacizumab for neovascular age related macular degeneration (ABC Trial): multicentre randomised double masked study. BMJ. 2010;340:c2459. doi:10.1136/bmj.c2459.

Wang JJ, Rochtchina E, Lee AJ, Chia EM, Smith W, Cumming RG, Mitchell P. Ten-year incidence and progression of age-related maculopathy: the Blue Mountains Eye Study. Ophthalmology. 2007;114(1):92–8. doi:10.1016/j.ophtha.2006.07.017.

Wang VM, Rosen RB, Meyerle CB, Kurup SK, Ardeljan D, Agron E, Tai K, Pomykala M, Chew EY, Chan CC, Tuo J. Suggestive association between PLA2G12A single nucleotide polymorphism rs2285714 and response to anti-vascular endothelial growth factor therapy in patients with exudative age-related macular degeneration. Mol Vis. 2012;18:2578–85.

Wickremasinghe SS, Xie J, Lim J, Chauhan DS, Robman L, Richardson AJ, Hageman G, Baird PN, Guymer R. Variants in the APOE gene are associated with improved outcome after anti-VEGF treatment for neovascular AMD. Invest Ophthalmol Vis Sci. 2011;52(7):4072–9. doi:10.1167/iovs.10-6550. iovs.10-6550 [pii].

Yamashiro K, Tomita K, Tsujikawa A, Nakata I, Akagi-Kurashige Y, Miyake M, Ooto S, Tamura H, Yoshimura N. Factors associated with the response of age-related macular degeneration to intravitreal ranibizumab treatment. Am J Ophthalmol. 2012;154(1):125–36. doi:10.1016/j.ajo.2012.01.010.

Ying GS, Huang J, Maguire MG, Jaffe GJ, Grunwald JE, Toth C, Daniel E, Klein M, Pieramici D, Wells J, Martin DF. Baseline predictors for one-year visual outcomes with ranibizumab or bevacizumab for neovascular age-related macular degeneration. Ophthalmology. 2013;120(1):122–9. doi:10.1016/j.ophtha.2012.07.042.

Yonekawa Y, Andreoli C, Miller JB, Loewenstein JI, Sobrin L, Eliott D, Vavvas DG, Miller JW, Kim IK. Conversion to aflibercept for chronic refractory or recurrent neovascular age-related macular degeneration. Am J Ophthalmol. 2013;156(1):29–35. doi:10.1016/j.ajo.2013.03.030.

Zhao L, Grob S, Avery R, Kimura A, Pieramici D, Lee J, Rabena M, Ortiz S, Quach J, Cao G, Luo H, Zhang M, Pei M, Song Y, Tornambe P, Goldbaum M, Ferreyra H, Kozak I, Zhang K. Common variant in VEGFA and response to anti-VEGF therapy for neovascular age-related macular degeneration. Curr Mol Med. 2013;13(6):929–34.

AREDS Supplementation and the Progression Towards Exudative AMD

4

David J. Valent and Emily Y. Chew

4.1 Introduction

Age-related macular degeneration (AMD) is a neurodegenerative disease of the eye and, according to the World Health Organization, is the third leading cause of blindness in the world (WHO 2012). AMD affects between 25 and 30 million people worldwide (Chopdar et al. 2003; Friedman et al. 2004), and with an aging population, this number is projected to increase markedly. The neovascular or "wet" form of the disease has effective therapies with intravitreal injections of anti-vascular endothelial growth factor (VEGF) agents (Brown et al. 2006; Heier et al. 2012; Kaiser et al. 2007; Rosenfeld et al. 2006). There are no treatments currently for the atrophic or "dry" form of the disease leading to several studies investigating treatments that attempt to prevent the progression of geographic atrophy associated with AMD (Borrelli et al. 2012; Studnicka et al. 2013; Yehoshua et al. 2014). This idea of preventing progression of disease is paramount and can significantly reduce morbidity. One hypothesis regarding the pathogenesis and progression of AMD involves damage to the retina secondary to oxidative stress.

D.J. Valent • E.Y. Chew (✉)
National Institutes of Health, National Eye Institute,
10 Center Drive, Building 10, 10D45, Bethesda, MD
20892-1166, USA
e-mail: dv299204@ohio.edu; echew@nei.nih.gov

With the retina's high concentration of polyunsaturated fatty acids and exposure to both sunlight and high oxygen content, the retina is particularly susceptible to production of oxidative radicals. This hypothesis, along with other supportive studies, led to the advent of Age-Related Eye Disease Study (AREDS).

4.2 Age-Related Eye Disease Study

The AREDS was a large, multicentered, phase III, randomized, double-masked placebo-controlled clinical trial (Age-Related Eye Disease Study Research Group 1999). The primary goal of this study was to assess the clinical course, prognosis, and risk factors including the role of nutrition for the development and progression of both AMD and cataracts. The rational for this study was multifactorial. With limited data regarding the natural history of both cataract formation and AMD, further studies were deemed necessary. Additionally, study results suggested that antioxidant vitamins and supplements may reduce the risk of cardiovascular disease (Stampfer et al. 1993) and eye diseases including the development of cataracts (Gerster 1989; Robertson et al. 1989) and macular degeneration (Newsome et al. 1988). A randomized double-masked placebo-controlled trial involving 151 patients with the diagnosis of macular degeneration, defined as the presence of drusen and pigmentary changes, showed that those participants who received zinc supplementation of 100 mg, had less visual acuity loss than those in the placebo group at 12 and 24 months (Newsome et al. 1988). In addition, when examining color fundus photographs, those participants in the zinc group were more likely to remain stable or accumulate less drusen than those in the placebo group (Newsome et al. 1988). It has been shown in the pigmented rat model that zinc deficiency leads to an increase of lipofuscin accumulation in the RPE when compared with controls (Julien et al. 2011). However, findings from population-based trials and observational data investigating antioxidant use in AMD were inconsistent and consisted of varying types and doses of antioxidants and other micronutrients (Christen et al. 1999; Eye Diseases Prevalence Research Group 1993; Goldberg et al. 1988; Seddon et al. 1994; VandenLangenberg et al. 1998). With at least some supportive trials on nutritional supplementation and eye health, commercially available vitamins were being used by patients both with and without macular degeneration without strong efficacy (Sperduto et al. 1990). In addition to providing valuable information regarding the natural history of two very common eye conditions, AREDS attempted to establish efficacy and safety for antioxidant vitamins in decreasing the progression of AMD and/or cataracts.

AREDS recruited 4757 participants aged 55–80 years, between 1992 and 1998, and these participants were enrolled into different AMD severity categories based on their fundus findings. Table 4.1 describes the ocular findings and the number of participants in each category. These participants were randomly assigned to receive either daily oral tablets of (1) high-dose antioxidants, (2) zinc and copper, (3) high-dose antioxidants plus zinc, or (4) placebo (Age-Related Eye Disease Study Research Group 1999). The formulation for the AREDS vitamins can be seen in Table 4.2 (Age-Related Eye Disease Study Research Group 1999). The dosages of the different vitamins and supplements were determined by a panel of expert biochemists, nutritionists, and ophthalmologists after reviewing the basic science and published litera-

Table 4.1 Baseline ocular characteristics from participants from the Age-Related Eye Disease Study (1999)

Category	Definition	Number of participants
1	Few if any drusen	1117
2	Extensive small drusen, pigment abnormalities, or at least 1 intermediate size druse	1063
3	Extensive intermediate drusen, GA not involving the center of the macula, or at least 1 large druse	1621
4	Advanced AMD or visual acuity less than 20/32 due to AMD in 1 eye	956

Table 4.2 Study formulation of the antioxidants used in the Age-Related Eye Disease Study (1999)

Study formulation	Daily dose
Antioxidants	
Vitamin C	500 mg
Vitamin E	400 IU
Beta-carotene	15 mg
Zinc (zinc oxide)	80 mg
Copper (cupric oxide)	2 mg

ture (Age-Related Eye Disease Study Research Group 1999). Lutein and zeaxanthin were known to be present in the retina however, were not included in the AREDS supplements because they were not commercially available at the time of study. The primary outcome measure was progression to or treatment for advanced AMD and moderate visual acuity loss (>15 letters) from baseline. Secondary outcomes included the development of neovascular macular degeneration, incidence of geographic atrophy, progression to advanced AMD with an associated 15 letter decrease in visual acuity, and worsening of AMD classification category 2 participants to category 3 or 4 during follow-up.

Advanced AMD was defined as either photocoagulation or other treatment for choroidal neovascularization (CNV) or photographic documentation of any of the following: nondrusenoid retinal pigment epithelial detachment, serous or hemorrhagic retinal detachment, hemorrhage under the retina or the retinal pigment epithelium and/or subretinal fibrosis (Age-

Related Eye Disease Study Research Group 2001). Another definition of advanced AMD was the development of geographic atrophy involving the center of the macula.

These participants were followed every 6 months during the course of the clinical trial and then annually. Each study visit included a complete ophthalmic examination. Best corrected visual acuity was obtained using the Early Treatment Diabetic Retinopathy Study protocol at every annual visit. Stereoscopic fundus photographs of the macula were taken both at baseline and then annually starting at year 2. These photographs were evaluated by certified personnel using standardized grading protocols at the Fundus Photograph Reading center. Fundus photographs were also taken if there was a decrease in visual acuity of 10 or more letter from baseline. Demographic information, smoking history, medical history, nutrition, and medication use were also obtained at baseline (Age-Related Eye Disease Study Research Group 1999).

4.3 Outcomes

Four thousand seven hundred fifty seven participants were evaluated for a median duration of 6.5 years. Only 2.4 % of the AREDS participants were lost to follow-up (Age-Related Eye Disease Study Research Group 2001). Of the over 4700 AREDS participants, 1117 participants had few if any drusen. In this group, only 5 (0.004 %) progressed to advanced AMD during the study while 1.3 % in category 2 progressed to advanced disease at 5 years. Those with eyes assigned to category 3, the probability to progression to advanced AMD was 18 %. However, when looking exclusively at those patients with either non-central GA in at least 1 eye or those that had bilateral large drusen, these participants were four times as likely to progress to advanced AMD when compared to the rest of the category three participants. Those with advanced AMD in 1 eye, defined as category 4, had a 43 % expected probability of progression to advanced AMD in the fellow eye at 5 years (Age-Related Eye Disease Study Research Group 2001).

At 5 years in those with more severe AMD (categories 3 and 4), there was a 25 % reduction in the risk of progressing to advanced disease in the antioxidants plus zinc group when compared with the placebo group (Odds Ratio (OR) 0.66; 99 % confidence interval (CI), 0.47–0.91). As for visual acuity in those in categories 3 and 4, there was a statistically significant reduction in the risk of 15 or more letter loss in the antioxidant plus zinc group when compared with the placebo group (OR 0.73; 99 % CI, 0.54–0.99) (Age-Related Eye Disease Study Research Group 2001).

One secondary outcome measure was the likelihood of progression to neovascular disease. There were 592 participants that developed neovascular disease in AREDS. There was a statistically significant benefit for those participants in category 3 and 4 in the antioxidant plus zinc group when compared to placebo for the development of CNV (OR 0.62 99 % CI, 0.43–0.90). The effect on the development of CNV of zinc vs. no zinc was statistically significant as well (OR 0.76; 99 % CI, 0.58–0.98) and was suggestive for the zinc arm when compared with placebo (OR 0.73; 99 % CI, 0.51–1.04) (Age-Related Eye Disease Study Research Group 2001). However, this finding was not significant for the antioxidant alone group when compared with placebo (OR, 0.79; 99 % CI, 0.56–1.13) (Age-Related Eye Disease Study Research Group 2001).

Risk factors for the development for advanced disease in AREDS based off the 5 year data has been evaluated (Clemons et al. 2005). Using multivariable models while controlling for age, gender, and treatment group, risk factors associated with advancement to neovascular AMD included race (OR, white vs. black, 6.77; 95 % CI, 1.24–36.9) and larger amount smoked (OR, >10 vs. ≤10 pack years, 1.55; 95 % CI, 1.15–2.09). Smoking was also a statistically significant risk factor for the development of geographic atrophy. In those persons at risk of developing advanced AMD in one eye, as defined as those patients having unilateral advanced AMD, diabetes was associated with an increased incidence of neovascular AMD (Clemons et al. 2005).

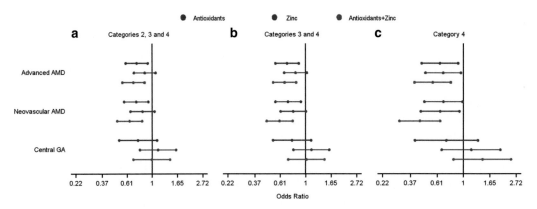

Fig. 4.1 Odds ratio (*central dot*) and 95 % confidence intervals for each original treatment assignment compared with placebo for participants in the following Age-Related Eye Disease Study age-related macular degeneration (AMD) categories. *A*: Categories 2, 3, and 4; *B*: Categories 3 and 4; and *C*: Categories 4. *GA* geographic atrophy. Modified from Chew EY et al. Long-term effects of vitamins C and E, β-carotene, and zinc on age-related macular degeneration: AREDS report no. 35. Ophthalmology. 2013, Aug; 120 (8): 1604-11. With permission from Elsevier

Ten year data regarding risk factors for progression to neovascular disease has also been published on this population (Chew et al. 2014). Increasing age, female sex (Hazard ratio (HR), 1.23; $p=0.005$) and current smoking (HR 1.56; $p<0.001$) were all associated with development of neovascular AMD (Chew et al. 2014). Forty-eight percent of those participants between the ages of 75 and 80 and in categories 3 or 4 at baseline went on to develop neovascular AMD at 10 years. As Fig. 4.1 shows, assignment to antioxidants plus zinc formulation in the original clinical trial appeared to decrease the probability of developing neovascular AMD but not central geographic atrophy (Chew et al. 2013, 2014).

After the clinical trial had been completed, participants were invited to continue in a long-term observational study (Chew et al. 2013). This constituted a comprehensive eye examination including assessment of visual acuity using the EDTRS standardized protocol and color fundus photographs. In addition, when the AREDS formulation became available, participants in AREDS category 3 or 4 were offered the antioxidant plus zinc formulation. The observational study enrolled 3549 of the 4203 surviving participants (Chew et al. 2013).

The proportion of the participants in categories 3 and 4 taking the AREDS formulation during the follow-up study was approximately 70 % in the last year of participation. Approximately 5 years after the clinical trial was completed, those in the antioxidant plus zinc formulation continued to have statistically significant reduced odds of developing advanced AMD when compared with those in the placebo group for those in categories 2, 3, or 4 (OR, 0.69; 95 % CI 0.56–0.86 $P=0.001$) (Chew et al. 2013). There was also a statistically significant reduction in the odds for the development of neovascular disease (OR, 0.64; 95 % CI 0.50–0.82 $P<0.001$) for those in the antioxidant plus zinc group when compared with the placebo arm. Those participants in categories 2, 3, and 4 who were randomly assigned to the antioxidant at baseline, also showed statistically significant reduction in the likelihood for developing advanced AMD, especially the development on neovascular disease (Chew et al. 2013).

When looking exclusively at those with category 4 disease, there was a significant reduction in the odds of developing both advanced AMD (OR 0.56; 95 % CI, 0.40–0.79; $P<0.001$) and neovascular AMD (OR 0.44; 95 % CI 0.30–0.65; $p<0.001$) in those assigned to the antioxidant plus zinc formulation when compared with controls. Estimates when examining exclusively category 3 disease trended in the beneficial direction but were not statistically significant (Chew et al. 2013).

The impact of the AREDS supplementation on public health is quite significant. Statistical models estimate that if all high-risk patients were able to receive AREDS supplementation, it could potentially prevent 300,000 patients from developing advanced AMD at 5 years (Bressler et al. 2003). This would have a huge impact on health care costs. This includes both direct costs, which include doctor visits and medications, and indirect costs, such as caregiver-related costs. Direct costs for just the treatment for wet macular degeneration can range between $385 and $23,400 per year depending on the medication and frequency of injections (CATT Research Group et al. 2011).

4.4 Age-Related Eye Disease Study 2

With the significant cost savings in the prevention of advanced macular degeneration, additional studies provided rational for investigating additional supplements for the prevention of advanced AMD. One area of focus was carotenoids. Carotenoids, specifically the xanthophylls, lutein, and zeaxanthin are the major component of the macular pigment (Landrum and Bone 2001). As stated previously, these were not available as supplements for use at the start of AREDS, but became commercially available and sparked much interest. These xanthophylls are thought to provide some protection against light-induced damage and possibly AMD (Krinsky et al. 2003; Landrum and Bone 2001). The proposed mechanism for protection by lutein and zeaxanthin include the ability to absorb blue light and the elimination of free radicals (Schalch 1992; Snodderly 1995). Omega-3 long chain poly-unsaturated fatty acids (LCPUFAs) are also thought to play an important role within the retina, including a role in ganglion cell function (Nguyen et al. 2008), making up some of the constituents of the photoreceptor outer segments (Bazan et al. 1992; Litman and Mitchell 1996) modulation of rhodopsin (Bush et al. 1994) and may have a neuroprotective effect (Bazan et al. 2013).

At baseline, the original AREDS participants took a semiquantitative food frequency questionnaire and those reporting the highest intake of omega-3 LCPUFAs (Sangiovanni et al. 2009b; SanGiovanni et al. 2007) and lutein/zeaxanthin (Age-Related Eye Disease Study Research Group 2007) were less likely to progress to advanced disease when compared to those with lower intake of these compounds. Those in the group with the highest intake of omega 3 LCPUFA (Sangiovanni et al. 2009b) or lutein and zeaxanthin (Age-Related Eye Disease Study Research Group et al. 2007) were less likely to develop neovascular AMD when compared with those with the lowest intake. In addition, higher fish consumption was also associated with lower risk of developing neovascular AMD (Sangiovanni et al. 2009b). Additional observational studies also demonstrated a similar correlation between higher dietary consumption of lutein/zeaxanthin and omega-3 LCPUFAs (Augood et al. 2008; Chua et al. 2006; Moeller et al. 2006; SanGiovanni et al. 2008, 2009a; Seddon et al. 2006; Swenor et al. 2010; Tan et al. 2008) and decreased progression to advanced disease. In a prospective study involving fifteen patients with AMD treated with lutein/zeaxanthin, functional improvement was seen on electroretinograms at 1 year when compared with age-matched controls (Parisi et al. 2008). Because of these supportive findings, the Age-Related Eye Disease Study 2 (AREDS2) was performed to investigate the safety and efficacy of adding lutein/zeaxanthin and omega 3 LCPUFAs to the AREDS supplements for persons at high risk for progression to advanced disease. In addition, AREDS2 also evaluated the outcome of reducing the concentration of zinc and omitting beta-carotene.

AREDS2 was a large, phase III, randomized, double-masked, placebo-controlled clinical trial involving 82 clinical sites across the United States (AREDS2 Research Group 2012). For the primary analysis, there were 4203 participants enrolled between the ages of 50–85 years. All participants were considered at risk for the development of advanced AMD, with the majority of the patients having bilateral large drusen (65 %) at baseline. The remaining participants had advanced AMD in one eye and large drusen in the fellow eye. The primary outcome for AREDS2 was the comparison of the three active treatment arms to placebo on progression to advanced AMD. Advanced AMD was defined as atrophic or neovascular changes of AMD that include one or more of the following: definite geographic atrophy involving the center of the macula or evidence suggesting CNV. Secondary analysis included progression to moderate vision loss ($\geq$15 letter loss), progression of lens opacity and moderate vision loss, or improvement in participants with advanced AMD (AREDS2 Research Group 2012).

The AREDS2 participants were randomly assigned, with equal probability, to one of four study formulations daily: lutein (10 mg)/zeaxanthin (2 mg), omega-3 LCPUFAs in the form of docosahexaenoic acid (DHA) 350 mg and eicosapentaenoic acid (EPA) 650 mg, both lutein/zeaxanthin and DHA/EPA or placebo. Of the 4203 participants, 1167 (28 %) opted to take the AREDS supplement, while 3036 (72 %) agreed to the secondary randomization, which was performed to evaluate the effect of removing betacarotene and/or lowering the level of zinc from the original AREDS formulation. The reasoning for eliminating beta-carotene is the increased risk for developing lung cancer in those persons who are smokers and taking beta-carotene (Albanes et al. 1995; Omenn et al. 1996). The interest in lower the levels of zinc was that evidence suggested that the maximal level of zinc absorbed was closer to 25 mg than 80 mg (Hambidge 2003; Newsome et al. 1988). The four treatment formulations are shown in Table 4.3. In those participants that were current or former smokers who discontinued their tobacco use within the previous year were assigned to one of the two arms that excluded beta-carotene. Participants were followed at annual study visits, which included a complete eye examination with best corrected visual acuity using an electronic version of the ETDRS technique. Standardized fundus photographs were obtained at each visit and evaluated at a central reading center (AREDS2 Research Group 2012). Participants were contacted by telephone 3 months after randomization and at 6 months between study visits to acquire

Table 4.3 Four treatment formulations in the second randomization in AREDS2 (2012)

	Vitamin C (mg)	Vitamin E (IU)	Beta carotene	Zinc (mg)	Cupric oxide (mg)
1	500	400	15 mg	80	2
2	500	400	0	80	2
3	500	400	15 mg	25	2
4	500	400	0	25	2

information regarding any additional therapies for their AMD.

4.5   Results

The primary analysis of AREDS2 demonstrated no beneficial or harmful effects of adding lutein/zeaxanthin (HR 0.90 98.7 % CI 0.76–1.07; $P=0.12$), omega-3 LCPUFAs (HR 0.97; 98.7 % CI 0.82–1.16; $P=0.70$), or both (HR 0.89, 95 % CI 0.75–1.05, $P=0.10$) to the original AREDS formulation on the progression to advanced AMD when compared with the placebo (Age-Related Eye Disease Study 2 Research Group 2013). However, the pre-specified analyses of the main effects (taking accounts of all those taking lutein/zeaxanthin vs. no lutein/zeaxanthin), there was an incremental increase in the effect of reducing the risk of progression to advanced AMD. When examining those participants in the lowest quintile of dietary intake of lutein and zeaxanthin, comparing those that had received lutein/zeaxanthin to those that did not, those receiving lutein/zeaxanthin were less likely to progress to advanced disease (HR: 0.74; 95 % CI 0.59–0.94; $P=0.01$) (Age-Related Eye Disease Study 2 Research Group 2013) Secondary analysis was performed comparing the lutein/zeaxanthin group vs. the beta-carotene group, the hazard ratios were 0.82 (95 % CI, 0.64–0.94; $P=0.02$) for progression to advanced disease and 0.78 (95 % CI, 0.64–0.94; $p=0.01$) for developing neovascular AMD (Age-Related Eye Disease Study AREDS2 Research Group 2014). When comparing those assigned to the lutein/zeaxanthin and beta-carotene vs. beta-carotene only, the results were: significant for the development of advanced AMD (HR 0.82; 95 % CI, 0.69–0.97;

$P = 0.02$) and for the progression to neovascular AMD (HR 0.72; 95 % CI, 0.59–0.89; $P = 0.002$) (Age-Related Eye Disease Study AREDS2 Research Group 2014).

An important adverse effect emerged when evaluating the treatment with beta-carotene in those AREDS2 participants who were former smokers and those who had never smoked. There were more participants that were diagnosed with lung cancer in the beta-carotene group when compared with the no beta-carotene group (23 (2.0 %) vs. 11 (0.9 %), $P = 0.04$) (Age-Related Eye Disease Study 2 Research Group 2013). Of those who developed lung cancer, 91 % were former smokers (Age-Related Eye Disease Study 2 Research Group 2013).

In regard to visual acuity, lutein/zeaxanthin or omega 3 LCPUFAs had no effects on moderate visual acuity loss, defined as a loss of 15 or more letters from baseline (Age-Related Eye Disease Study 2 Research Group 2013). Lowering zinc and eliminating beta-carotene had no significant effect on the progression to advanced AMD (Age-Related Eye Disease Study 2 Research Group 2013). These findings, in addition to the potential risks in smokers, have led to the recommendation of substituting lutein/zeaxanthin for beta-carotene in the AREDS formulation. Additionally, when analysis was limited to those just with bilateral large drusen at baseline, the comparison of supplements containing lutein/zeaxanthin vs. beta-carotene produced a hazard ratio of 0.76 (95 % CI 0.61–0.96; $P = 0.02$) for the progression to advanced AMD and 0.65 (95 % CI, 0.49–0.85; $P = 0.002$) for the progression to neovascular AMD (Age-Related Eye Disease Study AREDS2 Research Group 2014). A significant reduction in the risk of geographic atrophy was not identified.

4.6 Discussion

Both AREDS and AREDS2 clearly demonstrated the role of antioxidants for the progression of advanced disease in those with intermediate AMD. Both AREDS and in subgroup analysis in AREDS2, the supplements appear to be protective against the formation of neovascular disease;

however, there was no treatment effect on the development of geographic atrophy. The exact mechanism for this beneficial effect is unknown. It may be that the two processes have different cellular signaling which, in the formation of CNV, may more responsive to the potential antioxidative or immune-modulatory effects of supplements. This is purely speculation and this question cannot be answered based on the clinical or basic science data available at this time. In addition, as 34 % of patients with GA in one eye and neovascular AMD in the fellow eye will develop neovascularization in the eye with GA at 4 years (Sunness et al. 1999), treatment with AREDS/AREDS2 supplementation in this group should be considered.

Could the addition of other supplements or vitamins be protective against the progression to advanced AMD? Perhaps AREDS2 supplementation did not include every known retinal carotenoid. To date, there are as many as 25 dietary carotenoids identified; some of these could provide added benefit to the current AREDS supplementation. As shown by Bernstein et al. (2001), the RPE and choroid have not only lutein and zeaxanthin, but several other carotenoids which could assist in protecting against oxidative damage. There are ongoing studies attempting to evaluate three carotenoids in a double-blinded randomized placebo-controlled trial (Akuffo et al. 2014). In addition, the Women's Antioxidant and Folic Acid Cardiovascular Study (Christen et al. 2009) showed daily supplementation of B vitamins, folic acid, pyridoxine, and cyanocobalamin may decrease the risk of AMD in a secondary analysis. Vitamin D may also play a role as there is supportive evidence that it too may protect against the AMD (Millen et al. 2011; Montgomery et al. 2010).

Could the supplementation of lutein and zeaxanthin given at an earlier time point in the patient's care have an effect on the development of AMD? One study which was an off shoot of the Woman's Health Initiative evaluated 1787 women aged 50–79 years of age and examined their dietary intake of lutein plus zeaxanthin (Moeller et al. 2006). There was no statistically difference between those with low and high intake of lutein and zeaxanthin in the development of intermediate or advanced AMD. However, when evaluating the participants less than 75 years of age, without a history chronic disease and stable dietary intake of lutein and zeaxanthin, this did become statistically significant. In addition, there was a trend that higher intake of lutein and zeaxanthin was protective against advanced disease (Moeller et al. 2006). Another study investigated a link, independent of dietary consumption, between genetic determinates for macular xanthophylls and AMD (Meyers et al. 2014). How these genes influence the onset and severity of AMD is yet to be determined.

4.7   Conclusions

AREDS and AREDS2 have shown that supplementation with antioxidants and zinc may decrease the risk of developing advanced AMD, especially neovascular AMD. This risk reduction appears greatest for those at highest risk for advanced disease, categories 3 and 4. The totality of evidence from the pre-planned secondary analyses as well as post hoc AREDS2 did demonstrate an incremental benefit of lutein/zeaxanthin on progression to advanced AMD, especially for those in the lowest quintile of lutein dietary intake, those with bilateral large drusen and those advancing to neovascular AMD. Given this data, and the concerns associated with beta-carotene, consideration for substituting lutein/zeaxanthin in place of beta-carotene in AREDS supplements was recommended. Future considerations include the addition of other vitamins or supplements to further decrease the risk of progression to advanced disease.

Compliance with Ethical Requirements
David Valent declares that he has no conflict of interest.

Emily Chew declares that she has no conflict of interest.

Informed Consent and Animal Studies disclosures are not applicable to this review.

References

Age-Related Eye Disease Study (AREDS2) Research Group. Antioxidant status and neovascular age-related macular degeneration. Eye Disease Case-Control Study Group. Arch Ophthalmol. 1993;111:104–9.

Age-Related Eye Disease Study (AREDS2) Research Group, Chew EY, Clemons TE, Sangiovanni JP, Danis RP, Ferris 3rd FL, Elman MJ, Antoszyk AN, Ruby AJ, Orth D, Bressler SB, Fish GE, Hubbard GB, Klein ML, Chandra SR, Blodi BA, Domalpally A, Friberg T, Wong WT, Rosenfeld PJ, Agrón E, Toth CA, Bernstein PS, Sperduto RD. Secondary analyses of the effects of lutein/zeaxanthin on age-related macular degeneration progression: AREDS2 report No. 3. JAMA Ophthalmol. 2014;132:142–9.

Age-Related Eye Disease Study 2 Research Group. Lutein + zeaxanthin and omega-3 fatty acids for age-related macular degeneration: the Age-Related Eye Disease Study 2 (AREDS2) randomized clinical trial. JAMA. 2013;309:2005–15.

Age-Related Eye Disease Study Research Group. The Age-Related Eye Disease Study (AREDS): design implications. AREDS report no. 1. Control Clin Trials. 1999;20:573–600.

Age-Related Eye Disease Study Research Group. A randomized, placebo-controlled, clinical trial of high-dose supplementation with vitamins C and E, beta carotene, and zinc for age-related macular degeneration and vision loss: AREDS report no. 8. Arch Ophthalmol. 2001;119:1417–36.

Age-Related Eye Disease Study Research Group, SanGiovanni JP, Chew EY, Clemons TE, Ferris 3rd FL, Gensler G, Lindblad AS, Milton RC, Seddon JM, Sperduto RD. The relationship of dietary carotenoid and vitamin A, E, and C intake with age-related macular degeneration in a case-control study: AREDS Report No. 22. Arch Ophthalmol. 2007;125:1225–32.

Akuffo KO, Beatty S, Stack J, Dennison J, O'Regan S, Meagher KA, Peto T, Nolan J. Central Retinal Enrichment Supplementation Trials (CREST): design and methodology of the CREST randomized controlled trials. Ophthalmic Epidemiol. 2014;21:111–23.

Albanes D, Heinonen OP, Huttunen JK, Taylor PR, Virtamo J, Edwards BK, Haapakoski J, Rautalahti M, Hartman AM, Palmgren J, et al. Effects of alpha-tocopherol and beta-carotene supplements on cancer incidence in the Alpha-Tocopherol Beta-Carotene Cancer Prevention Study. Am J Clin Nutr. 1995;62:1427S–30S.

AREDS2 Research Group, Chew EY, Clemons T, SanGiovanni JP, Danis R, Domalpally A, McBee W, Sperduto R, Ferris FL. The Age-Related Eye Disease Study 2 (AREDS2): study design and baseline characteristics (AREDS2 report number 1). Ophthalmology. 2012;119:2282–9.

Augood C, Chakravarthy U, Young I, Vioque J, de Jong PT, Bentham G, Rahu M, Seland J, Soubrane G,

Tomazzoli L, Topouzis F, Vingerling JR, Fletcher AE. Oily fish consumption, dietary docosahexaenoic acid and eicosapentaenoic acid intakes, and associations with neovascular age-related macular degeneration. Am J Clin Nutr. 2008;88:398–406.

Bazan NG, Gordon WC, Rodriguez de Turco EB. Docosahexaenoic acid uptake and metabolism in photoreceptors: retinal conservation by an efficient retinal pigment epithelial cell-mediated recycling process. Adv Exp Med Biol. 1992;318:295–306.

Bazan NG, Calandria JM, Gordon WC. Docosahexaenoic acid and its derivative neuroprotectin D1 display neuroprotective properties in the retina, brain and central nervous system. Nestle Nutr Inst Workshop Ser. 2013;77:121–31.

Bernstein PS, Khachik F, Carvalho LS, Muir GJ, Zhao DY, Katz NB. Identification and quantitation of carotenoids and their metabolites in the tissues of the human eye. Exp Eye Res. 2001;72:215–23.

Borrelli E, Diadori A, Zalaffi A, Bocci V. Effects of major ozonated autohemotherapy in the treatment of dry age related macular degeneration: a randomized controlled clinical study. Int J Ophthalmol. 2012;5:708–13.

Bressler NM, Bressler SB, Congdon NG, Ferris 3rd FL, Friedman DS, Klein R, Lindblad AS, Milton RC, Seddon JM, Age-Related Eye Disease Study Research Group. Potential public health impact of Age-Related Eye Disease Study results: AREDS report no. 11. Arch Ophthalmol. 2003;121:1621–4.

Brown DM, Michels M, Kaiser PK, Heier JS, Sy JP, Ianchulev T, ANCHOR Study Group. Ranibizumab versus verteporfin for neovascular age-related macular degeneration. N Engl J Med. 2006;355:1432–44.

Bush RA, Malnoe A, Reme CE, Williams TP. Dietary deficiency of N-3 fatty acids alters rhodopsin content and function in the rat retina. Invest Ophthalmol Vis Sci. 1994;35:91–100.

CATT Research Group, Martin DF, Maguire MG, Ying GS, Grunwald JE, Fine SL, Jaffe GJ. Ranibizumab and bevacizumab for neovascular age-related macular degeneration. N Engl J Med. 2011;364:1897–908.

Chew EY, Clemons TE, Agrón E, Sperduto RD, Sangiovanni JP, Kurinij N, Davis MD; Age-Related Eye Disease Study Research Group. Long-term effects of vitamins C and E, beta-carotene, and zinc on age-related macular degeneration: AREDS report no. 35. Ophthalmology 2013; 120: 1604–11 e1604.

Chew EY, Clemons TE, Agrón E, Sperduto RD, Sangiovanni JP, Davis MD, Ferris 3rd FL, Age-Related Eye Disease Study Research Group. Ten-year follow-up of age-related macular degeneration in the age-related eye disease study: AREDS report no. 36. JAMA Ophthalmol. 2014;132:272–7.

Chopdar A, Chakravarthy U, Verma D. Age related macular degeneration. BMJ. 2003;326:485–8.

Christen WG, Ajani UA, Glynn RJ, Manson JE, Schaumberg DA, Chew EC, Buring JE, Hennekens CH. Prospective cohort study of antioxidant vitamin supplement use and the risk of age-related maculopathy. Am J Epidemiol. 1999;149:476–84.

Christen WG, Glynn RJ, Chew EY, Albert CM, Manson JE. Folic acid, pyridoxine, and cyanocobalamin combination treatment and age-related macular degeneration in women: the Women's Antioxidant and Folic Acid Cardiovascular Study. Arch Intern Med. 2009;169: 335–41.

Chua B, Flood V, Rochtchina E, Wang JJ, Smith W, Mitchell P. Dietary fatty acids and the 5-year incidence of age-related maculopathy. Arch Ophthalmol. 2006;124:981–6.

Clemons TE, Milton RC, Klein R, Seddon JM, Ferris 3rd FL, Age-Related Eye Disease Study Research Group. Risk factors for the incidence of Advanced Age-Related Macular Degeneration in the Age-Related Eye Disease Study (AREDS) AREDS report no. 19. Ophthalmology. 2005;112:533–9.

Friedman DS, O'Colmain BJ, Munoz B, Tomany SC, McCarty C, de Jong PT, Nemesure B, Mitchell P, Kempen J, Eye Diseases Prevalence Research Group. Prevalence of age-related macular degeneration in the United States. Arch Ophthalmol. 2004;122:564–72.

Gerster H. Antioxidant vitamins in cataract prevention. Z Ernahrungswiss. 1989;28:56–75.

Goldberg J, Flowerdew G, Smith E, Brody JA, Tso MO. Factors associated with age-related macular degeneration. An analysis of data from the first National Health and Nutrition Examination Survey. Am J Epidemiol. 1988;128:700–10.

Hambidge M. Underwood Memorial Lecture: human zinc homeostasis: good but not perfect. J Nutr. 2003;133: 1438S–42S.

Heier JS, Brown DM, Chong V, Korobelnik JF, Kaiser PK, Nguyen QD, Kirchhof B, Ho A, Ogura Y, Yancopoulos GD, Stahl N, Vitti R, Berliner AJ, Soo Y, Anderesi M, Groetzbach G, Sommerauer B, Sandbrink R, Simader C, Schmidt-Erfurth U, VIEW 1 and VIEW 2 Study Groups. Intravitreal aflibercept (VEGF trap-eye) in wet age-related macular degeneration. Ophthalmology. 2012;119:2537–48.

Julien S, Biesemeier A, Kokkinou D, Eibl O, Schraermeyer U. Zinc deficiency leads to lipofuscin accumulation in the retinal pigment epithelium of pigmented rats. PLoS One. 2011;6, e29245.

Kaiser PK, Brown DM, Zhang K, Hudson HL, Holz FG, Shapiro H, Schneider S, Acharya NR. Ranibizumab for predominantly classic neovascular age-related macular degeneration: subgroup analysis of first-year ANCHOR results. Am J Ophthalmol. 2007;144:850–7.

Krinsky NI, Landrum JT, Bone RA. Biologic mechanisms of the protective role of lutein and zeaxanthin in the eye. Annu Rev Nutr. 2003;23:171–201.

Landrum JT, Bone RA. Lutein, zeaxanthin, and the macular pigment. Arch Biochem Biophys. 2001;385:28–40.

Litman BJ, Mitchell DC. A role for phospholipid polyunsaturation in modulating membrane protein function. Lipids. 1996;31(Suppl):S193–197.

Meyers KJ, Mares JA, Igo Jr RP, Truitt B, Liu Z, Millen AE, Klein M, Johnson EJ, Engelman CD, Karki CK, Blodi B, Gehrs K, Tinker L, Wallace R, Robinson J, LeBlanc ES, Sarto G, Bernstein PS, SanGiovanni JP, Iyengar SK. Genetic evidence for role of carotenoids in age-related macular degeneration in the Carotenoids in Age-Related Eye Disease Study (CAREDS). Invest Ophthalmol Vis Sci. 2014;55:587–99.

Millen AE, Voland R, Sondel SA, Parekh N, Horst RL, Wallace RB, Hageman GS, Chappell R, Blodi BA, Klein ML, Gehrs KM, Sarto GE, Mares JA, CAREDS Study Group. Vitamin D status and early age-related macular degeneration in postmenopausal women. Arch Ophthalmol. 2011;129:481–9.

Moeller SM, Parekh N, Tinker L, Ritenbaugh C, Blodi B, Wallace RB, Mares JA, CAREDS Research Study Group. Associations between intermediate age-related macular degeneration and lutein and zeaxanthin in the Carotenoids in Age-related Eye Disease Study (CAREDS): ancillary study of the Women's Health Initiative. Arch Ophthalmol. 2006;124:1151–62.

Montgomery MP, Kamel F, Pericak-Vance MA, Haines JL, Postel EA, Agarwal A, Richards M, Scott WK, Schmidt S. Overall diet quality and age-related macular degeneration. Ophthalmic Epidemiol. 2010;17:58–65.

Newsome DA, Swartz M, Leone NC, Elston RC, Miller E. Oral zinc in macular degeneration. Arch Ophthalmol. 1988;106:192–8.

Nguyen CT, Vingrys AJ, Bui BV. Dietary omega-3 fatty acids and ganglion cell function. Invest Ophthalmol Vis Sci. 2008;49:3586–94.

Omenn GS, Goodman GE, Thornquist MD, Balmes J, Cullen MR, Glass A, Keogh JP, Meyskens Jr FL, Valanis B, Williams Jr JH, Barnhart S, Cherniack MG, Brodkin CA, Hammar S. Risk factors for lung cancer and for intervention effects in CARET, the Beta-Carotene and Retinol Efficacy Trial. J Natl Cancer Inst. 1996;88:1550–9.

Parisi V, Tedeschi M, Gallinaro G, Varano M, Saviano S, Piermarocchi S, Group CS. Carotenoids and antioxidants in age-related maculopathy Italian study: multifocal electroretinogram modifications after 1 year. Ophthalmology. 2008;115(324–333), e322.

Robertson JM, Donner AP, Trevithick JR. Vitamin E intake and risk of cataracts in humans. Ann N Y Acad Sci. 1989;570:372–82.

Rosenfeld PJ, Brown DM, Heier JS, Boyer DS, Kaiser PK, Chung CY, Kim RY, MARINA Study Group. Ranibizumab for neovascular age-related macular degeneration. N Engl J Med. 2006;355:1419–31.

SanGiovanni JP, Chew EY, Clemons TE, Davis MD, Ferris FL, Gensler GR, Kurinij N, Lindblad AS, Milton RC, Seddon JM, Sperduto RD, Age-Related Eye Disease Study Research Group. The relationship of dietary lipid intake and age-related macular degeneration in a case-control study: AREDS Report No. 20. Arch Ophthalmol. 2007;125:671–9.

SanGiovanni JP, Chew EY, Agrón E, Clemons TE, Ferris 3rd FL, Gensler G, Lindblad AS, Milton RC, Seddon JM, Klein R, Sperduto RD, Age-Related Eye Disease Study Research Group. The relationship of dietary omega-3 long-chain polyunsaturated fatty acid intake with incident age-related macular degeneration: AREDS report no. 23. Arch Ophthalmol. 2008;126:1274–9.

SanGiovanni JP, Agron E, Clemons TE, Chew EY. Omega-3 long-chain polyunsaturated fatty acid intake inversely associated with 12-year progression to advanced age-related macular degeneration. Arch Ophthalmol. 2009a;127:110–2.

Sangiovanni JP, Agrón E, Meleth AD, Reed GF, Sperduto RD, Clemons TE, Chew EY, Age-Related Eye Disease Study Research Group. {Omega}-3 Long-chain polyunsaturated fatty acid intake and 12-y incidence of neovascular age-related macular degeneration and central geographic atrophy: AREDS report 30, a prospective cohort study from the Age-Related Eye Disease Study. Am J Clin Nutr. 2009b;90:1601–7.

Schalch W. Carotenoids in the retina—a review of their possible role in preventing or limiting damage caused by light and oxygen. EXS. 1992;62:280–98.

Seddon JM, Ajani UA, Sperduto RD, Hiller R, Blair N, Burton TC, Farber MD, Gragoudas ES, Haller J, Miller DT, et al. Dietary carotenoids, vitamins A, C, and E, and advanced age-related macular degeneration. Eye Disease Case-Control Study Group. JAMA. 1994;272:1413–20.

Seddon JM, George S, Rosner B. Cigarette smoking, fish consumption, omega-3 fatty acid intake, and associations with age-related macular degeneration: the US Twin Study of Age-Related Macular Degeneration. Arch Ophthalmol. 2006;124:995–1001.

Snodderly DM. Evidence for protection against age-related macular degeneration by carotenoids and antioxidant vitamins. Am J Clin Nutr. 1995;62:1448S–61S.

Sperduto RD, Ferris 3rd FL, Kurinij N. Do we have a nutritional treatment for age-related cataract or macular degeneration? Arch Ophthalmol. 1990;108:1403–5.

Stampfer MJ, Hennekens CH, Manson JE, Colditz GA, Rosner B, Willett WC. Vitamin E consumption and the risk of coronary disease in women. N Engl J Med. 1993;328:1444–9.

Studnicka J, Rencova E, Blaha M, Rozsival P, Lanska M, Blaha V, Nemcansky J, Langrova H. Long-term outcomes of rheohaemapheresis in the treatment of dry form of age-related macular degeneration. J Ophthalmol. 2013;2013:135798.

Sunness JS, Gonzalez-Baron J, Bressler NM, Hawkins B, Applegate CA. The development of choroidal neovascularization in eyes with the geographic atrophy form of age-related macular degeneration. Ophthalmology. 1999;106:910–9.

Swenor BK, Bressler S, Caulfield L, West SK. The impact of fish and shellfish consumption on age-related macular degeneration. Ophthalmology. 2010;117:2395–401.

Tan JS, Wang JJ, Flood V, Rochtchina E, Smith W, Mitchell P. Dietary antioxidants and the long-term incidence of age-related macular degeneration: the Blue Mountains Eye Study. Ophthalmology. 2008;115:334–41.

VandenLangenberg GM, Mares-Perlman JA, Klein R, Klein BE, Brady WE, Palta M. Associations between antioxidant and zinc intake and the 5-year incidence of early age-related maculopathy in the Beaver Dam Eye Study. Am J Epidemiol. 1998;148:204–14.

WHO. Global data on visual impairments 2010. Geneva: WHO; 2012.

Yehoshua Z, de Amorim Garcia CA, Filho RP, Nunes G, Gregori FM, Penha AA, Moshfeghi K, Zhang S, Sadda WF, Rosenfeld PJ. Systemic complement inhibition with eculizumab for geographic atrophy in age-related macular degeneration: the COMPLETE study. Ophthalmology. 2014;121: 693–701.

VEGF-Inhibition in Macular Telangiectasia Type 2

5

Peter Charbel Issa and Frank G. Holz

5.1 Introduction

Macular telangiectasia (MacTel) type 2 is a macular degenerative disease characterized by slowly progressing photoreceptor atrophy and peculiar vascular alterations within the central retina (Charbel Issa et al. 2013). The disease usually presents bilaterally and has no gender predilection. A genetic component has been suggested due to occurrence in monozygotic twins and other family members (Gillies et al. 2009; Charbel Issa et al. 2013). However, the exact genetic cause and the pathophysiology of MacTel type 2 currently remain unknown.

Gass and Blodi (1993) proposed five consecutive disease stages: stage 1 is characterized by a diffuse paracentral (juxtafoveolar) hyperfluorescence in late phase fluorescein angiography. In stage 2, a reduced parafoveolar retinal transparency becomes evident ophthalmoscopically. The hallmark of stage 3 are dilated right-angled venules and of stage 4 plaque-like pigmentation

("pigment-plaques"), probably due to intraretinal proliferation of pigment epithelial cells along right-angled vessels. Stage 5 is characterized by secondary neovascular membranes, the so-called "proliferative MacTel type 2." However, it should be noted that neovascular membranes may develop at any time point and should rather be seen as a complication during the disease course than as the natural end point of the disease process (Charbel Issa et al. 2013). Neovascular membranes develop mostly from retinal vessels, i.e., not from the choroid as in age-related macular degeneration and many other retinal diseases with secondary choroidal neovascularization.

In all disease stages, visualization of the vascular alterations is enhanced on fluorescein angiography, which may show ectatic capillaries in early frames and leakage from these vessels in later angiographic phases. The functionally relevant natural end point of the disease is an atrophy of the photoreceptor layer in the macular area (Charbel Issa et al. 2013) which is best visualized on spectral-domain optical coherence tomography (SD-OCT). All morphological changes predominantly manifest temporal to the foveal center, but an area extending by about 2 disc diameters across the central retina may eventually be affected.

First symptoms experienced by patients with MacTel type 2 commonly are reading problems and/or metamorphopsia (Heeren et al. 2013). Reading difficulties have been explained by the

Parts of the text of this chapter have been modified from Charbel Issa P, Gillies MC. Macular telangiectasia type 2. Prog Retin Eye Res. 2013;34:49–77. doi:10.1016/j.preteyeres.2012.11.002.Epub2012Dec3.

P. Charbel Issa, M.D., D.Phil. (✉) • F.G. Holz, M.D.
Department of Ophthalmology, University of Bonn, Ernst Abbe Strasse 2, Bonn 53127, Germany
e-mail: peter.issa@ukb.uni-bonn.de;
frank.holz@ukb.uni-bonn.de

© Springer International Publishing Switzerland 2016
A. Stahl (ed.), *Anti-Angiogenic Therapy in Ophthalmology*,
Essentials in Ophthalmology, DOI 10.1007/978-3-319-24097-8_5

presence of paracentral scotomata, which represent the characteristic functional defect in this disease (Finger et al. 2009). Initially, such scotomata develop in the nasal paracentral visual field, in correspondence to the predominant localization of morphological alterations in the temporal paracentral area. Because the scotomata initially are very small, they may be missed on conventional functional testing using static perimetry and visual acuity testing. Due to their sharp delineation from normally functioning retina, visual acuity may be unimpaired even in the presence of an absolute scotoma. Functional deterioration beyond those related to degenerative changes may occur due to the development of secondary neovascular membranes as well as partial- or full-thickness macular holes (Charbel Issa et al. 2009, 2013).

Through increased research efforts stimulated by the Macular Telangiectasia Project ("MacTel Project"; http://www.mactelresearch.org), it has become evident that certain novel imaging modalities have a high diagnostic value and might also be relevant for longitudinal disease monitoring. Specifically, optical coherence tomography (OCT) commonly shows alterations within the central retina and may be the most sensitive noninvasive imaging technology to diagnose MacTel type 2. Characteristic alterations on OCT imaging include a disruption of the ellipsoid zone, hyporeflective cavities at the level of the inner or outer retina, and atrophy of the photoreceptor layer in later disease stages (Charbel Issa et al. 2013; Gaudric et al. 2006). Although OCT findings are not included in the classification by Gass and Blodi, these atrophic changes appear to be the functionally limiting natural end point of the disease.

Fundus autofluorescence is another imaging modality that reveals characteristic alterations in patients with MacTel type 2. Typical changes include a relatively increased signal within the affected area due to loss of macular pigment (Charbel Issa et al. 2013). Such new noninvasive imaging techniques may aid as an objective measure to assess therapeutic effects and to complement fluorescein angiography.

Therapeutic effects for MacTel type 2 may depend upon the presence or absence of a proliferative disease stage. Thus, we separately report potential therapeutic options in non-proliferative and proliferative (i.e., with a neovascular membrane) disease. In any case, the potential benefit of any therapy will depend upon the presence of atrophic changes, irreversible cell death, in the photoreceptor layer at the time of intervention and during follow-up.

5.2 Non-proliferative Stage of Macular Telangiectasia Type 2

In disease stages without neovascular membranes (i.e., stages 1–4), argon laser photocoagulation (Chopdar 1978; Hutton et al. 1978; Friedman et al. 1993; Gass and Blodi 1993; Park et al. 1997), photodynamic therapy (De Lahitte et al. 2004), intravitreal injection of steroids alone (Alldredge and Garretson 2003; Martinez 2003; Cakir et al. 2006), or in combination with indocyanine green-mediated photothrombosis (Arevalo et al. 2007) and posterior juxtascleral administration of steroids (Eandi et al. 2006) have been tried. All these therapeutic approaches have been shown to be ineffective or even to potentially accelerate disease progression. For instance, there may be an increased risk for the development of new fibrovascular membranes after focal argon laser photocoagulation in MacTel type 2 (Gass and Blodi 1993; Park et al. 1996, 1997; Engelbrecht et al. 2002). For other therapies, only very few cases have been reported so that no conclusion can be drawn with regard to effectiveness or safety.

The eponymous ectatic and leaking capillaries within the macular area have led to the hypothesis that vascular endothelial growth factor (VEGF) might play a role in the pathophysiology of this disease. In a first report on *intravitreal inhibition of VEGF*, it was shown that intravitreal injection of bevacizumab resulted in a marked decrease of vascular leakage; however, without significant improvement in visual acuity (Charbel

Issa et al. 2007). This observation confirmed the hypothesis on a role of VEGF in the pathophysiology of MacTel type 2 and stimulated further therapeutic investigations in small case series. A report on short-term effects in six non-proliferative eyes revealed that intravitreal injections of bevacizumab with an interval of 4 weeks resulted in a decrease in macular thickness on SD-OCT imaging and a reduction of angiographically visible vascular changes in all eyes (Charbel Issa et al. 2007). However, visual acuity improved in only a subset of patients. Two subsequent studies reported a longer follow-up (18 and 32 months, respectively) after intravitreal bevacizumab injections (Charbel Issa et al. 2008; Matt et al. 2010). These studies showed that the effect of anti-VEGF treatment, monitored by fluorescein angiography and OCT imaging, abated after 3–4 months. Additional treatments within the reported review period showed similar morphological effects as the initial injections.

In two prospective studies including ten and five patients, respectively, treatment with intravit-

really administered ranibizumab was performed monthly for 1 year. In both studies, there was no significant change in visual acuity. Of note, paracentral photoreceptor atrophy and corresponding scotomata progressed slowly despite a marked effect on the vascular pathological changes (Figs. 5.1, 5.2 and 5.3) (Charbel Issa et al. 2010, 2011; Toy et al. 2012). These findings prompted us to conclude that regular intravitreal injections of VEGF-inhibitors should not be recommended for patients with non-proliferative MacTel type 2. Nine of the ten patients included in one of these studies were examined again after a mean follow-up of 6.0±0.4 years (Kupitz et al. 2015). More eyes of the treatment group had lost two or more lines on BCVA testing (4 versus 1), although mean visual acuity at baseline was similar in treated and control eyes. In addition, more eyes had developed an absolute paracentral scotoma (7 versus 2; Fig. 5.4) and a secondary neovascular membrane had formed in four of the treated and in none of the untreated fellow eyes (Kupitz et al. 2015). Thus, although the worse outcome in

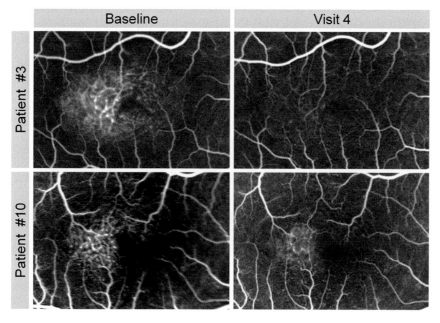

Fig. 5.1 Early fluorescein angiography in two different patients with non-proliferative macular telangiectasia type 2 before (*left column*) and after (*right column*) three intravitreal injections of ranibizumab in monthly intervals. The telangiectatic capillaries show a marked reduction after therapy. Reproduced from Charbel Issa, P., R. P. Finger, et al. Monthly ranibizumab for nonproliferative macular telangiectasia type 2: a 12-month prospective study. Am J Ophthalmol (2011) 151(5): 876-886 e871, with permission of Elsevier

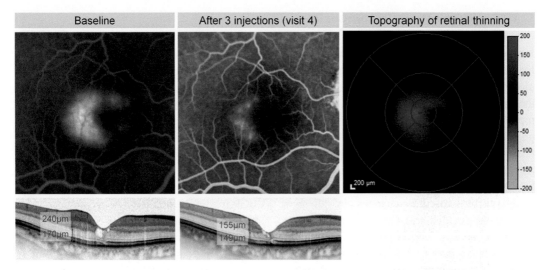

Fig. 5.2 Reduction of late phase fluorescein angiographic leakage in a patient with non-proliferative macular telangiectasia type 2 before (*left column*) and after (*right column*) three intravitreal injections of ranibizumab in monthly intervals. Topographic (*green coding*) and cross-sectional localization of retinal thinning is also shown. Reproduced from Charbel Issa, P., R. P. Finger, et al. Monthly ranibizumab for nonproliferative macular telangiectasia type 2: a 12-month prospective study. Am J Ophthalmol (2011) 151(5): 876-886 e871, with permission of Elsevier

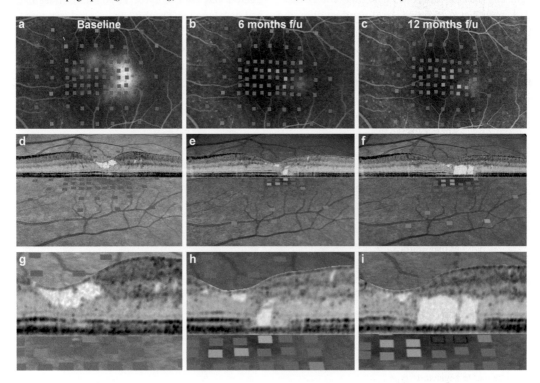

Fig. 5.3 Longitudinal structure–function correlation in macular telangiectasia type 2 treated with monthly injections of ranibizumab over 1 year. Retinal sensitivity of the individual testing points is color coded. Shown are images obtained at baseline (*left column*), after 6 (*middle column*) and 12 monthly treatments (*right column*). The *first row* shows functional maps superimposed on late-phase fluorescein angiography images. Treatment considerably reduced angiographic leakage (**a–c**). However, an absolute scotoma (*open red rectangles*) developed at the completion of the study period (**c**). The *second* and *third row* (enlarged cut-outs of the *middle row*) show corresponding SD-OCT images superimposed on back-tilted infrared cSLO images and the same functional map as shown in the *upper row*. A defect in the photoreceptor layer developed over time (panels **e**, **h**) despite normalization of the vascular changes visible on angiography. Damage of the outer retina was associated with a strong loss of retinal sensitivity (**f**, **i**). Visual acuity at baseline was 20/40 and remained unchanged over the study period despite the pronounced loss of paracentral visual function (reprint from Charbel Issa et al. 2010 under a Creative Commons license)

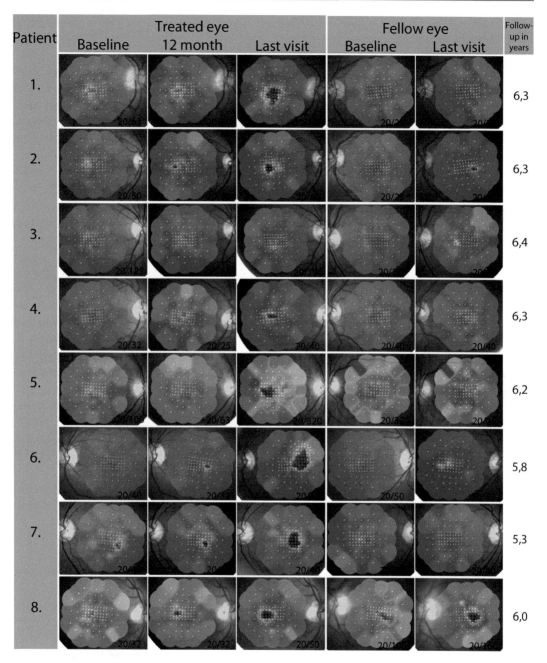

Fig. 5.4 Long-term microperimetric follow-up in patients with macular telangiectasia type 2 who received monthly injections of ranibizumab in one eye during the first year of the observational period. At baseline, no patient presented with an absolute scotoma. In the treated eye, an absolute scotoma (*red*) was present in 4/8 patients after 12 months (i.e., 1 month after 12 injections) and in 7/8 patients at last follow-up. An absolute scotoma developed in only 2/8 of the fellow eyes. Visual acuity at each time point is provided in the *right lower corner* of each microperimetry image. Time between baseline and last follow-up is shown on the *right*. One patient was excluded from functional assessment due to psychogenic vision loss (reprint from Kupitz et al. 2015, with permission of Wolters Kluwer)

treated eyes may have been due to selection bias or the small sample size, these results suggest that VEGF-inhibition has no long-term benefit in patients with non-proliferative MacTel type 2.

There might be exceptions from this conclusion for well-controlled and short-term use of VEGF-inhibition for foveal detachments associated with MacTel type 2. Maia Jr. and coworkers published an observation after intravitreal bevacizumab injection in three non-proliferative eyes with foveal detachment on OCT analysis (Maia et al. 2007). The foveal anatomy regained a normal configuration and visual acuity significantly increased after a single intravitreal injection of bevacizumab.

5.3 Proliferative Stage of Macular Telangiectasia Type 2

Development of secondary neovascularizations represents a major cause for severe vision loss in MacTel type 2 (Gass and Blodi 1993; Engelbrecht et al. 2002). Therapeutic approaches including focal laser photocoagulation (Lee 1996; Watzke et al. 2005), photodynamic therapy alone (Potter et al. 2002, 2006; Hershberger et al. 2003; Snyers et al. 2004; Hussain et al. 2005; Shanmugam and Agarwal 2005), or combined with intravitreal injection of triamcinolone (Smithen and Spaide 2004), transpupillary thermotherapy (Shukla et al. 2004), posterior juxtascleral administration of steroids (Eandi et al. 2006), and recently, intravitreal injection of VEGF-inhibitors (Charbel Issa et al. 2007; Jorge et al. 2007; Maia et al. 2007; Mandal et al. 2007; Shanmugam et al. 2007) have been tried to limit the consequences of this complicated disease course. Park and coworkers found little change in the size of the fibrovascular tissue over time and consequently questioned the usefulness for treatment in stage 5 eyes (Park et al. 1996). Therefore, interventions appear to be most beneficial in early and active proliferative disease stages (i.e., while a neovascular membrane grows) before the development of fibrotic membranes.

Visual stabilization as well as deterioration has been reported after *argon laser photocoagulation* in stage 5 MacTel type 2 (Lee 1996; Watzke et al. 2005). Although this treatment approach seems to be relatively safe in terms of recurrence of the membranes, large subsequent parafoveal scars may severely interfere with reading ability. However, this functional outcome measure was not reported.

Photodynamic therapy (PDT) with verteporfin has been shown to be beneficial for the treatment of subfoveal choroidal neovascularization secondary to age-related macular degeneration and other diseases. The largest series, a retrospective analysis, encompassed seven eyes of six patients. Patients received on average 2.4 treatments and mean follow-up after the last treatment was 21 months. Median initial and final visual acuity was 20/80. More than two lines decrease or increase in visual acuity was observed in one eye each while the other five eyes remained stable. There is the theoretical concern that the photosensitizing drug may leak out of the retinal vessels in the macula and is potentially associated with adverse effects (Potter et al. 2002; Hussain et al. 2005). Indeed, Shanmugam et al. showed atrophy of the retinal pigment epithelium corresponding to the size of the laser spot (Shanmugam and Agarwal 2005). However, others did not observe complications attributed to the treatment (Potter et al. 2002, 2006).

The use of *intravitreal applicationofbevacizumab* for proliferative MacTel type 2 was first described by Jorge and coworkers (2007). A single injection in their patient presenting with an extrafoveal membrane resulted in the absence of signs of activity and significant improvement of visual acuity within a follow-up period of 6 months. Similar observations of significant functional and anatomical improvement in a proliferative disease stage were reported in individual patients and case series with or without accompanying foveal detachment (Roller et al. 2011; Mandal et al. 2007; Shanmugam et al. 2007). In a patient with a larger subfoveal membrane, no increase in visual acuity despite anatomical improvement was achieved, again

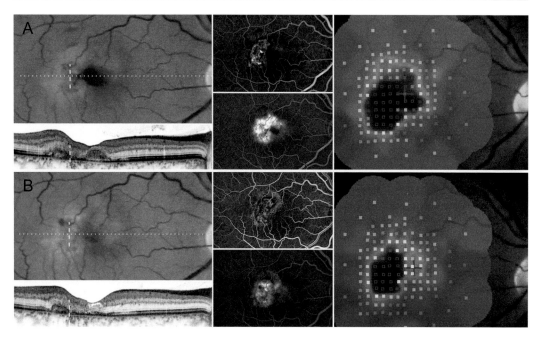

Fig. 5.5 Effects of intravitreal bevacizumab therapy in neovascular MacTel type 2. (**a**) Findings at baseline visit: Foveal hemorrhage (*left*) from an actively leaking neovascular membrane (*middle*; *top*, early phase; *bottom*, late phase). On microperimetry testing, there is a large absolute scotoma which encompasses the foveal center (*right*). (**b**) Four months after one single treatment with intravit-real bevacizumab, the hemorrhage had been resorbed and leakage was reduced. The foveal center after treatment shows only a relative defect and visual acuity has improved from 20/80 to 20/50. Reproduced from Charbel Issa, P., M. C. Gillies, et al. (2013). "Macular telangiectasia type 2." Prog Retin Eye Res 34: 49-77, with permission of Elsevier

suggesting that early intervention seems to be essential (Charbel Issa et al. 2007). In another retrospective case series, 16 treatment-naïve eyes of 16 patients were treated with intravitreal ranibizumab or bevacizumab monotherapy (Narayanan et al. 2012). A mean of 1.9 injections (range, 1–3 injections) were needed during a mean follow-up time of 12 months (range, 3–43 months). Mean visual acuity improved significantly from 20/120 to 20/70. Figure 5.5 shows the functional and morphological disease course under anti-VEGF treatment in a right eye of a patient with proliferative MacTel type 2 over a period of 2 months.

There are two reports on *subretinal surgery* with removal of subfoveal vascular membranes in two eyes with MacTel type 2 (Berger et al. 1997; Davidorf et al. 2004). Due to the adherence of the membranes to the neurosensory retina, removal was obviously difficult and subsequent visual outcome was poor.

5.4 Conclusions from Clinical Observations

In summary, patients with MacTel type 2 who develop an active neovascular membrane and recent loss in visual function appear to benefit from timely therapy with intravitreally applied VEGF-antagonists. There is yet insufficient evidence for following specific treatment regimens. However, a single initial injection with subsequent treatment on a pro re nata basis may be sufficient, similar to the current approach in myopic choroidal neovascularization.

The situation appears different in patients with non-proliferative disease stages. If MacTel type 2 is a progressive neurodegenerative disease with secondary changes of macular vessels due to altered VEGF levels, the long-term success of treatments targeting VEGF may be limited. Indeed, long-term observations after monthly intravitreal

VEGF-inhibition over one year were unfavorable, with an even worse functional and morphological outcome in treated versus untreated fellow eyes.

Müller cells have been implicated in the pathophysiology of MacTel type 2. The involvement of Müller cells in supporting both neurons and vasculature suggests that their dysfunction may be a central, although not necessarily primary, feature of MacTel type 2, which is characterized mainly by dysfunction of these two retinal elements. Two clinicopathological studies of eyes from patients with MacTel type 2 suggested a depletion of Müller cells (Powner et al. 2010, 2013) and, thus, support this hypothesis.

Disease characteristics similar to MacTel type 2 have recently been shown in an animal model with conditional Müller cell ablation (Shen et al. 2012). Impairment of Müller cells resulted in upregulation of VEGF and photoreceptor degeneration. VEGF-inhibition attenuated vascular alterations that occurred after Müller cell death, but had no effect on photoreceptor death. Because VEGF has a role in the maintenance of cones (Kurihara et al. 2012) and Müller cells (Wurm et al. 2008), there is the possibility of a protective upregulation of VEGF in the retina of patients with MacTel type 2. Moreover, the rather high rate of incident neovascular membranes (four out of nine) might also suggest a rebound effect with higher VEGF levels after VEGF suppression with subsequent development of a neovascular membrane (Kupitz et al. 2015). Hence, prolonged VEGF-inhibition in non-proliferative disease stages might predispose to a worse functional and morphological outcome and neuroprotective treatment strategies might be a more promising treatment approach (Chew et al. 2015).

Compliance with Ethical Requirements

Informed Consent and Animal Studies disclosures are not applicable to this review. The authors have received research grants from the Lowy Medical Research Institute as a clinical center of the MacTel research consortium, and a research grant from Novartis for an investigator initiated trial on anti-VGEF therapy in MacTel type 2.

References

Alldredge CD, Garretson BR. Intravitreal triamcinolone for the treatment of idiopathic juxtafoveal telangiectasis. Retina. 2003;23(1):113–6.

Arevalo JF, Sanchez JG, et al. Indocyanine-green-mediated photothrombosis (IMP) with intravitreal triamcinolone acetonide for macular edema secondary to group 2A idiopathic parafoveal telangiectasis without choroidal neovascularization: a pilot study. Graefes Arch Clin Exp Ophthalmol. 2007;245(11):1673–80.

Berger AS, McCuen 2nd BW, et al. Surgical removal of subfoveal neovascularization in idiopathic juxtafoveolar retinal telangiectasis. Retina. 1997;17(2):94–8.

Cakir M, Kapran Z, et al. Optical coherence tomography evaluation of macular edema after intravitreal triamcinolone acetonide in patients with parafoveal telangiectasis. Eur J Ophthalmol. 2006;16(5):711–7.

Charbel Issa P, Holz FG, et al. Findings in fluorescein angiography and optical coherence tomography after intravitreal Bevacizumab in Type 2 idiopathic macular telangiectasia. Ophthalmology. 2007a;114(9):1736–42.

Charbel Issa P, Scholl HPN, et al. Short-term effects of intravitreal bevacizumab in Type II idiopathic macular telangiectasia. Retin Cases Brief Rep. 2007b;1(4):189–91. doi:10.1097/ICB.0b013e31802efef2.

Charbel Issa P, Finger RP, et al. Eighteen-month follow-up of intravitreal bevacizumab in type 2 idiopathic macular telangiectasia. Br J Ophthalmol. 2008;92(7):941–5.

Charbel Issa P, Scholl HP, et al. Macular full-thickness and lamellar holes in association with type 2 idiopathic macular telangiectasia. Eye. 2009;23(2):435–41.

Charbel Issa P, Troeger E, et al. Structure-function correlation of the human central retina. PLoS One. 2010;5(9):e12864.

Charbel Issa P, Finger RP, et al. Monthly ranibizumab for nonproliferative macular telangiectasia type 2: a 12-month prospective study. Am J Ophthalmol. 2011;151(5):876–86. e871.

Charbel Issa P, Gillies MC, et al. Macular telangiectasia type 2. Prog Retin Eye Res. 2013;34:49–77.

Chew EY, Clemons TE, et al. Ciliary neurotrophic factor for macular telangiectasia type 2: results from a phase 1 safety trial. Am J Ophthalmol. 2015;159(4):659–66. e651.

Chopdar A. Retinal telangiectasis in adults: fluorescein angiographic findings and treatment by argon laser. Br J Ophthalmol. 1978;62(4):243–50.

Davidorf FH, Pressman MD, et al. Juxtafoveal telangiectasis-a name change? Retina. 2004;24(3):474–8.

De Lahitte GD, Cohen SY, et al. Lack of apparent short-term benefit of photodynamic therapy in bilateral, acquired, parafoveal telangiectasis without subretinal neovascularization. Am J Ophthalmol. 2004;138(5):892–4.

Eandi CM, Ober MD, et al. Anecortave acetate for the treatment of idiopathic perifoveal telangiectasia: a pilot study. Retina. 2006;26(7):780–5.

Engelbrecht NE, Aaberg Jr TM, et al. Neovascular membranes associated with idiopathic juxtafoveolar telangiectasis. Arch Ophthalmol. 2002;120(3):320–4.

Finger RP, Charbel Issa P, et al. Reading performance is reduced due to parafoveal scotomas in patients with macular telangiectasia type 2. Invest Ophthalmol Vis Sci. 2009;50(3):1366–70.

Friedman SM, Mames RN, et al. Subretinal hemorrhage after grid laser photocoagulation for idiopathic juxtafoveolar retinal telangiectasis. Ophthalmic Surg. 1993;24(8):551–3.

Gass JD, Blodi BA. Idiopathic juxtafoveolar retinal telangiectasis. Update of classification and follow-up study. Ophthalmology. 1993;100(10):1536–46.

Gaudric A, Ducos de Lahitte G, et al. Optical coherence tomography in group 2A idiopathic juxtafoveolar retinal telangiectasis. Arch Ophthalmol. 2006;124(10):1410–9.

Gillies MC, Zhu M, et al. Familial asymptomatic macular telangiectasia type 2. Ophthalmology. 2009;116(12): 2422–9.

Heeren TF, Holz FG, et al. First symptoms and their age of onset in macular telangiectasia Type 2. Retina. 2013;34(5):916–9.

Hershberger VS, Hutchins RK, et al. Photodynamic therapy with verteporfin for subretinal neovascularization secondary to bilateral idiopathic acquired juxtafoveolar telangiectasis. Ophthalmic Surg Lasers Imaging. 2003;34(4):318–20.

Hussain N, Das T, et al. Bilateral sequential photodynamic therapy for sub-retinal neovascularization with type 2A parafoveal telangiectasis. Am J Ophthalmol. 2005;140(2):333–5.

Hutton WL, Snyder WB, et al. Focal parafoveal retinal telangiectasis. Arch Ophthalmol. 1978;96(8):1362–7.

Jorge R, Costa RA, et al. Intravitreal bevacizumab (Avastin) associated with the regression of subretinal neovascularization in idiopathic juxtafoveolar retinal telangiectasis. Graefes Arch Clin Exp Ophthalmol. 2007;245(7):1045–8.

Kupitz EH, Heeren TFC et al. (2015). Long-term poor outcome of anti-VEGF therapy in non-proliferative macular telangiectasia type 2. Retina [in press].

Kurihara T, Westenskow PD, et al. Targeted deletion of Vegfa in adult mice induces vision loss. J Clin Invest. 2012;122(11):4213–7.

Lee BL. Bilateral subretinal neovascular membrane in idiopathic juxtafoveolar telangiectasis. Retina. 1996;16(4): 344–6.

Maia Jr OO, Bonanomi MT, et al. Intravitreal bevacizumab for foveal detachment in idiopathic perifoveal telangiectasia. Am J Ophthalmol. 2007;144(2):296–9.

Mandal S, Venkatesh P, et al. Intravitreal bevacizumab (Avastin) for subretinal neovascularization secondary to type 2A idiopathic juxtafoveal telangiectasia. Graefes Arch Clin Exp Ophthalmol. 2007;245(12):1825–9.

Martinez JA. Intravitreal triamcinolone acetonide for bilateral acquired parafoveal telangiectasis. Arch Ophthalmol. 2003;121(11):1658–9.

Matt G, Sacu S, et al. Thirty-month follow-up after intravitreal bevacizumab in progressive idiopathic macular telangiectasia type 2. Eye (Lond). 2010;24(10):1535–41.

Narayanan R, Chhablani J, et al. Efficacy of anti-vascular endothelial growth factor therapy in subretinal

neovascularization secondary to macular telangiectasia type 2. Retina. 2012;32(10):2001–5.

Park D, Schatz H, et al. Fibrovascular tissue in bilateral juxtafoveal telangiectasis. Arch Ophthalmol. 1996; 114(9):1092–6.

Park DW, Schatz H, et al. Grid laser photocoagulation for macular edema in bilateral juxtafoveal telangiectasis. Ophthalmology. 1997;104(11):1838–46.

Potter MJ, Szabo SM, et al. Photodynamic therapy of a subretinal neovascular membrane in type 2A idiopathic juxtafoveolar retinal telangiectasis. Am J Ophthalmol. 2002;133(1):149–51.

Potter MJ, Szabo SM, et al. Photodynamic therapy for subretinal neovascularization in type 2A idiopathic juxtafoveolar telangiectasis. Can J Ophthalmol. 2006; 41(1):34–7.

Powner MB, Gillies MC, et al. Perifoveal Müller cell depletion in a case of macular telangiectasia type 2. Ophthalmology. 2010;117(12):2407–16.

Powner MB, Gillies MC, et al. Loss of Muller's cells and photoreceptors in macular telangiectasia type 2. Ophthalmology. 2013;120(11):2344–52.

Roller AB, Folk JC, et al. Intravitreal bevacizumab for treatment of proliferative and nonproliferative type 2 idiopathic macular telangiectasia. Retina. 2011;31(9): 1848–55.

Shanmugam MP, Agarwal M. RPE atrophy following photodynamic therapy in type 2A idiopathic parafoveal telangiectasis. Indian J Ophthalmol. 2005; 53(1):61–3.

Shanmugam MP, Mythri HM, et al. Intravitreal bevacizumab for parafoveal telangiectasia-associated choroidal neovascular membrane. Indian J Ophthalmol. 2007;55(6):490–1.

Shen W, Fruttiger M, et al. Conditional Müller cell ablation causes independent neuronal and vascular pathologies in a novel transgenic model. J Neurosci. 2012;32(45):15715–27.

Shukla D, Singh J, et al. Transpupillary thermotherapy for subfoveal neovascularization secondary to group 2A idiopathic juxtafoveolar telangiectasis. Am J Ophthalmol. 2004;138(1):147–9.

Smithen LM, Spaide RF. Photodynamic therapy and intravitreal triamcinolone for a subretinal neovascularization in bilateral idiopathic juxtafoveal telangiectasis. Am J Ophthalmol. 2004;138(5):884–5.

Snyers B, Verougstraete C, et al. Photodynamic therapy of subfoveal neovascular membrane in type 2A idiopathic juxtafoveolar retinal telangiectasis. Am J Ophthalmol. 2004;137(5):812–9.

Toy BC, Koo E, et al. Treatment of nonneovascular idiopathic macular telangiectasia type 2 with intravitreal ranibizumab: results of a phase II clinical trial. Retina. 2012;32(5):996–1006.

Watzke RC, Klein ML, et al. Long-term juxtafoveal retinal telangiectasia. Retina. 2005;25(6):727–35.

Wurm A, Pannicke T, et al. Glial cell-derived glutamate mediates autocrine cell volume regulation in the retina: activation by VEGF. J Neurochem. 2008;104(2): 386–99.

Diabetic Retinopathy

6

Focke Ziemssen and Hansjürgen T. Agostini

6.1 Nomenclature, Classification, and Epidemiology

6.1.1 Incidence and Prevalence

Diabetic retinopathy (DR) is still the leading cause of vision loss in the working-aged adults worldwide (Yau et al. 2012), thereby causing a significant impairment in utility and quality of life. Forty years ago, persons with diabetes were 25 times more likely to become blind than people without diabetes (Kahn and Hiller 1974). However, over the last decades, lower incidences of diabetic retinopathy (DR) and rates of progression to proliferative retinopathy (PRD) were seen than historically (Ding and Wong 2012). The risk of severe visual loss has slightly decreased in the Western countries, which may reflect better control of glucose, blood pressure, and serum lipids as well as earlier diagnosis (Kempen et al. 2004).

F. Ziemssen (✉)
Center for Ophthalmology, Eberhard-Karl University Tübingen, Schleichstr. 12, Tübingen 72076, Germany
e-mail: focke.ziemssen@med.uni-tuebingen.de

H.T. Agostini
Eye Center, Albert-Ludwigs-University Freiburg, Killianstr. 5, Freiburg im Breisgau 79106, Germany
e-mail: hansjuergen.agostini@uniklinik-freiburg.de

Nevertheless, blindness is not only the fear No. 1 in persons affected. Diabetic retinopathy still is a growing disease. The current epidemic of diabetes and growing numbers in the world are linked to a changing lifestyle—in the Western world as well as in the developing countries (Scanlon et al. 2013). The International Diabetes Federation (IDF) predicts a further rise from 382 million in 2013 to 552 million people affected in 2030. Diabetes according to most recent estimates affects 8.3 % of adults. Yet, with 175 million persons (45.8 %) currently undiagnosed, a large amount of people are progressing globally towards complications while being unaware of their disease (Beagley et al. 2014). An estimated 83.8 % of all undiagnosed cases are in low- and middle-income countries. The lifetime risk of developing diabetes is approx. 30 %, but decisively influenced by the body weight (Narayan et al. 2003, 2007).

6.1.2 Worldwide Incidence and Prevalence

Type 1 diabetes shows a heterogeneous distribution, being more common in the Northern countries. Globally, the age-standardized prevalence of DR is assumed to be 10 % for the vision-threatening disease, with diabetic macular edema and/or proliferative DR each accounting for approx. 7 % (Yau et al. 2012). Diabetes still is a common cause of blindness, especially in the working age adults.

© Springer International Publishing Switzerland 2016
A. Stahl (ed.), *Anti-Angiogenic Therapy in Ophthalmology*,
Essentials in Ophthalmology, DOI 10.1007/978-3-319-24097-8_6

Even in developed countries, DR is responsible for 10 % of new blindness (Congdon et al. 2004; Finger et al. 2011), in dependence of race and living conditions. One in 11 adults has diabetes, one of two adults with diabetes is undiagnosed (IDF 2015). Conservative estimations lead to the rate of one person becoming blind every minute.

A genetic predisposition has been shown to affect the lifetime risk of retinopathy. After controlling for other independent risk factors some polymorphisms have been found to be either protective or deleterious (Grassi et al. 2012; Schwartz et al. 2013).

The Wisconsin Epidemiologic Study of Diabetic Retinopathy (WESDR) underlined the influence of the duration of disease on the development of DR (Klein et al. 1984, 2009). The incidence of DR increases with the duration of diabetes (Fig. 6.1). While almost none of the affected persons with type 1 diabetes had macular edema within the first 5 years of onset, reti-

nopathy increased to 60 % after 10 years and even 80 % after 15 years. It is noteworthy that the risk of severe retinopathy seems to be reduced in more recent studies (LeCaire et al. 2013).

The Los Angeles Latino Eye Study (LALES) described a prevalence of 18 % of proliferative diabetic retinopathy, with no difference between those with type 1 vs. type 2 diabetes (Varma et al. 2004). A pooled analysis in China reported a prevalence of DR of 29 % for the rural areas. The frequency was slightly higher in the Northern region (Liu et al. 2012). In the Middle East, most patients presented with mild nonproliferative DR (up to 65 %), but the proliferative disease varied between 2.3 and 10 % among affected persons (Zabetian et al. 2013). These discrepancies point also to the higher risk of some racial groups.

The Gutenberg Health study found a total prevalence of DR of 24 % in a German cross-sectional cohort (Raum et al. 2014). The rate of diabetes was 7.5 % within the age between 35

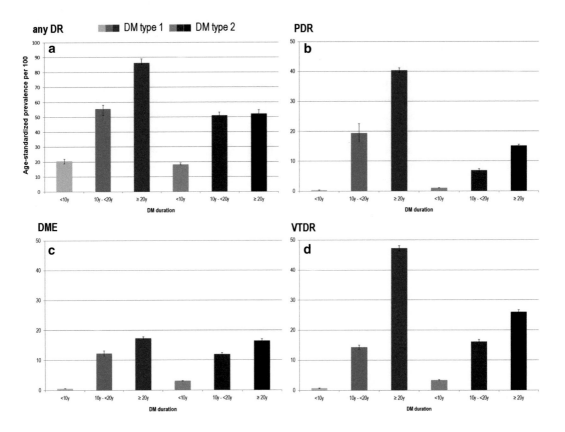

Fig. 6.1 Influence of diabetes duration on frequency of diabetic eye disease (Yau et al. 2012). VTDR = vision-threatening diabetic retinopathy

and 74 years of age. Only 5 % of these suffered from sight-threatening DR. Other studies indicate the frequent unawareness of disease, in early phases similarly to vision-threatening stages (Huang et al. 2009; Silva et al. 2010).

Persistent severe visual loss was an infrequent observation in the Early Treatment of Diabetic Retinopathy Study (ETDRS) and most commonly caused by vitreous or preretinal hemorrhage, followed by macular edema or macular pigmentary changes (Fong et al. 1999). The influence of modifiable risk factors for progression makes it difficult to project the exact incidences of the advanced stages or blindness for the future.

6.1.3 Prevention and Health Costs

Even in the absence of other major complications DR has a major impact on the quality of life (Alcubierre et al. 2014). Early detection and treatment of DR can avoid and considerably reduce the economic costs of the most frequent diabetic complication. Reducing the burden and follow-up costs, the effectiveness of screening and treatment is dependent on the subtype of DR (Javitt and Aiello 1996). Therefore, prevention programs aimed at improving eye care for diabetic persons result in substantial federal budgetary savings and are highly cost-effective health investments for society. Besides the improvement of quality of life, the main benefit is the prevention of further medical costs (Pelletier et al. 2009). A Swedish study calculated annual DR-related costs of 106.000€ per 100.000 inhabitants (Heintz et al. 2010).

6.2 Clinical Entities

6.2.1 Nonproliferative Diabetic Retinopathy

Vascular changes and exudation are the hallmark of early diabetic retinopathy. On ophthalmoscopic examination, the characteristic features of nonproliferative diabetic retinopathy (NPDR) are microaneurysms (MAs), intraretinal hemorrhages, and hard exudates.

Retinal capillary microaneurysms (MAs) are usually the first visible sign of diabetic retinopathy. The characteristics of MAs are the appearance of round deep-red dots, a size of 15–60 µm and a spatial preference for the macula, located in the inner nuclear layer and the capillary network (Byeon et al. 2012). The saccular outpouchings of the capillary wall are a consequence of a loss of pericytes and precede capillary closure (Fig. 6.2). There is recent evidence that the structural variability is higher when examined by adaptive optics imaging (Dubow et al. 2014). Mechanistically, a weakness of the capillary wall from the early loss of pericytes and changes of the vascular endothelium or the intraluminal pressure are discussed as contributing factors. Rupture of larger aneurysms can lead to extensive intraretinal or vitreous hemorrhage.

In fluorescein angiography (FLA), MAs exhibit bright hyperfluorescence, distinguishable from small hemorrhages (Hellstedt et al. 1996; Ito et al. 2013; Jalli et al. 1997; Kohner and Henkind 1970; Schiffman et al. 2005; Wang et al. 2012a). Although increased density is associated with an area of leakage, the presence or absence of MAs alone is not of clinical significance and therefore does not in itself warrant the need for the invasive FLA procedure (Fig. 6.3). Nevertheless, it is important to be aware of the *prognostic value* of the turnover occurrence of MAs, respectively (Nunes et al. 2009). Regarding the dynamic nature of MAs, it is noteworthy that older or regressing MAs are not necessarily identified in FLA (Goatman et al. 2003; Leicht et al. 2014). When compared to color photography, FLA examinations allow a modest increase in sensitivity of DR (DCCT Research Group 1987; Agardh and Cavallin-Sjoberg 1998) (Table 6.1). Therefore, an implementation of the procedure in addition to biomicroscopy remains reserved for predefined scenarios (Banerjee et al. 2007; Khalaf et al. 2007; Olsen et al. 2014).

Hemorrhages within the macular area usually originate from ruptured small vessels and MAs. Small pinpoint bleedings occur early in maculopathy. In contrast, hemorrhages in the periphery are more frequently an indication of other concomitant diseases or extensive isch-

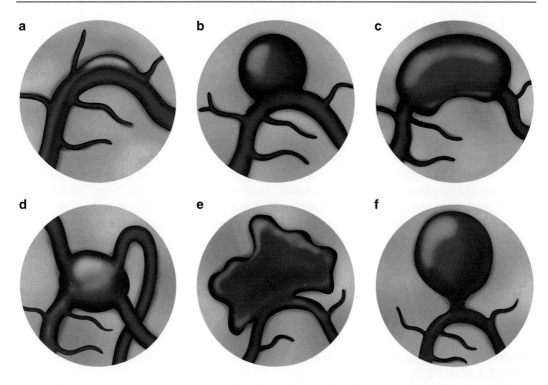

Fig. 6.2 *Retinal microaneurysms* appear as *round red dots* (Dubow et al. 2014)

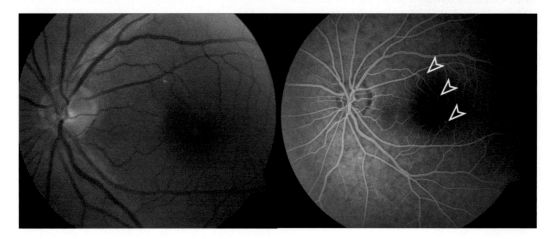

Fig. 6.3 Clinical image of microaneurysms (*right*: *arrow* in fluorescein angiogram)

Table 6.1 Rational for the performance of FLA

Scenarios to perform fluorescein angiography (FLA)		
Essential	Helpful	Not appropriate
• Clarification of unexplained vision loss	• Differential diagnosis in unusual findings	• Screening at no or minimal DR
• Identification of capillary nonperfusion	• Support of laser treatment	

emia. In cases of preretinal bleeding, PRD should be excluded.

Hard exudates can represent the extracellular accumulation of lipids, proteins, and lipoproteins. There is a huge variation in size and structure, from tiny precipitates and circinate atolls to confluent arrangements and large lipid plaques. Hard exudates can indicate the extent and location of vascular leakage and transiently increase, if edema diminishes.

In the course of the disease, the *closure of retinal capillaries* is a major feature and reflects retinal ischemia. While there are early preclinical signs such as dysfunction of photoreceptors (Verma et al. 2012) and/or vascular inflammation (Daley et al. 1987; Lung et al. 2012), capillary obliteration and nonperfusion are the hallmarks of the advanced diabetic retinopathy (Li et al.

2014; Lombardo et al. 2013). On histopathological examination, endothelial proliferation and pericyte damage in the small vessels (Ashton 1958) are more and more accompanied by vasoregression (Cunha-Vaz et al. 2014b).

Initially smaller patches of acellular capillaries can become confluent over time. Tortuous cluster of MAs and intraretinal microvascular abnormalities (IRMA) develop, often coinciding. The areas of capillary nonperfusion enlarge as the disease progresses (Sim et al. 2013a), while associated with retinal thinning (Sim et al. 2014). Although visual acuity can be preserved during mild grades of ischemia, more severe stages are associated with a loss of visual acuity, especially if the papillomacular nerve fiber bundle is affected (Arden and Sivaprasad 2011; Sim et al. 2013b) (Fig. 6.4). Rarefication of vascular branches leads to the

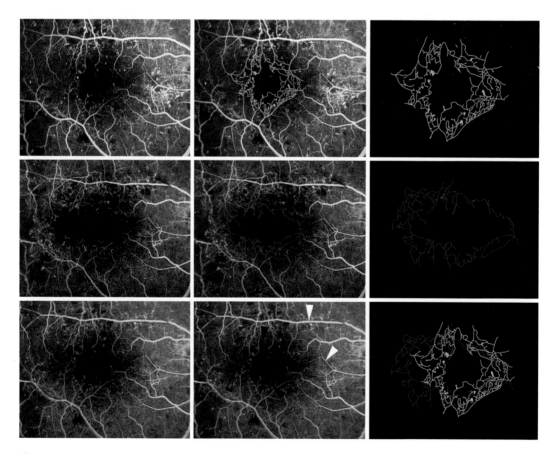

Fig. 6.4 Progression of foveal ischemia (*first row*: perifoveal capillary in *green* after 2 years, *second row*: perifoveal capillaries in *red*, and *third row*: merged angiograms) shown by Sim et al. (2013a)

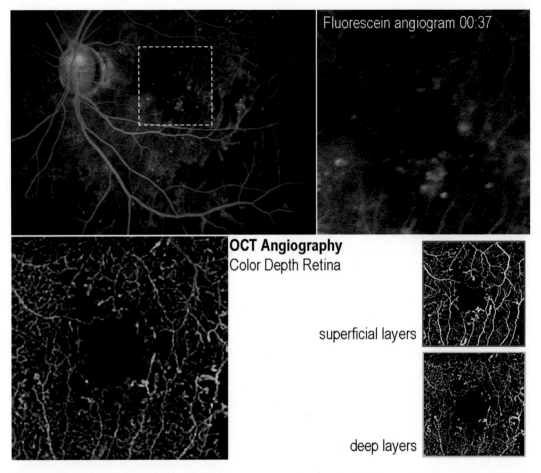

Fig. 6.5 Differential layers of the perifoveal morphology can be detected by OCT Angiography (*Courtesy*: Dr. Scott Lee, Oakland; Prototype Zeiss SD-Angio-OCT)

typical appearance of pruning (ETDRS Research Group 1991b).

Venous beading and loops, intraretinal microvascular changes and areas of nonperfusion indicate an increased risk of progression of the retinopathy to more severe stages (Benson et al. 1988) (Fig. 6.5).

6.2.2 Proliferative Diabetic Retinopathy

Proliferative changes, affecting approximately 7 % of persons with DR, are considered to be mainly induced by ischemia (Liu et al. 2013; Miller et al. 2013; Rodrigues et al. 2013; Yau

et al. 2012). Proliferative diabetic retinopathy (PDR) is much more frequently seen in younger persons with type 1 diabetes (Klein et al. 1992). Hyperglycemia, longer duration of diabetes, and more severe retinopathy at baseline were associated with an increased 4-year risk of developing PDR.

The accompanying inflammation and chronic disruption of the blood–retina barrier contribute to the reduced perfusion (Klaassen et al. 2013; Lang 2013; Silva et al. 2007) (Fig. 6.6). Retinal nonperfusion was reported to affect predominantly the midperiphery (Cardillo et al. 1987). However, it has to be mentioned that wide-angle imaging nowadays does allow a much better assessment of the far periphery. There have been

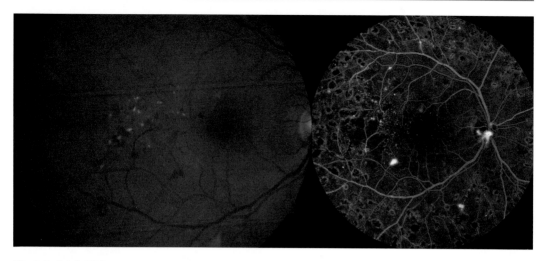

Fig. 6.6 Subtle NVD can be delineated by fluorescein angiography

different hypothesis that a disc-centered pattern might be a sign of a more important role of hypertension, while peripheral patterns might be attributed to the presence of additional systemic diseases. Chronic ischemia contributes in turn to a localized low-grade inflammatory response within the vessels, subsequent migration, and stimulation of immunogenic cells in the tissue (Sebag 1993).

While VEGF is the most prominent proangiogenic factor (Ishida et al. 2003), other growth factors like TGFβ are important for the clinically relevant processes of membrane formation and fibrovascular contraction (Deissler et al. 2006; Nawaz et al. 2013; Sohn et al. 2012).

The risk for conversion to PDR increases with the severity of NPDR. Peripheral lesions seen by 200° ultrawide field imaging might be predictive (Silva et al. 2015). However, due to the transient nature of hemorrhages and vessel abnormalities, it is not possible in all cases to correctly identify the severity of NPDR based on fundoscopy alone (Danis and Davis 2008).

Two out of three subjects with PDR, the neovascularization is first detected on or adjacent to the optic disc (DRS Group 1981b; Taylor and Dobree 1970). Such neovascularization of the optic disc (NVD) starts as fine loops or networks of vessels on the surface of the disc or bridging across the physiologic cup (Fig. 6.6).

Initially, new vessels may be very subtle (Li et al. 2010). Wheel-like networks, an irregularity in shape or adjacent hemorrhages are common. The growth rate of neovessels is very variable. Regarding concomitant proliferative vitreopathy or fibrovascular proliferations, early membranes can sometimes be overlooked or underestimated due to their translucency in the early phase. OCT imaging has a high sensitivity to better detect a fibrovascular reaction of the posterior pole.

If in doubt, FLA should be performed to confirm the diagnosis and determine the proliferative activity. FLA is also superior to fundoscopy differentiating between IRMAs and a neovascularization that is located outside the disc area, classified as neovascularization elsewhere (NVE).

If fibrovascular membranes contract and/or vitreous detachment occurs, hemorrhages are more frequently seen, otherwise important indicators of local ischemia. Vitreous hemorrhage is an important sight-threatening complication in DR. Depending on the extent and duration, it does not only cause serious loss of vision, but can also restrict the diagnostic possibilities (fundus details) and delay initiation of panretinal photocoagulation (PRP).

The contraction of fibrovascular proliferations can displace the retina or cause tractional detachment (Bresnick et al. 1979; Kampik et al. 1981). The extent of subretinal fluid under the detached retina and macular involvement are the most important predictors of function (Panozzo et al. 2004). However, subsequent thinning of the retina due to malperfusion of the detached retina as well as the high risk of re-proliferation of epiretinal membranes limits the functional and anatomical outcome, even after vitreoretinal surgery with silicon tamponade (Boynton et al. 2015).

6.2.3 Macular Disease

Macular edema (DME) is defined as retinal thickening due to an accumulation of fluid. The leakage of fluid is caused by a disruption of the blood–retinal barrier.

In former times, edema was detected with slit-lamp microscopy and/or stereoscopic photography. Nowadays, OCT is the diagnostic gold standard, not only to test for the presence of thickening, but to quantify retinal thickness and allow follow-up examinations in the same retinal location (Chalam et al. 2012; De et al. 2015; Dmuchowska et al. 2014; Fiore et al. 2013; Vujosevic et al. 2013) (Fig. 6.7). The introduction of OCT has reduced the need of the invasive FLA examination, as it can detect already subclinical macular edema, a precursor to significant DME (Bressler et al. 2012; Pires et al. 2013).

Although retinal thickness does not directly correlate with function, changes in retinal thickness are of importance when dosing medical treatment (Browning et al. 2007). The cautious prognosis of functional outcome after therapy is better delivered by evaluating the integrity of the outer retinal layers (i.e., the photoreceptors) (Maheshwary et al. 2010). In addition, spectral-domain OCT imaging is able to visualize the vitreoretinal interface or indicate inflammatory disease activity such as neurosensory detachment (Murakami et al. 2013; Sonoda et al. 2013).

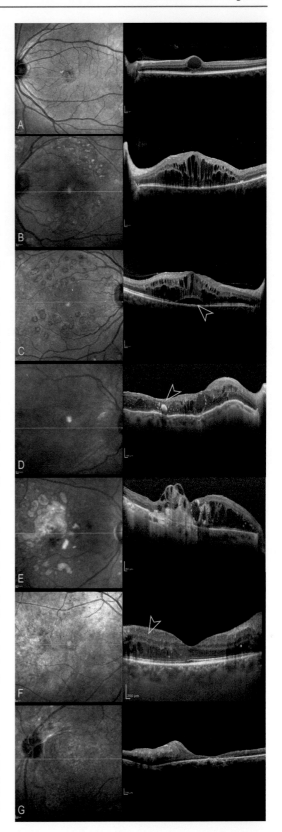

Fig. 6.7 OCT imaging allows classifying for different morphology patterns: (**a**) focal or multifocal cystic edema (**b**) non-focal capillary leakage (**c**) subretinal fluid (*arrow*) (**d**) lipid plaques (**e**) atrophic edema (**f**) diffuse thickening (**g**) ischemic atrophy

Although a consistent relationship between FLA and OCT has been described (e.g., petaloid pattern and large pseudocysts within the outer nuclear and plexiform layers, honeycomb-like pattern with involvement of the inner layers) (Bolz et al. 2009a; Byeon et al. 2012), the clinical relevance of the OCT findings has not been fully established in prospective trials, including such as subretinal fluid or hyperreflective dots. Previous analyses indicate that edema showing subretinal fluid have favorable outcome under anti-VEGF therapy (Sophie et al. 2015).

The concept of *clinically significant macular edema* (CSME) has been introduced by the ETDRS Research Group (1985). The term comprises clinical findings associated with an increased risk of visual loss. Therefore, it is important to identify the area and localization of retinal edema and lipid deposits with respect to the fovea. It should be remembered that the diagnosis of CSME was based on binocular ophthalmoscopy or stereoscopic photographs. In the era preceeding the resolution of SD-OCT, the images had to be stereoscopically recorded in order not to overlook retinal thickening. Future studies have to assess how OCT imaging changes the phenotyping (Bolz et al. 2009b).

The definition of CSME included the following findings (Fig. 6.8):

- Retinal thickening within a radius of 500 μm around the foveal center
- Lipid deposits within a radius of 500 μm around the fovea with an accompanying thickening

- Retinal thickening of an area of more than one disc area within a radius of one disc diameter around the fovea

The differentiation of *focal* and *diffuse edema* is not without problems, as the terms are not used in a consistent way (Browning et al. 2008). Physicians made use of different methods and definitions. Often the angiographic pattern and source of fluorescein leakage are described. Others grade on the base of extent and location of macular thickening, involvement of the center of the macula, and quantity and pattern of lipid exudates or grade the edema with respect to the modality of the planned photocoagulation technique (Callanan et al. 2013; Funatsu et al. 2009; Ophir 2014).

Although some scientists found a difference in treatment efficacy in dependence of the chronicity (Lee and Olk 1991), a general significance of the duration is questionable. In accordance to most definitions, every diffuse edema is a CSME, but in contrast a CSME can be located either extrafoveally or be of minimum size. With regard to the treatment options, it is useful to distinguish edema with and without involvement of the fovea.

The amount of foveal ischemia is of great relevance for clinical evaluation and treatment decision. Nevertheless, there is no uniform definition of *ischemic maculopathy*. The classic diagnosis is made based upon FLA examination. Most frequently, an outage of the perifoveolar capillary arcade and/or areas of capillary closure are considered to delimit the damage (Sim et al. 2013a; Zheng et al. 2014). The diameter and/or the area of the foveal avascular zone (FAZ) were often calculated

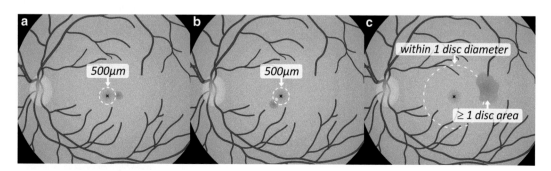

Fig. 6.8 Definition of clinically significant macular edema (CSME)

to quantify the extent of nonperfusion and the limited prognosis. The diameter of the regular FAZ is often defined to lie between 400 and 500 μm, while DR can lead to diameters of more than 1000 μm (Bresnick 1983). In future, the loss of ganglion cells or the reduced integrity of photoreceptors might be more easily detected by OCT imaging (Byeon et al. 2009; Sim et al. 2014); the size of the avascular zone may be imaged by Angio-OCT.

Vitreomacular traction reflects the involvement of the vitreous interface in DR (Haller et al. 2010). These alterations of the vitreomacular interface as well as epiretinal membranes can induce retinal thickening and complicate the treatment of DME (Buabbud et al. 2010; Giovannini et al. 1999; Ophir et al. 2010) (Fig. 6.9). As changes of the vitreomacular interface are frequent after chronic edema as detected by SD-OCT, it is sometimes difficult to judge their respective contribution to visual deterioration, respectively, the potential for visual acuity improvement through surgical membrane peeling (Ghazi et al. 2007).

6.2.4 ETDRS Severity Score

DR often worsens in unequal steps described by the ETDRS severity scale (ETDRS Research Group 1991a). The stage itself as well as the

velocity at which worsening occurs are both correlated to the risk of severe vision loss. Therefore, exact fundoscopic examination in mydriasis and correct classification of DR severity is clinically important (Fig. 6.10).

Future classification systems should also include the manifestations of DR that are visible on SD-OCT imaging. The more accurately DR severity is classified, the better the risk of subsequent worsening can be predicted and treatment and follow-up exams can be scheduled accordingly.

6.2.5 Screening for Diabetic Retinopathy

As sight-threatening retinopathy can be asymptomatic, screening has to be conducted in regular time intervals before the onset of symptoms (Klein 2003). Young patients are able to compensate for an edema by accommodation; subtle and thus subclinical DME is apparently not all that uncommon (Braun et al. 1995). The unknown date of onset is an important reason not to forget regular screening intervals in type 2 diabetes. In prediabetes or even "nondiabetes" DR was seen in up to 8 % of patients (DPP Research Group 2007). Treatment for DR may be 90 % effective in preventing severe vision loss using current strategies, but fewer persons

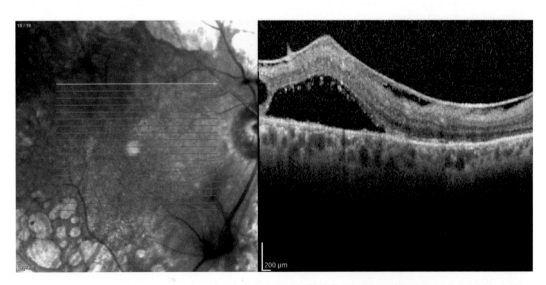

Fig. 6.9 Retinal folds and focal detachment due to vitreoretinal traction by epiretinal membrane

ETDRS severity score	10			20	35	43	47		60	89		
	no DR	DR questionable		MA	mild NPDR	moderate NPDR	moderate-to-severe NPDR		severe NPDR	PDR		Diabetic Macular Edema	pregnancy
		hard exudates cotton-wool spots			hard exudates cotton-wool spots ≥ 1 venous loop					retinal neovascularization		
RH		IRMA no MA	RH		RH present	severe ≥ 1 quadrant moderate ≥ 4 quadrants	severe ≥ 2 quadrants		severe ≥ 4 quadrants			
MA				no MA	MA	severe ≥ 1 quadrant moderate ≥ 4 quadrants			severe ≥ 4 quadrants			
IRMA					IRMA questionabl	IRMA	IRMA		IRMA ≥ 2 quadrants			
VB					VB questionable		VB		VB ≥ 2 quadrants			

Fig. 6.10 ETDRS severity scale. *RH* retinal hemorrhage, *IRMA* intraretinal microvascular abnormalities, *VB* venous beading, adapted from the ETDRS Research Group (1991d). Future classifications will also include ocular coherence tomography (OCT)

are referred for ophthalmic care than necessary in accordance to current guidelines (Ferris 1993; Paz et al. 2006).

Different factors are discussed that could explain the insufficient disease awareness of persons with diabetes that leads to an underuse of the healthcare system (Bressler et al. 2014; Maberley et al. 2002; Maclennan et al. 2014). Primary care physicians are not always familiar with the increasing incidence of DR during the course of metabolic changes and therefore preclude the implementation of treatment guidelines (Looker et al. 2014; Witkin and Klein 1984). 30–50 % of persons with diabetes still do not receive timely examinations, even within the framework of cost-free programs of NEI or NHS and despite extensive education of patients and physicians (Brechner et al. 1993).

The low utilization keeps most guideline commissions from extending the screening intervals (Hutchins et al. 2012; Nam et al. 2011; Romero-Aroca et al. 2010; Yuen et al. 2010). Longer screening intervals might increase the risk of an irreversible loss of vision due to nonappearance (Kristinsson et al. 1995). Recent experiences showed that adherence did not improve with longer control intervals (Misra et al. 2009). Sociocultural differences and individual risk profiles should be considered when discussing the best interval for the next visit in the individual patient (Do and Eggleston 2011; Garay-Sevilla et al. 2011; Gulliford et al. 2010).

Nevertheless, some economists find it acceptable to screen less and less frequently. The recommended interval for eye examinations was initially based on observations from epidemiological studies. Following cost-utility analyses, the rate of deterioration might not justify the costs and efforts of yearly examinations (Vijan et al. 2000). Due to interindividual differences, however, the time course of DR progression can be fast, even within these first years of DR. Essential framework conditions include the duration of disease, the type of diabetes, and all cardiovascular risk factors for the individual person (Mehlsen et al. 2012). Type 1 diabetes must not be mixed up with type 2 diabetes (Klonoff and Schwartz 2000). To achieve better knowledge of the individual risk factors, a good communication between primary physicians and ophthalmologists is essential.

Accurate and early diagnosis is of great importance for the successful treatment of DR (Fong et al. 2001). The stereoscopic capabilities of digital cameras are less important, since SD-OCT is much more sensitive to detect retinal thickening (Nisic et al. 2014). Imaging and discussing the obtained images with the persons screened might enhance the adherence to future examinations (Fonda et al. 2007). Some authors even argue in favor of a smartphone ophthalmoscopy though missing 5 % of the patients (Russo et al. 2015).

However, newer devices allow wide-angle imaging under non-mydriatic conditions. Further health care research studies have to prove whether these methods allow a sensitive detection of DR, thus equivalent efficacy at reasonable costs (Nam et al. 2011). Telemedicine using wide-angle cameras might be of even greater use if the access to ophthalmic care is limited.

6.3   Current Knowledge on Pathophysiology

Although hyperglycemia remains the key characteristic of DR, the huge differences between type 1 and type 2 diabetes with regard to DR progression underline the multiple factors involved (Campos 2012) (Fig. 6.11). Increasing the serum level of glucose has been shown to be sufficient to initiate the early retinopathy changes in animal models (Kern and Engerman 1996; Ly et al. 2014; Robinson et al. 2012). Several biochemical pathways have been discussed to link hyperglycemia and microvascular complications (Ahsan 2015; Kamoi et al. 2013; Ola et al. 2012; Tarr et al. 2013; Zhang et al. 2012).

The structural features of the central retina, in particular loose intercellular contacts and the absence of Mueller cells are considered to explain the predilection of the disease for the macular

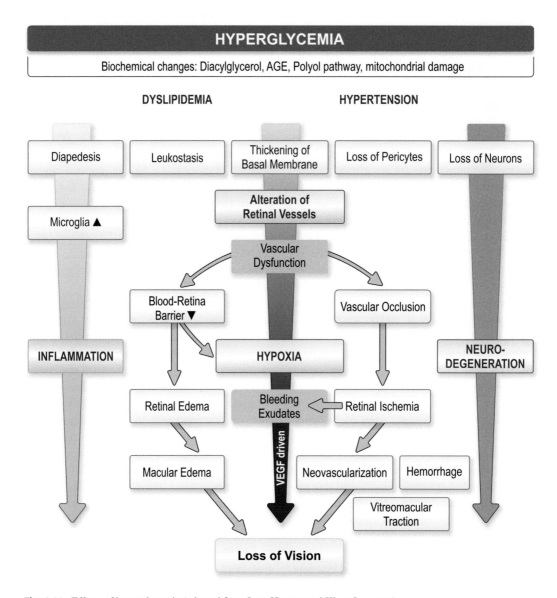

Fig. 6.11   Effects of hyperglycemia (adopted from Lutz Hansen and Klaus Lemmen)

area (Cunha-Vaz 2004). At an early stage, the crosstalk of glial cells, pericytes, and endothelial cells seems to be impaired (Antonetti et al. 2006). Later, a thickening of the basement membrane, loss of pericytes, and an altered endothelium contribute to focal areas of hypoxia (Ashton 1974; Ejaz et al. 2008; Lutty 2013). The exact relationship between vasoregression, primary neurodegeneration and the impairment of neurovascular coupling, however, still needs to be clarified (Clermont and Bursell 2007; Hammes et al. 2011a). Mechanisms of neurodegeneration have been identified, such as a loss of astrocytes, Müller cells, and retinal ganglion cells.

The distinct inflammatory component of DR is most clearly illustrated by the increased leukocytes adhesion and emigration (Matsuoka et al. 2007; Tang and Kern 2011). In addition, a marked increase in inflammatory cytokines can be measured (Rangasamy et al. 2014). It is very likely that the proinflammatory steps are not only coinciding phenomena, but part of sequential, interdependent pathways. In this context, it is noteworthy that Müller cells were found to show inflammation-linked responses if exposed to diabetic retinal milieu (Kern 2007; Zhong et al. 2012). The intercellular adhesion molecule ICAM-1, a transmembrane protein binding to integrins, was attributed to increased leukostasis (Ugurlu et al. 2013).

Long-lived glycosylated proteins (AGE) contribute to the generalized endothelial dysfunction (Kandarakis et al. 2014; Stitt 2010; Yamagishi et al. 2008). An increased transvascular passage of macromolecules has been documented and resembles the pathogenic mechanism of diabetic nephropathy and DR (Sander et al. 2003; Zandbergen et al. 2007). The oxygen consumption in the retina is very demanding. Toxic endproducts as peroxides, superoxides, and reactive oxygen species are released secondary to hyperglycaemia and the activation of alternative pathways (Madsen-Bouterse and Kowluru 2008; Santos et al. 2011). The activation of protein kinase C (PKC-β) and increased diacylglycerol are associated with vascular changes of different organs (Brownlee 2001).

Among all factors involved, VEGF A is the most investigated and certainly an important mediator of vascular permeability and proliferative endothelial activity (Klaassen et al. 2013; Pfeiffer et al. 1997). VEGF-induced breakdown of the blood–retinal barrier is mediated by a change of occluding and claudin-1, suggesting the latter to be potentially the most relevant tight junction protein (Lang 2012). Other factors than VEGF did not show such a strong effect on transendothelial resistance (Deissler et al. 2013). This does, of course, not preclude any other—to date uninvestigated factors—from being important additional effectors of DME formation.

6.4 Systemic Risk Factors in Diabetes

6.4.1 Risk Factors and Metabolic Control

Intensive lifestyle interventions can not only prevent or delay the onset of diabetes in high-risk individuals (Karam and McFarlane 2011; Palermo et al. 2014; Tahrani et al. 2011), but have an important influence on the course of the disease and the incidence of complications (Klein et al. 2002). Therefore, knowledge and management of medical and vascular parameters in persons with diabetes is of upmost importance (Kiire et al. 2013).

In *type 1 diabetes*, convincing data suggest a direct relationship between the occurrence of DR and the severity as well as the duration of diabetes (Hietala et al. 2010; Moss et al. 1994). Type 1 diabetes is characterized by an autoimmune destruction of beta cells leading to a deficiency of insulin. Very rarely DR becomes apparent before 6 years after diagnosis of diabetes, but increases fast with longer diabetes duration (Klein et al. 1984). Puberty can act as an accelerator of complications (Cho et al. 2014). Most guidelines recommend ophthalmic examination 5 years after the onset of type 1 diabetes.

The precise time of onset is often much more difficult to assess in *type 2 diabetes*, when an asymptomatic phase precedes diagnosis. The rate of preexisting DR is not negligible (DPP Research Group 2007). The variability of the type 2 diabetes is much larger ranging from slight insulin resistance to an absolute insulin deficiency. The majority of persons with type 2 diabetes are obese and the prevalence of type 2 diabetes increases with age.

Gestational diabetes is a special form seen in women at a preexisting predisposition or so far unknown diabetes of earlier onset. If it is the former (and previous disease is unlikely) the risk of retinopathy does not seem to be significantly increased (Gunderson et al. 2007). If DR is known, there is a high risk of worsening during pregnancy (DCCT Research Group 2000; Chew et al. 1995b; Hellstedt et al. 1997; Klein et al. 1990): persons with diabetes who plan to become pregnant or are in early pregnancy, should therefore undergo a comprehensive eye exam and be counseled about the risk of progression. Follow-up visits should be arranged depending on the severity of the retinopathy (Vestgaard et al. 2010).

6.4.2   Disease Duration

When assessing the risk of DR development, the duration of diabetes is an important parameter. The differences between type 1 and type 2 diabetes have to be considered.

In historic trials, DR was seen in 25 % of persons with type 1 diabetes after 5 years. The rate further increased to 60 % at 10 years and 80 % at 15 years (Hammes et al. 2011b; LeCaire et al. 2013). In type 2 diabetes, the rates of DR also rose in dependence of the duration of diabetes. The percentages of DR in those patients taking insulin were found considerably higher than in those on diet or oral drugs (5 years: 40 % and 19 years: 84 % vs. 5 years: 24 % and 19 years: 53 %, respectively).

There is only limited data available regarding the effects of changed treatment patterns. However, when appraising the different risk factors of each population the background of each ethnic group has to be considered (Mazhar et al. 2011; West et al. 2001).

6.4.3   Control of Blood Sugar

Glycemic control is an important effector when thinking of microvascular complications (Sander et al. 1994). The evidence of its impact is supported by epidemiologic studies and prospective clinical trials (Zhang et al. 2015).

Increased glucose levels are not only risk factors for developing DR, but also relevant for the progression to more advanced stages.

Traditionally, it was recommended to generally aim for a low target of glycemic control, thus preferring a target of 6.5 % instead of 7 % HbA_{1c} (ADA 2013). However, the ACCORD study raised concerns that a very aggressive HbA_{1c} management might increase the risk of dementia and macrovascular complications in older patients (Chew et al. 2014; Frank 2014). This is the more important as patients with type 2 diabetes and retinopathy represent a subgroup at higher risk for future cognitive decline (Hugenschmidt et al. 2014).

The DCCT and UKPDS showed that the development and progression of DR can be delayed when HbA_{1c} is optimized (DCCT Research Group 1995). Several studies indicated that each 1 % increase in hemoglobin above 7 % raises the incidence of DR by 50 % and the progression by 50 % (LeCaire et al. 2013). A 35 % risk reduction can be achieved with every percentage point of HbA1c decreased (The Diabetes Control and Complications Trial/Epidemiology of Diabetes Interventions and Complications Research Group 2000; Fullerton et al. 2014). There is no glycemic threshold when metabolic control becomes irrelevant. Furthermore, there is evidence of an "HbA1c memory effect" meaning that persons with good HbA1c management benefit not only during the times of tight glycemic control, but also over the following decades (The Diabetes Control and Complications Trial/ Epidemiology of Diabetes Interventions and Complications Research Group 2000; Hemmingsen et al. 2011; Kohner et al. 2001). It has to be considered, however, that after initiation of strict glycemic control a transient worsening has to be anticipated in particular in patients with preexisting advanced DR and high HbA_{1c} levels before therapy is initiated (Chantelau and Meyer-Schwickerath 2003). The overall effect of slowing the progression of DR by intensive treatment of glycemia alone was observed to be stronger in patients with mild DR (Chew et al. 2014).

Nevertheless, it has to be mentioned that the HbA1c gives only a rough estimate of the individual patient´s extreme values, more precisely representing the average peak values of the last 120 days (Inchiostro et al. 2013). Therefore, the value has its limitations with regard to interpretation of 24 h fluctuations and is influenced by other diseases such as anaemia. A lower HbA_{1c} can also indicate the risk of hypoglycemia (Tamborlane et al. 2008). The occurrence of extreme hypoglycemia is not only detrimental to DR, but increases the risk of falls and prohibits driving (Frier 2014).

In the clinical setting, a close partnership with the primary care physician is important in order to enhance the exchange of knowledge. Analyses showed that blood sugar and duration of diabetes explain only 11 % of the risk to develop retinopathy (Lachin et al. 2008). If the stage of DR is known, an individualized education of patients can be ensured. Newer drugs as inhibitors of the sodium/glucose cotransporter 2 (SGLT2) might provide another risk-benefit ratio than Insulin alone (Matsuda et al. 2015).

6.4.4 Blood Pressure

A tight blood pressure control was proven to lower the incidence of DR as well as the progression rate of already existing DR (Do et al. 2015; Ferrannini and Cushman 2012; Snow et al. 2003).

The UKPDS study randomly assigned patients to a "tight" blood pressure control group with a target of less than 150/85 mmHg or a "less tight" control group with a target of less than 180/105 mmHg (UKPDS Group 1998). It is important to know that these targets, described as "tight" and "less tight" control, do not conform with current standards from the Joint National Committee on Prevention, Detection, Evaluation, and Treatment of High Blood Pressure, in which a

blood pressure above 140/90 mmHg is considered uncontrolled. The achieved values in the UKPDS were 144/82 mmHg and 154/87 mmHg, respectively. Substantial reductions in risk for any diabetes end point, deaths related to diabetes, and stroke were seen in the "tight" control group.

Each reduction of 10 mmHg in blood pressure can lead to a 10 % reduction of DR incidence (UKPDS Group 1998). Even after 9 years of follow-up, the patients assigned to "tight" blood pressure control had a 34 % risk reduction with regard to the proportion of patients with deterioration of retinopathy by two steps and a 47 % risk reduction with regard to deterioration in visual acuity (three ETDRS-lines). Intervening on blood pressure solely to prevent diabetic retinopathy is not necessarily beneficial. Other comorbidities have to be considered, when the target pressure is defined (usual goal ≤130/80 mmHg).

6.4.5 Dyslipidemia

Epidemiologic data showed only a very little effect of serum lipids or lipid-lowering statins on the incidence of PDR or DME (Klein et al. 2015). Some interventional studies failed to prove any significant influence of statins on microvascular complications. This does not question the role of statins in the context of macrovascular events. However, the decision of their use should not be made in dependence of DR.

In contrast, there is growing evidence that the (additional) intake of fibrates has a moderate impact on DR progression. The FIELD study showed a 30 % reduction for the need of laser treatment and progression of albuminuria (Keech et al. 2007). In ACCORD-Eye, the addition of fenofibrate to a basal statin therapy resulted in a significant decrease in the progression of diabetic retinopathy, in a similar manner as that observed with intensifying blood glucose control (Chew et al. 2010, 2014). However, a strong degree of retardation of DR progression was only seen in study participants with mild retinopathy at baseline. Only very limited conclusions were possible regarding the incidence of DME. The small MacuFen study showed minor effects on the macular volume in DME (Massin et al. 2014).

The mode of action of fenofibrate might be based more on its activation of the peroxisome proliferator-activated receptor (PPAR), independently of any lipid-lowering effects (Simo et al. 2013).

Concerning the traditional lipid markers as total cholesterol and low-density lipoprotein cholesterol, these parameters might be associated with the presence of hard exudates in patients with DR (Chang and Wu 2013). The level of apolipoprotein A1 (ApoA1) might be negatively related to DR.

6.4.6 Nephropathy and Retinopathy

Nephropathy is the other significant microvascular complication of diabetes (Kaul et al. 2010; Wong et al. 2014). The renal damage is characterized by a decreased glomerular filtration rate (GFR) and microalbuminuria and frequently coincides with DR (Fig. 6.12).

In some patients, the eye can be an indicator of an imminent kidney disease. Similarly, extensive capillary nonperfusion was associated with an increased risk of chronic kidney disease (Lee et al. 2014). Besides the function of retinal vascular calibers as early sign of preclinical target organ damage (Daien et al. 2013; Edwards et al. 2005), association between nephropathy (defined by microalbuminuria) and retinopathy have been well recorded (Wong et al. 2014). The bidirectional relationship let suggest a common but still poorly understood pathogenic pathway (Grunwald et al. 2014).

It has also been speculated that the diabetic nephropathy may lead to an increased vascular damage and might provoke/intensify DME as a result of a change in osmotic balance. That possibly is the reason why microalbuminuria was identified as an independent risk factor for DME. The WESDR described an increased risk for developing DME with gross albuminuria (Klein et al. 2009). Within type 1 diabetes, microalbuminuria and macroalbuminuria were found to be associated with an increased risk of developing

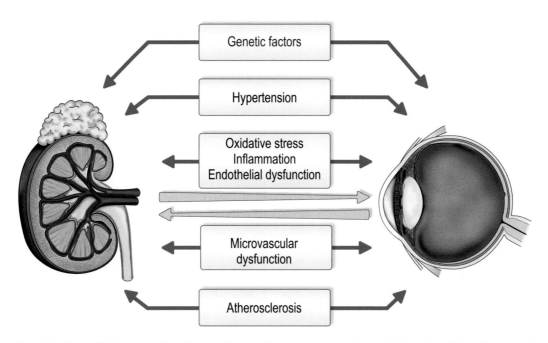

Fig. 6.12 Strong link between the microvascular complications, nephropathy, and DR (adopted from Wong et al. (2014))

DME (Roy and Klein 2001). However, smaller studies did not find a significant correlation when adjusting for confounding factors.

There are reports on a potential clinical improvement of DME under dialysis (Matsuo 2006; Tokuyama et al. 2000). However, these reports are contradictory and even when using OCT imaging to quantify retinal thickness, the findings of DME patients undergoing dialysis are not consistent (Theodossiadis et al. 2012; Tokuyama et al. 2000).

6.4.7 Mortality

Several studies suggest that the presence of DR is an indicator of increased mortality risk (Hayes et al. 2013). Already incidental findings of mild DR have to remind the physicians that the microvascular alterations point towards the risk profile of severely ill patients, being at an increased risk of many other serious events (Stamler et al. 1993). In comparison to healthy subjects, people with diabetes have a greater than fourfold risk of cardiovascular diseases and a life expectancy shortened by up to 8 years (Gu et al. 1998). The presence of DME increases the risk of being hospitalized by 98 % after adjustment for other comorbidities (Nguyen-Khoa et al. 2012).

6.4.8 Pregnancy

Pregnancy is a known risk factor for progression of diabetic retinopathy (DCCT Research Group 2000; Klein et al. 1990; Phelps et al. 1986). The responsible mechanisms discussed to lead to disease acceleration are hemodynamic changes, increased release of growth factors (e.g., IGF1), and hormonal influences (Lauszus et al. 2003; Loukovaara et al. 2003).

The stage of disease prior to conception is an important predictor of the disease progression, including the time after delivery (Chew et al. 1995b). That explains why patients with moderate-to-severe NPDR have to be watched very closely. Additional risk factors of progression are hypertension and poor glycemic control

prior to conception (Rahman et al. 2007; Rasmussen et al. 2010; Schultz et al. 2005; Vestgaard et al. 2010).

Preferably, women who are planning to become pregnant should have their eyes examined before they attempt to conceive and be counselled about the risks of worsening (Ringholm et al. 2012). PRP for severe NPDR or PDR should be considered. In unstable disease, patients should be advised to postpone conception until these conditions are properly treated.

An exam in early pregnancy has been recommended anyway, at the latest soon after conception. The findings of the first trimester grading determine the time of the next eye examination: Pregnant women with less than severe NPDR should be examined every 3 months, whereas those with more severe stages should be seen more frequently, e.g., every 1–3 months. Intensive glycemic control before and during pregnancy gives considerable benefits to pregnant women and their offspring. Severe hypoglycemia occurs most frequently in the first trimester, but should be possibly avoided (Nielsen et al. 2008). Early worsening has been reported after intensification of insulin. The therapy should be managed as a collaborative effort between obstetricians, endocrinologists, dieticians, and ophthalmologists.

Thy typical gestational diabetes is not considered to be associated with DR and does not require regular check-up examinations (Gunderson et al. 2007). According to current guidelines, women also have to be followed up after delivery (Chen et al. 2004). During the postnatal period, the mother´s need for insulin declines to approximately 60 % of the pregnancy dose, owing to the lack of placental hormonal influence, and the risk of fluctuating glucose levels are associated with an increased risk of maternal hypoglycemia during breastfeeding. Facing a high risk of progression, meticulous retinal surveillance is mandatory.

6.4.9 Systemic Treatment

Therapeutic exercise, weight loss, and smoking cessation are important lifestyle changes influencing DR risk (Klein et al. 2014; Loprinzi et al.

2014; Perreault et al. 2012). Newer drugs such as injectable incretin mimetics, Glucagon-like peptide analogs/agonists, and dipeptidyl peptidase-4 Inhibitors may have their role, but currently there is not sufficient data to evaluate their effect on DR. The theoretical benefits of glucosurics like SGLT-2 inhibitors similarly still need to be verified (Dziuba et al. 2014). Previous expectations in relation to the efficacy of PKCβ inhibitors or somatostatin replacement therapy ended disappointingly (Shah et al. 2010; Sheetz et al. 2013).

At this point, we want to remind of the previous experiences proving that aspirin and rheological therapy is ineffective (ETDRS Research Group 1991c). Aspirin therapy at a dose of 650 mg per day was shown to be ineffective by the ETDRS, although not causing more severe or frequent hemorrhages in PDR (Chew et al. 1995a). Data of epidemiologic studies and small case series is the only hint that anemia might be associated with the progression of DR (Davis et al. 1998; Qiao et al. 1997; Shorb 1985).

6.5   Treatment of DR

The treatment of DR depends on the presence or absence of clinically significant or center—involving macular edema and peripheral disease. The current treatment recommendations are based on the results of two major randomized landmark trials, the Diabetic Retinopathy Study (DRS), and the ETDRS. While the treatment algorithm of severe NPDR accords with that of PDR regarding their "high-risk profile", the approach will be presented together following the strategies in DME.

6.6   Treatment of DME

6.6.1   Focal/Grid Laser Coagulation

The efficacy of laser treatment was discussed to be partly due to its ability to occlude leaking microaneurysms. But as grid treatment alone was shown to be effective, indirect effects have

to be considered. Some pioneers have suggested that, following the reduction in tissue associated with photocoagulation, the retinal autoregulation might decrease the retinal blood flow to the macula, attributable to improvements in the oxygenation of the outer retina (Stefansson 2006; Wilson et al. 1988). Changes of the retinal pigment epithelium (RPE) characterize the response mechanisms, concomitant to the resolution of the DME (Ogata et al. 2001). Restoration of the outer blood–retina barrier and a better pump function of the RPE are also discussed (Klaassen et al. 2013).

The ETDRS was the first trial, describing the various manifestations of CSME (ETDRS Research Group 1985). All these constellations are associated with an increased risk of visual loss. The effect of focal laser photocoagulation on DME was analyzed in eyes with a broad range of edema severity at baseline (ETDRS Research Group 1995). The extent and intensity of the effect were independent of the size of edema, the type of leakage pattern (focal, diffuse) or the extent of concomitant ischemia. Prompt treatment was advised in eye with edema involving the center of the macular or large plaques of hard exudate threatening the center. The main benefit of the central photocoagulation as identified in ETDRS was the reduction of visual loss (Fong et al. 1999).

A later modification of the initial laser protocol was evaluated in 840 eyes with a retinal thickness of more than 250 μm by the DRCR.net (2008). The laser spot size was limited to 50–80 μm (Fong et al. 2007) (see below table). Besides the "focal" sources of leakage such as microaneurysms, every retinal thickening was targeted by an additional "grid" with a pattern of laser spots applied at a distance of two laser spot diameters to each other. An FLA was taken at baseline and follow-up treatments. The parameters of laser spots (energy, exposure) were chosen in order to generate very faint, but still visible spots. The wavelength of the lasers was green or yellow. The focal/grid laser resulted in a modest stabilization of visual acuity which was superior to repeated injections of triamcinolone (Fong et al. 2007).

Settings of focal/grid laser	
Spot size	50–80 μm
Laser energy/exposure	(Barely) visible spots
Distance of laser spots (grid)	2 spots
Retreatment interval	4 months

Drawbacks of the focal/grid laser are a decrease in retinal sensitivity. This has an impact on the reading ability or reading speed of treated patients (Comyn et al. 2014; Pearce et al. 2014). Regarding its impact on reading, the central area to the left should be spared if possible. Older studies did only include a limited documentation of visual fields following laser treatment. This is important, since later laser spots can enlarge and become confluent over time (Kang et al. 2010; Lovestam-Adrian and Agardh 2000; Maeshima et al. 2004). When comparing the amount and intensity of the laser treatment used in various studies, a large variety has to be noted. The number of laser treatments ranges even within controlled DME studies from 1.1x to 3.1x (DRCR.net 2008; Mitchell et al. 2011).

Today, monitoring noncentral edema with SD-OCT and having alternative drug treatments at hand, the observation—instead of laser treatment—has to be reevaluated. Therefore, some patients with noncentral DME might be spared the downsides of laser treatment and for those that do expand into the fovea; drug therapy (when delivered timely) can still prevent visual deterioration or achieve improvement.

6.6.2 Subthreshold Micropulse Laser

In contrast to conventional lasers, devices delivering short pulses are intended to cause less thermal damage to the tissue (Park et al. 2014). Shorter exposure times are considered to cause less harm to the neural retina and the choriocapillaries than the "continuous-wave" lasers, while still reaching the RPE (Framme et al. 2009). One practical consequence is that the laser spots of subthreshold micropulse diode laser remain invisible, using ophthalmic imaging methods as biomicroscopy, fundus auto-

fluorescence, OCT or FLA. The use of the 532 nm-wavelength promises less pain during the treatment, a wavelength of the diode laser of 810 nm might have a better penetration (blood, cataract).

Some authors reported a good response to subthreshold micropulse laser treatment, measured by visual acuity or electrophysiology (Friberg and Karatza 1997; Venkatesh et al. 2011). Prospective trials showed at least a non-inferiority to conventional lasers, including the promise of a better safety profile (Figueira et al. 2009; Pei-Pei et al. 2015).

6.6.3 Selective Laser Therapy

By using a wavelength of 527 nm and even shorter pulses than the micropulse lasers (1.7 μs), the selective retina therapy (SRT) was described to be absorbed to a greater extent by the melanosomes of the RPE. High peak temperatures that develop around melanosomes during irradiation create short-lived microbubbles that can mechanically disrupt RPE cells as the cell volume rises (Brinkmann et al. 2000). SRT showed promising results in early pilot and phase II studies, providing follow-up periods of 6 months (Roider et al. 2000, 2010). As the effects are invisible, the implementation of optoacoustic systems and reflectometry was used to allow dosimetry and ensure the safety of the applied energy.

6.6.4 Navigated or Targeted Laser

Newer laser machines implement technical enhancements, such as the possibility of noncontact imaging or eye-tracking (Kozak et al. 2011; Liegl et al. 2014) (Fig. 6.13). The procedure still has to be conducted by an attentive user, as variations in fundus pigmentation require adjustment of the laser energy during the treatment, but the strategy for the laser treatment becomes more independent on the experience of the treating physicians. At present, the applied parameters as retreatment intervals still need to be established in larger conclusive trials (Neubauer et al. 2013). A standardized procedure and the complete

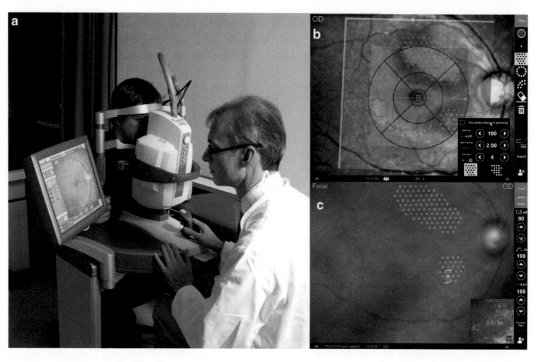

Fig. 6.13 Navigated laser treatment is easily possible without contact lens (**a**) Location and density of the laser pattern can be preplanned in the photograph (**b**) The progression is indicated during the implementation ((**c**), *Courtesy*: Michael Ulbig, wearing reading glasses)

documentation of target localization and energy used are important advantages, especially when considering the large variability of older trials. This might be more important for newer laser modalities, invisible to the eye of the examiners.

It has been recommended not only to laser on the basis of biomicroscopy or angiograms, but to use the information of OCT examinations to plan the laser protocol (Kozak et al. 2014). The question of combination therapy is addressed in the abstract of the particular drug.

> **Important to remind**
> Focal/grid laser can deliver a considerable risk reduction of a visual loss in CSME.
> By affecting the central visual field, focal/grid laser may cause (growing) retinal sensitivity defects and reading problems.
> Micropulse lasers have shown equal efficacy to conventional lasers in small, but prospective trials. However, longer follow-up data is needed.

6.6.5   Intravitreal Steroids

As many inflammatory cytokines were identified in the vitreous of patients with DME, the pleiotropic mechanisms of corticosteroids have been discussed to be beneficial for DME treatment (Zhang et al. 2011).

The intravitreous route of steroid administration is thought to minimize systemic side effects. The modalities of the different steroid formulations, however, have not been directly compared in a clinical trial (Al Dhibi and Arevalo 2013).

6.6.6   Triamcinolone Acetate

Triamcinolone therapy has been reported to be quite effective in the short term, but to be inferior to focal/grid laser therapy over 3 years in the DRCR.net study protocol B (Elman et al. 2011). Glaucoma surgery was described to be necessary in 1.6 % of treated patients. A subgroup analysis of the protocol I study showed a much greater amount of visual improvement, when combining laser and triamcinolone in pseudophakic eyes (Elman et al. 2015). However, in the overall group the probability of anatomic restoration of retinal thickness after 2 years was only 16 % with triamcinolone, compared to 34 % by ranibizumab (Elman et al. 2010). Thus, the long-term benefits of triamcinolone treatment do not seem to persist, even after repeated injections (Table 6.2).

Throughout all published studies, the cumulative risk of subsequent cataract surgery (83 %) or

Table 6.2 Important landmark studies of DR and DME treatment

Abbreviation	Study name	Key findings
DRS	Diabetic Retinopathy Study	Risk reduction for loss of vision by laser photocoagulation in severe NPDR (13–4 % < 5/200) and PDR (44–20 % < 5/200)
ETDRS	Early Treatment of Diabetic Retinopathy Study	Risk reduction for loss of vision by laser photocoagulation in clinically significant macular edema (33–14 %)
DRVS	Diabetic Vitrectomy Study	Early vitrectomy beneficial in eyes <5/200 and severe hemorrhage >4 weeks with type 1 diabetes (≥20/40: 36 vs. 12 %)
		Vitrectomy beneficial in eyes ≥20/400 if severe neovascularization, fibrous proliferation, and moderate vitreous hemorrhage or moderate neovascularization with severe fibrous proliferation (≥20/40: 44 vs. 28 %)
FIELD	Fenofibrate Intervention and Event Lowering in Diabetes	In spite of a baseline imbalances (statins) addition of fenofibrate positive impact on progression of DR
ACCORD-EYE	Action to Control Cardiovascular Risk in Diabetes	Retardation of DR by fenofibrate seen in mild and early DR stages from 10 to 6 %
		Tight blood sugar control with HbA1c ≤6.4 decreased progression of DR from 10 to 7 %
Drug therapy DME		
RESTORE	0.5 mg ranibizumab as monotherapy and/or adjunctive to laser treatment vs. laser therapy	0.5 mg ranibizumab monotherapy (similar to adjunctive therapy to laser photocoagulation) provided superior benefits as compared to laser monotherapy
		37–43 % of 0.5 mg ranibizumab-treated patients improved vision by ≥10 letters compared to 16 % with laser therapy
REVEAL	Ranibizumab in the TrEatment of Visual Impairment in DiabEtic MAcuLar Edema	More Asian patients gained 15 letters with 0.5 mg ranibizumab (18.8 %) and combined laser (17.8 %) compared with laser (7.8 %)
RIDE and RISE	Monthly intravitreal ranibizumab (0.5 or 0.3 mg) vs. sham	Mean visual acuity shows an increase beyond 12 months
		Significant differences between the twin studies indicate the need on confirmatory studies
BOLT	Prospective randomized trial of intravitreal Bevacizumab Or Laser Therapy	Superiority of bevacizumab (n=42) over laser (n=38) in pretreated patients with CSME
VISTA and VIVID	Aflibercept 2 mg every 4 weeks (2q4), aflibercept 2 mg every 8 weeks after 5 initial monthly doses (2q8) vs. macular laser	More patients gained 15 letters with 2q4 (VISTA: 41.6 %, VIVID: 32.4 %) and 2q8 (VISTA: 31.1 %, VIVD: 33.3 %) compared with laser (VISTA: 7.8 %, VIVID: 9.1 %)
MEAD	Dexamethasone implant (0.7 mg or 0.35 mg) vs. sham	More patients gained 15 letters with the 0.7 mg implant (22.2 %, 4.1 tx) and 0.35 mg implant (18.4 %, 4.4 tx) compared with sham (12.0 %, 3.3tx) over 3 years
		Indications of undertreatment with 6-months retreatment intervals of dexamethasone implants
		Better functional outcomes of pseudophakic patients
		High rate of study discontinuation due to the study protocol

(continued)

Table 6.2 (continued)

Abbreviation	Study name	Key findings
DRCR.net	*The Diabetic Retinopathy Clinical Research Network*	
Protocol B	Randomized Trial Comparing Intravitreal Triamcinolone Acetonide and Laser Photocoagulation for DME	
Protocol H	Subclinical Diabetic Macular Edema	
Protocol I	Randomized Trial Evaluating Ranibizumab Plus Prompt or Deferred Laser or Triamcinolone Plus Prompt Laser for Diabetic Macular Edema	
Protocol M	Effects of Diabetes Education during Retinal Ophthalmology Visits on Diabetes Control	
Protocol R	A Phase II Evaluation of Topical NSAIDs in Eyes with Noncentral-Involved DME	
Protocol S	Prompt panretinal photocoagulation vs. intravitreal ranibizumab with Deferred panretinal photocoagulation for PDR	
Protocol T	A comparative effectiveness study of intravitreal aflibercept, bevacizumab, and ranibizumab for DME	
Protocol V	Treatment for Central-involved DME in eyes with very good visual acuity	

increased intraocular pressure (IOP, >10 mmHg: 33 %) after triamcinolone have been reported invariably high (Kiddee et al. 2013; Yilmaz et al. 2009). There are some indications that the risk of an increase in intraocular pressure depends on the applied dosage (2 mg < 4 mg < 10 mg).

None of the available triamcinolone drugs has been approved for the use in DME. The crystalloid triamcinolone has large variability in resorption, though the intravitreal administration seems to be superior to subtenonal injections (Qi et al. 2012). After intravitreal injection, however, crystalloid particles or remnants of conservatives can induce the unpleasant complication of pseudo-endophthalmitis which can be confused with infectious endophthalmitis and sometimes needs removal of the drug by vitrectomy (Marticorena et al. 2012). In addition, intravitreal triamcinolone should be used with caution in eyes after removal of the inner limiting membrane (ILM) due to potential toxicity (Jaissle et al. 2004).

6.6.7 Dexamethasone Implants

The dexamethasone drug delivery system (Ozurdex®, Allergan, Irvine, California, USA) consists of dexamethasone bound with a biodegradable copolymer of lactic and glycolic acids (Nehme and Edelman 2008). The implant is injected through the pars plana using a 22G injection system, before releasing 700 µg of dexamethasone as the polymer degrades (Chang-Lin et al. 2011; Fialho et al. 2006). Single case series showed efficacy in eyes more resistant to other treatment modalities (Kuppermann et al. 2007; Zucchiatti et al. 2012) (Fig. 6.14).

The approval of the dexamethasone implant is based on a prospective randomized comparison with sham injections (including rescue laser) (Boyer et al. 2014). The MEAD study design was influenced by the hope that the effect of the delivery device always lasts for 6 months. Fixed retreatments were planned twice a year, unless resolution was seen or one of the many discontinuation criteria (rise of IOP, lack of efficacy, etc.) was fulfilled. Less than 60 % of patients (607 of 1048) completed the study. This constellation limits the evaluation of the ITT-analysis. The main study publication described a mean VA increase of 6.5 ETDRS letters for pseudophakic patients after 3 years. Study participants received a mean number of 4.1 treatments with the 700 µg implant. The saw tooth pattern of central retinal thickness seen on OCT examinations suggests that the treatment interval was too long for most of the patients. Mean visual acuity started to worsen after the 6-week examination. The maximum gain in visual acuity was achieved after the first injection and was stabilized by the following treatments. There is room for speculation about the results if an individualized PRN dosing would have been used.

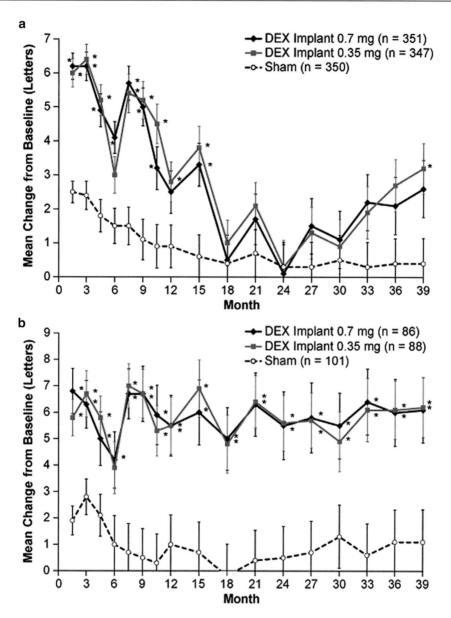

Fig. 6.14 While the initial gain in best-corrected visual acuity from baseline could not be maintained for the total study population (**a**) by 6-monthly retreatment with dexa-methasone implants, the subgroup of pseudophakic patients (**b**) achieved a mean improvement of 6.1 ETDRS letters (Boyer et al. 2014)

An IOP of ≥ 25 mmHg was found to occur in 32 % of treated patients. 5 out of 347 patients had undergone glaucoma surgery. Meanwhile, there are many case series reported, showing shorter retreatment intervals and a better efficacy of naïve patients when compared with pretreated DME (Escobar-Barranco et al. 2015; Guigou et al. 2014; Scaramuzzi et al. 2015).

One study found comparable treatment efficacies when comparing bevacizumab and the 22-Gauge dexamethasone implant in a randomized trial over 12 months (Gillies et al. 2014). The implant exhibits some variability in dissolving; sometimes, the biologic activity is decreasing though patient and physician still clearly notice the "bar" consisting of the remaining

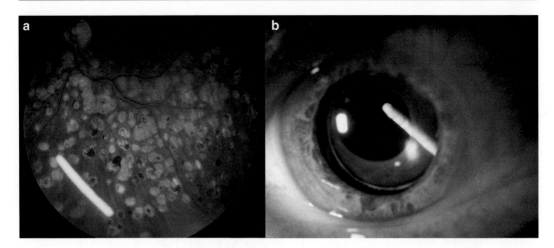

Fig. 6.15 The resorption of the intravitreal PLGA implant into a translucent matrix usually takes 6–8 weeks and can be monitored in the inferior vitreous (**a**). Dislocation in the anterior chamber in pseudophakic and in particular aphakic patients can lead to corneal decompensation (**b**)

PLGA shell (Fig. 6.15). Corneal problems have been reported, when displacement of the implant into the anterior chamber occurs in aphakic or pseudophakic patients (Voykov and Bartz-Schmidt 2012).

6.6.8   Fluocinolone Implants

Fluocinolone was first evaluated in a study with surgically implanted, nonbiodegradable intravitreal insert (Messenger et al. 2013). The breakdown of the central polymer–drug matrix leads to a release of 0.59 µg fluocinolone per day over a time period of approximately 3 years. The Retisert® (Bausch & Lomb) implant which received initial FDA approval for the treatment of chronic, posterior uveitis was also investigated for its efficacy in DME (Pearson et al. 2011). Two trials showed an increase in visual acuity of more than three lines in about 30 % of patients after 3 years, however also a considerable amount of side effects.

The other delivery system was analyzed in two double-masked trials (FAME A, FAME B) that recruited 951 participants with persistent DME (Campochiaro et al. 2011). Two different dosages were tested, releasing 0.2 or 0.5 µg of drug per day. The prospective design allowed concomitant treatments with anti-VEGF drugs; over a quarter of recruited patients received off-protocol treatment and 40 % additional laser therapy (Campochiaro et al. 2012). Therefore, it is not possible to directly assign the change of visual acuity to the implant alone. Both fluocinolone dosages showed similar numbers of patients with 15-letter improvements at month 24 (28.7 %, 28.6 %) sham-treated patients achieved a 15-letter VA improvement only in 15 % of the cases. Glaucoma requiring surgery was necessary in 3.7 and 7.6 % of patients in the two fluocinolone groups. In addition, almost 90 % of phakic patients required cataract surgery after fluocinolone implant treatment. Further post hoc analyses found a more pronounced difference between chronic edema (defined as edema of at least 3 years duration) and non-chronic DME (Cunha-Vaz et al. 2014a). A similar stratification was not investigated for any other treatment modality.

After the approval of the 190 µg implant (0.2 µg/d over 18 months) head-to-head comparisons to other treatment modalities or laser treatment alone are still missing (Kane et al. 2008). The cylindrical tubes (3.5 × 0.37 mm), injected through a transconjunctival self-sealing wound with a

25-gauge needle, have the disadvantage to be non-biodegradable. Facing the safety profile discussed above, fluocinolone implants might be considered if prior treatments have failed and long duration of persistent DME has been verified.

> **Important to remind**
>
> In the absence of direct head-to-head comparisons, only indirect conclusions can be drawn regarding potentially different efficacies between different steroid agents. The broadest evidence is available for dexamethasone implants, although open questions exist regarding retreatment intervals, the need of long-term treatment as well as complications.
>
> The rapid and profound steroid action is limited by the complications of cataract formation and steroid-induced glaucoma, which lead to their attribution in most guidelines as a second-line treatment.
>
> The need of regular control examinations (in order not to miss any significant rise in IOP) limits the advantage of longer duration and treatment intervals.
>
> Very limited experience exists regarding the switching between different steroid drugs and the efficacy of combination therapy of steroids with other modalities.

6.6.9 Intravitreal Anti-VEGF Therapy

The inhibitors of the vascular endothelial growth factor (VEGF) have brought the treatment of DME to a new era (Rosberger 2013). Since a meta-analysis in 2009 questioning the evidence large RCTs have not only proven the treatment efficacy but also its long-term safety (Abouammoh 2013; Parravano et al. 2009; Regnier et al. 2014; Schwartz et al. 2014; Virgili et al. 2014). Anti-VEGF treatment was shown to be superior to the focal/grid laser treatment, regarding the primary outcome of visual acuity (Table 6.3).

A recent head-to-head study described a better response to aflibercept in comparison to bevacizumab, when picking out those patients with a visual acuity of 20/50 or worse (Wells et al. 2015). The difference might be more pronounced, if treating a macular edema with retinal thickness ≥ 400 µm (Wells et al. 2015). Most studies focused on DME involving the center of the macula by defining inclusion criteria, either a decrease of visual acuity related to center involvement or a minimum thickness of the fovea when measured with OCT (Aiello et al. 2011). Therefore, it is still unclear, whether watch and wait (for later anti-VEGF treatment) might be an alternative to focal/grid laser in CSME fovea-sparing.

The evidence is low regarding the best retreatment approach (Treat&Extend vs. Pro re nata). There is only one unpublished study comparing two different regimens for the same drug (RETAIN, NCT01171976): After an uniform upload phase ranibizumab 0.5 mg was administered either in a T&E regimen or an as-needed retreatment (PRN). Non-inferior results were reported for T&E to PRN over 24 months. The T&E regimen might lead to a reduction in the number of treatment visits, although having some issues related to its implementation in a bilateral disease.

A marked improvement of the DR severity has been reported in most of the prospective trials (Korobelnik et al. 2014; Stewart 2014). Moreover, eyes receiving anti-VEGF drugs were significantly more likely to improve by ≥ 2 or ≥ 3 on the ETDRS severity scale. However, caution seems to be necessary regarding the end or cessation of treatment (Ip et al. 2015). The shortness of follow-up might not allow completely assessing the possibility of reverting worsening. As vasoconstriction of retinal vessels was described to be induced by the inhibition of VEGF (Sacu et al. 2011), a change of the perfusion and vascular remodeling have been discussed to cause a reduction of treatment burden over time (Elman et al. 2015). Although pro-

Table 6.3 Visual improvement as seen after the first year of treatment (Ishibashi et al. 2015; Korobelnik et al. 2014; Mitchell et al. 2011; Nguyen et al. 2012; Rajendram et al. 2012; Wells et al. 2015)

	Mean initial BCVA	Prior anti-VEGF	Mean number of treatments		Increase in BCVA ≥ 15 ETDRS letters	
			1 year	2 years	1 year	2 years
Ranibizumab 0.5 mg						
PRN + prompt laser Prot I (n = 187)	Median 66	13 %	Median 8	Median 2	30	26
PRN + deferred laser Prot I (n = 188)	Median 66	11 %	Median 9	Median 3	28	29
Sham + prompt laser (n = 293)	Median 65	9 %			15	17
PRN RESTORE (n = 116)	64.8 (10.1)	–	7.0	10.0	22	28.9
Laser/sham (n = 110)	62.4 (11.1)	–	2.1 (+1.1)		8	18.9
PRN REVEAL (n = 133)	58.6	–				
Laser/sham (n = 131)	56.6	–				
FIXED RISE (n = 125)	56.9 (11.6)	17 %				39.2
Sham (n = 127)	57.2 (11.1)	17 %				18.1
FIXED RIDE (n = 125)	56.9 (11.8)	20 %				45.7
Sham (n = 130)	57.3 (11.3)	16 %				12.3
Aflibercept 2 mg						
2q8 VISTA (n = 151)	59.4 (10.9)	45 %	8.4		31	
Laser/sham (n = 154)	59.7 (10.9)	41 %	31.2 %*		8	
2q8 VIVID (n = 135)	60.8 (10.6)	11 %	8.7		33	
Laser/sham (n = 132)	58.8 (11.2)	10 %	24.1 %*		9	
PRN Protocol T (n = 224)	65.0 (11.8)	11 %	9.2		42	
Bevacizumab 1.25 mg						
PRN BOLT (n = 37)	55.8 (9.7)	n.d.	9	13	12	32
Laser (n = 28)	55.4 (7.9)	n.d.			5	4
PRN Protocol T (n = 206)	64.8 (11.2)	13 %	9.4		32	

spective studies were running at longest over 5 years, the marked decrease of necessary treatments does further reinforce the cost efficacy of the expensive drugs (Pershing et al. 2014). While more than eight treatments were considered during the first year for the majority of patients (>2/3), the reduction of intraretinal fluid is accompanied by only very little treatments after year 3, even though a regular combination with a deferred focal/grid laser was applied (Fig. 6.16). More than half of the eyes in which laser treatment is deferred may avoid laser for at least 5 years; however, such eyes may need slightly more injections.

Retinal thinning remains an imminent part of the underlying disease (Douvali et al. 2014; Shin et al. 2014). In spite of the limited experience, the ocular safety of intravitreal injections seems to be convincing (Virgili et al. 2014; Zechmeister-Koss and Huic 2012).

Facing the high comorbidity and reduced life expectancy due to the cardiovascular risk profile of DME patients, there have been valid concerns about the systemic safety of anti-VEGF

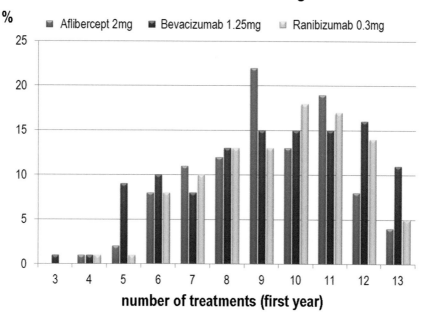

Fig. 6.16 Injection frequency during the first year of anti-VEGF treatment (DRCR.net PRN retreatment algorithm) (Wells et al. 2015)

treatment (Lim et al. 2011). So far, there are no threatening safety signals in the prospective studies which are different to the sham groups. The phase III trials were not powered to detect small differences. Therefore, more investigations are necessary, while some patients with a recent cardiovascular event had been excluded and study cohorts are known to be healthier than the general population in real life (Thulliez et al. 2014). Due to the different duration and extent of use, the body of evidence regarding the clinical safety differs between the available drugs.

6.6.10 Combination

So far, no convincing evidence exists that a fixed combination of different treatment modalities (anti-VEGF and laser, anti-VEGF and steroids) might further increase the efficacy (Chen et al. 2014; Liegl et al. 2014). Especially, the combination of focal/grid laser has extensively been studied (Schmidt-Erfurth et al. 2014). Furthermore, most of the studies investigating monotherapy have included patients with a considerable amount of previous laser treatment. A sequential combination frequently occurs in the daily routine.

A substantial difference in the number of laser treatments was found as difference of a prompt against a deferred laser combination (Elman et al. 2015). Nevertheless, the need or burden of anti-VEGF could not be significantly reduced. It is unclear whether the absence of any additional improvement is influenced by the low standardization of laser. One smaller trial used a navigated laser and reported a potential reduction of injection number (Liegl et al. 2014). Before this experience of a single center has not been confirmed, a routine co-administration cannot be recommended.

Important to remind

Frequent anti-VEGF treatment is necessary during the first year of initiation. The need for retreatment considerably decreases during the following years.

One recent head-to-head trial showed a more pronounced response to aflibercept in a subgroup of patients with visual acuity of 20/50 or worse.

The usefulness of a combined laser treatment with anti-VEGF therapy has not yet been fully established. Though implemented in some studies, a marked reduction of treatment burden or other advantages have not been found.

Do not forget to evaluate the peripheral retina when treating DME patients. Progression of DR might occur, especially during longer therapy-free intervals.

Before appraising nonresponders (and switching drugs), careful follow-up examinations and adherence to predefined retreatment algorithms allow a better evaluation of the action in the individual patient.

In DME with foveal involvement anti-VEGF therapy should be preferred over focal/grid laser therapy.

6.7 Antiangiogenic Treatment of PDR

While new vessels were found to respond to anti-VEGF drugs (Avery 2006), their temporary use have been discussed as adjunct or therapeutic agents to achieve regression of retinal neovascularizations or at least decrease the risk of later vitreous hemorrhage during vitreoretinal surgery (Gunduz and Bakri 2007; Martinez-Zapata et al. 2014). In contrast to case series and single reports, the evidence—apart from the effects on DME—is still limited (Martinez-Zapata et al. 2014).

There have been some randomized studies verifying a reduction of postoperative hemorrhages for vitrectomy in proliferative vitreoretinopathy. The improvement of DR severity seen in DME trials does not yet justify leaving the panretinal scatter laser. Trials (NCT01594281, NCT01489189) addressing this issue are either still recruiting or ongoing.

Vitreous hemorrhage accumulates depending on the position and gravity, patients with dense vitreous hemorrhage can be advised to sleep with the head elevated so that the blood can settle in the inferior periphery and not restrict the optical axis by deposition in the macula.

6.7.1 Panretinal Photocoagulation

The development of retinal laser photocoagulation by Meyer-Schwickerath did achieve a remarkable decrease in visual loss by PDR (Meyer-Schwickerath 1977). Successfully at preventing blindness, PRP still is the most widespread treatment for PDR (DRS Group 1981a). Recent analyses of visual outcome suggest that the recommendation to consider PRP in severe NPDR or non-high-risk PDR before the development of high-risk PDR is particularly appropriate for persons with type 2 diabetes and older age (Ferris 1996). However, the clinical application and its reported efficacy vary markedly (Luo et al. 2015).

PRP leads to a regression of neovascularization within several weeks after treatment, presumably due to a reduction of the metabolic demand of the lasered retina (Doft and Blankenship 1984). While the initial pathomechanistic concept of PRP was based on destruction of poorly perfused cells in the neurosensory retina, the retinal pigment epithelium and the photoreceptor layers of the peripheral retina are now thought the key targets in order to reduce the angiogenic signaling. Monitoring of the choroidal thickness demonstrates a redistribution of choroidal blood flow after PRP indicating an altered metabolic demand of the lasered retina in the outer retinal layers and/or RPE (Zhu et al. 2015).

It has to be kept in mind that PRP treatment causes collateral damage to the retina, associated with a constriction of visual fields, impaired dark adaption, and a decrease in contrast sensitivity (Boynton et al. 2015). A focal retinochoroidal atrophy at the laser spots and a progressive scar formation is seen. There are attempts to reduce the visual field defects by the spatial localization of laser burns (Wang et al. 2014). Patients treated with PRP demonstrate increased photostress recovery time and dark adaptation speed. After PRP, a diffuse thickening of the retinal nerve fiber layers and thinning of the retinal pigment epithelium layers is observed. Ultimately, the unwanted side effects can lead to reduced driving abilities, especially under low light conditions (Gardner et al. 2002).

Another caveat is that following PRP an increase in macular edema was noticed in some patients. No difference of the risk, however, was found whether the PRP was conducted in one or four sittings (Brucker et al. 2009). Panretinal scatter coagulation remains the first-line treatment in severe NPDR and PDR, as the evidence of medical treatment has not been provided with regard to longevity of the effect (Evans et al. 2014).

6.7.2 Intravitreal Anti-VGEF Therapy

There is a growing body of evidence that intravitreal drugs might be - at least in the short term - an alternative to panretinal lasercoagulation. The DRCR.net provided data of the protocol S study indicating non-inferior visual acuity of ranibizumab (DRCR.net 2015). However, during the follow-up of two years, a large portion of the laser arm (53 %) did also receive ranibizumab treatment. Without laser, a larger extent of the visual fields was found to be preserved. The different rate of vitrectomy (laser: 15 %, ranibizumab: 4 %) might be influenced by the reserved attitude of surgeons to perform surgery in eyes without any laser pretreatment. Regardless of costs, the short follow-up of the study feeds the doubts about the sustainability of anti-VEGF

treatment in PDR. Ischemic retinal area, the key trigger of proliferations, are unlikely to disappear (within a short time).

6.7.3 Vitreomacular Traction

The high incidence of vitreomacular traction in DR is caused by an increased glycosylation of collagen fibers and the accumulation of proliferative factors in the vitreous causing vascular hyperpermeability and augmented cell migration (Khan and Haller 2015). Traction at the vitreomacular interface has been considered to be an important contributing factor for DME. The attachment of the vitreous might increase the frequency of barrier disturbance (Jackson et al. 2013). Similarly, epiretinal membranes might weaken the efficacy of laser and medical treatment (Snead et al. 2008).

There have been reports about eyes with DME and vitreomacular traction showing benefits from the removal of epiretinal membranes (Laidlaw 2008; Simunovic et al. 2014). Regarding pharmacological vitreolysis, no data is available beyond a theoretic concept (de and Castilla 2013). Spontaneous resolution of vitreomacular traction seems to occur very rarely in the context of DR.

In a prospective study, a marked reduction of retinal thickness was achieved by vitrectomy with removal of the posterior vitreous and peeling of epiretinal membranes (if present). However, the functional results were less convincing: Visual acuity after 6 months was improved in 28–49 % of cases, but worsened in 13–31 % of patients (Haller et al. 2010).

Inconsistent results are available regarding vitrectomy with or without peeling of the ILM in DME devoid of vitreomacular traction. Some authors report on functional improvement, others on a reduction/normalization of retinal thickness only (Kumagai et al. 2009; Patel et al. 2006). The low quality of report leads to a low level of evidence, not justifying a general recommendation (Yamamoto et al. 2007). A multivariate analysis of the DRCR.net described a significant decrease of edema, but without functional benefit in 241 eyes. Worse visual acuity and the removal of epiretinal membranes increased the probability to gain (Flaxel et al. 2010).

The known risks of vitrectomy have to be reminded, in spite of theoretical thoughts about a better oxygenation (Navarro et al. 2010; Park et al. 2009). Besides the formation of cataract and retinal holes, the development of secondary proliferative vitreoretinopathy (PVR) and an increased risk of endophthalmitis are relevant postoperative problems. In addition, it has to be kept in mind, that vitrectomy might change the pharmakokinetics of intravitreally injected drugs

6.7.4 Tractional Retinal Detachment

Fibrovascular tissue-induced retinal elevation is an important cause of visual loss in PDR (Imai et al. 2001). Membranes frequently develop along the temporal vascular arc, while the interface of the attached vitreous might serve as "guide rail". The whole complex can cause a localized distance. Macular elevation is seen in tractional retinal detachment and tractional retinoschisis (Su et al. 2014).

If the visual acuity is good and stable in spite of a localized traction, an observant approach including regular control examinations is possible after a sufficient laser treatment. But at latest in the case of a progression, tractional forces have been removed during vitrectomy (Helbig 2007). The dissection of tractional membranes has to be done very carefully, as retinal breaks may determine the need of permanent endotamponade (Fortun and Hubbard 2011; Wang et al. 2012b). Good outcomes have been reported, if the indication has taken into account visual prognosis and systemic treatment (Gupta et al. 2012; Kumar et al. 2014; Ostri et al. 2014; Zenoni et al. 2010). Anti-VEGF drugs prior to vitrectomy might not necessarily facilitate the surgery, but prevent intra- and postoperative bleeding (Pokroy et al. 2011; Romano et al. 2009).

6.7.5 Neovascular Glaucoma

Neovascular glaucoma is a blinding, intractable complication of late PDR (Hayreh 2007). The glaucoma may occur without retinal or optic disc neovascularization, however it is more commonly seen in association with PDR (Fig. 6.17).

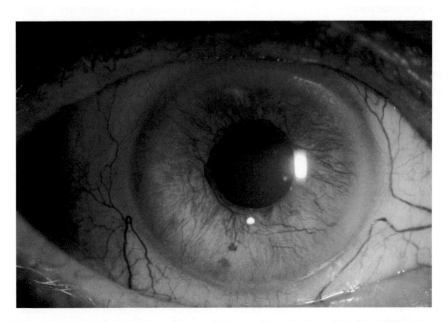

Fig. 6.17 It has to be reminded that the first changes of iris neovascularization can be seen in the iridocorneal angle. Leaking vessels can be detected around the pupil by angiography far earlier than additional vessel trunks have been formed

In the patients affected, differentiation of the various diseases (retinal vascular occlusive diseases, ocular ischemic syndrome) might be difficult, but important. Early on, the disease can present with subtle findings. A thorough examination of the iris and angle are essential before pupil dilation, since up to 30 % of the neovascular changes are limited to the angle.

Once neovascular glaucoma develops and the intraocular pressure is high, the major aspect of management is to control the high intraocular pressure, which is almost invariably the main factor in irreversible and massive visual loss in addition to PDR. The care includes retinal ablation by laser or cryocoagulation and control of the increased intraocular pressure with medical and surgical therapy (DRS Group 1976; Sivak-Callcott et al. 2001). Besides topical therapy cycloablative procedures promise to be more successful (Bloom et al. 1997; Delgado et al. 2003). If filtering surgery becomes necessary, the high risk of failure might be reduced by the use of drainage devices (Yalvac et al. 2007).

If the neovascularizations of the angle are detected early, anti-VEGF treatment might achieve some temporary regression (Luke et al. 2013). But even in the presence of synechiae and pretrabecular fibrovascular membranes, the drugs might offer a decrease in barrier disturbance (Andreoli and Miller 2007). The limited short-term experience does not justify the usage of VEGF-inhibitors only (Simha et al. 2013), but to try a combination treatment with conventional measures of pressure release (Jacobson et al. 1979).

References

Abouammoh MA. Ranibizumab injection for diabetic macular edema: meta-analysis of systemic safety and systematic review. Can J Ophthalmol. 2013;48(4):317–23.

Agardh E, Cavallin-Sjoberg U. Peripheral retinal evaluation comparing fundus photographs with fluorescein angiograms in patients with diabetes mellitus. Retina. 1998;18(5):420–3.

Ahsan H. Diabetic retinopathy—biomolecules and multiple pathophysiology. Diabetes Metab Syndr. 2015;9(1):51–4.

Aiello LP, Beck RW, Bressler NM, et al. Rationale for the diabetic retinopathy clinical research network treatment protocol for center-involved diabetic macular edema. Ophthalmology. 2011;118(12):e5–14.

Al Dhibi HA, Arevalo JF. Clinical trials on corticosteroids for diabetic macular edema. World J Diabetes. 2013;4(6):295–302.

Alcubierre N, Rubinat E, Traveset A, et al. A prospective cross-sectional study on quality of life and treatment satisfaction in type 2 diabetic patients with retinopathy without other major late diabetic complications. Health Qual Life Outcomes. 2014;12:131.

American Diabetes Association (ADA). Standards of medical care in diabetes—2013. Diabetes Care. 2013;36 Suppl 1:S11–66.

Andreoli CM, Miller JW. Anti-vascular endothelial growth factor therapy for ocular neovascular disease. Curr Opin Ophthalmol. 2007;18(6):502–8.

Antonetti DA, Barber AJ, Bronson SK, et al. Diabetic retinopathy: seeing beyond glucose-induced microvascular disease. Diabetes. 2006;55(9):2401–11.

Arden GB, Sivaprasad S. Hypoxia and oxidative stress in the causation of diabetic retinopathy. Curr Diabetes Rev. 2011;7(5):291–304.

Ashton N. Diabetic microangiopathy. Bibl Ophthalmol. 1958;12(52):1–84.

Ashton N. Vascular basement membrane changes in diabetic retinopathy. Montgomery lecture, 1973. Br J Ophthalmol. 1974;58(4):344–66.

Avery RL. Regression of retinal and iris neovascularization after intravitreal bevacizumab (Avastin) treatment. Retina. 2006;26(3):352–4.

Banerjee S, Ghosh US, Biswas G, et al. Comparative evaluation of ophthalmoscopy and angiography for the assessment of retinopathy in type 2 diabetes mellitus. J Indian Med Assoc. 2007;105(1):33–6.

Beagley J, Guariguata L, Weil C, et al. Global estimates of undiagnosed diabetes in adults. Diabetes Res Clin Pract. 2014;103(2):150–60.

Benson WE, Brown GC, Tasman W. Diabetes and its ocular complications. Philadelphia: Saunders; 1988.

Bloom PA, Tsai JC, Sharma K, et al. "Cyclodiode". Trans-scleral diode laser cyclophotocoagulation in the treatment of advanced refractory glaucoma. Ophthalmology. 1997;104(9):1508–19.

Bolz M, Ritter M, Schneider M, et al. A systematic correlation of angiography and high-resolution optical coherence tomography in diabetic macular edema. Ophthalmology. 2009a;116(1):66–72.

Bolz M, Schmidt-Erfurth U, Deak G, et al. Optical coherence tomographic hyperreflective foci: a morphologic sign of lipid extravasation in diabetic macular edema. Ophthalmology. 2009b;116(5):914–20.

Boyer DS, Yoon YH, Belfort Jr R, et al. Three-year, randomized, sham-controlled trial of dexamethasone intravitreal implant in patients with diabetic macular edema. Ophthalmology. 2014;121(10):1904–14.

Boynton GE, Stem MS, Kwark L, et al. Multimodal characterization of proliferative diabetic retinopathy reveals alterations in outer retinal function and structure. Ophthalmology. 2015;122:957–67.

Braun CI, Benson WE, Remaley NA, et al. Accommodative amplitudes in the Early Treatment Diabetic Retinopathy Study. Retina. 1995;15(4):275–81.

Brechner RJ, Cowie CC, Howie LJ, et al. Ophthalmic examination among adults with diagnosed diabetes mellitus. JAMA. 1993;270(14):1714–8.

Bresnick GH. Diabetic maculopathy. A critical review highlighting diffuse macular edema. Ophthalmology. 1983;90(11):1301–17.

Bresnick GH, Haight B, de VG. Retinal wrinkling and macular heterotopia in diabetic retinopathy. Arch Ophthalmol. 1979;97(10):1890–95.

Bressler NM, Miller KM, Beck RW, et al. Observational study of subclinical diabetic macular edema. Eye (Lond). 2012;26(6):833–40.

Bressler NM, Varma R, Doan QV, et al. Underuse of the health care system by persons with diabetes mellitus and diabetic macular edema in the United States. JAMA Ophthalmol. 2014;132(2):168–73.

Brinkmann R, Huttmann G, Rogener J, et al. Origin of retinal pigment epithelium cell damage by pulsed laser irradiance in the nanosecond to microsecond time regimen. Lasers Surg Med. 2000;27(5):451–64.

Browning DJ, Glassman AR, Aiello LP, et al. Relationship between optical coherence tomography-measured central retinal thickness and visual acuity in diabetic macular edema. Ophthalmology. 2007;114(3):525–36.

Browning DJ, Altaweel MM, Bressler NM, et al. Diabetic macular edema: what is focal and what is diffuse? Am J Ophthalmol. 2008;146(5):649–55.

Brownlee M. Biochemistry and molecular cell biology of diabetic complications. Nature. 2001;414(6865):813–20.

Brucker AJ, Qin H, Antoszyk AN, et al. Observational study of the development of diabetic macular edema following panretinal (scatter) photocoagulation given in 1 or 4 sittings. Arch Ophthalmol. 2009;127(2):132–40.

Buabbud JC, Al-latayfeh MM, Sun JK. Optical coherence tomography imaging for diabetic retinopathy and macular edema. Curr Diab Rep. 2010;10(4):264–9.

Byeon SH, Chu YK, Lee H, et al. Foveal ganglion cell layer damage in ischemic diabetic maculopathy: correlation of optical coherence tomographic and anatomic changes. Ophthalmology. 2009;116(10):1949–59.

Byeon SH, Chu YK, Hong YT, et al. New insights into the pathoanatomy of diabetic macular edema: angiographic patterns and optical coherence tomography. Retina. 2012;32(6):1087–99.

Callanan DG, Gupta S, Boyer DS, et al. Dexamethasone intravitreal implant in combination with laser photocoagulation for the treatment of diffuse diabetic macular edema. Ophthalmology. 2013;120(9):1843–51.

Campochiaro PA, Brown DM, Pearson A, et al. Long-term benefit of sustained-delivery fluocinolone acetonide vitreous inserts for diabetic macular edema. Ophthalmology. 2011;118(4):626–35.

Campochiaro PA, Brown DM, Pearson A, et al. Sustained delivery fluocinolone acetonide vitreous inserts provide benefit for at least 3 years in patients with diabetic macular edema. Ophthalmology. 2012;119(10):2125–32.

Campos C. Chronic hyperglycemia and glucose toxicity: pathology and clinical sequelae. Postgrad Med. 2012;124(6):90–7.

Cardillo PF, Zingirian M, Mosci C. Classification of proliferative diabetic retinopathy. Graefes Arch Clin Exp Ophthalmol. 1987;225(4):245–50.

Chalam KV, Bressler SB, Edwards AR, et al. Retinal thickness in people with diabetes and minimal or no diabetic retinopathy: Heidelberg Spectralis optical coherence tomography. Invest Ophthalmol Vis Sci. 2012;53(13):8154–61.

Chang YC, Wu WC. Dyslipidemia and diabetic retinopathy. Rev Diabet Stud. 2013;10(2–3):121–32.

Chang-Lin JE, Burke JA, Peng Q, et al. Pharmacokinetics of a sustained-release dexamethasone intravitreal implant in vitrectomized and nonvitrectomized eyes. Invest Ophthalmol Vis Sci. 2011;52(7):4605–9.

Chantelau E, Meyer-Schwickerath R. Reversion of 'early worsening' of diabetic retinopathy by deliberate restoration of poor metabolic control. Ophthalmologica. 2003;217(5):373–7.

Chen YJ, Kuo HK, Huang HW. Retinal outcomes in proliferative diabetic retinopathy presenting during and after pregnancy. Chang Gung Med J. 2004;27(9):678–84.

Chen G, Li W, Tzekov R, et al. Ranibizumab monotherapy or combined with laser versus laser monotherapy for diabetic macular edema: a meta-analysis of randomized controlled trials. PLoS One. 2014;9(12):e115797.

Chew EY, Klein ML, Murphy RP, et al. Effects of aspirin on vitreous/preretinal hemorrhage in patients with diabetes mellitus. Early Treatment Diabetic Retinopathy Study report no. 20. Arch Ophthalmol. 1995a;113(1):52–5.

Chew EY, Mills JL, Metzger BE, et al. Metabolic control and progression of retinopathy. The Diabetes in Early Pregnancy Study. National Institute of Child Health and Human Development Diabetes in Early Pregnancy Study. Diabetes Care. 1995b;18(5):631–7.

Chew EY, Ambrosius WT, Davis MD, et al. Effects of medical therapies on retinopathy progression in type 2 diabetes. N Engl J Med. 2010;363(3):233–44.

Chew EY, Davis MD, Danis RP, et al. The effects of medical management on the progression of diabetic retinopathy in persons with type 2 diabetes: the Action to Control Cardiovascular Risk in Diabetes (ACCORD) Eye Study. Ophthalmology. 2014;121(12):2443–51.

Cho YH, Craig ME, Donaghue KC. Puberty as an accelerator for diabetes complications. Pediatr Diabetes. 2014;15(1):18–26.

Clermont AC, Bursell SE. Retinal blood flow in diabetes. Microcirculation. 2007;14(1):49–61.

Comyn O, Sivaprasad S, Peto T, et al. A randomized trial to assess functional and structural effects of ranibizumab versus laser in diabetic macular edema (the LUCIDATE study). Am J Ophthalmol. 2014;157(5):960–70.

Congdon N, O'Colmain B, Klaver CC, et al. Causes and prevalence of visual impairment among adults in the United States. Arch Ophthalmol. 2004;122(4):477–85.

Cunha-Vaz JG. The blood-retinal barriers system. Basic concepts and clinical evaluation. Exp Eye Res. 2004;78(3):715–21.

Cunha-Vaz J, Ashton P, Iezzi R, et al. Sustained delivery fluocinolone acetonide vitreous implants: long-term benefit in patients with chronic diabetic macular edema. Ophthalmology. 2014a;121(10):1892–903.

Cunha-Vaz J, Ribeiro L, Lobo C. Phenotypes and biomarkers of diabetic retinopathy. Prog Retin Eye Res. 2014b;41:90–111.

Daien V, Kawasaki R, Villain M, et al. Retinal vascular caliber is associated with renal function in apparently healthy subjects. Acta Ophthalmol. 2013;91(4):e283–8.

Daley ML, Watzke RC, Riddle MC. Early loss of blue-sensitive color vision in patients with type I diabetes. Diabetes Care. 1987;10(6):777–81.

Danis R, Davis M. Proliferative diabetic retinopathy. In: Duh E, editor. Diabetic retinopathy. Totowa: Humana Press; 2008. p. 29–65.

Davis MD, Fisher MR, Gangnon RE, et al. Risk factors for high-risk proliferative diabetic retinopathy and severe visual loss: Early Treatment Diabetic Retinopathy Study Report #18. Invest Ophthalmol Vis Sci. 1998;39(2):233–52.

Diabetes Control and Complications Trial (DCCT) Research Group. Color photography vs fluorescein angiography in the detection of diabetic retinopathy in the diabetes control and complications trial. Arch Ophthalmol. 1987;105(10):1344–51.

DCCT Research Group. The relationship of glycemic exposure (HbA1c) to the risk of development and progression of retinopathy in the diabetes control and complications trial. Diabetes. 1995;44(8):968–83.

DCCT Research Group. Effect of pregnancy on microvascular complications in the diabetes control and complications trial. Diabetes Care. 2000;23(8):1084–91.

de S, Castilla M. Ocriplasmin for diabetic retinopathy. Expert Opin Biol Ther. 2013;13(12):1741–47.

De BU, Sacconi R, Pierro L, et al. Optical coherence tomographic hyperreflective foci in early stages of diabetic retinopathy. Retina. 2015;35(3): 449–53.

Deissler H, Deissler H, Lang GK, et al. TGFbeta induces transdifferentiation of iBREC to alpha SMA-expressing cells. Int J Mol Med. 2006;18(4):577–82.

Deissler HL, Deissler H, Lang GK, et al. VEGF but not PlGF disturbs the barrier of retinal endothelial cells. Exp Eye Res. 2013;115:162–71.

Delgado MF, Dickens CJ, Iwach AG, et al. Long-term results of noncontact neodymium:yttrium-aluminum-garnet cyclophotocoagulation in neovascular glaucoma. Ophthalmology. 2003;110(5):895–9.

Diabetes Prevention Program (DPP) Research Group. The prevalence of retinopathy in impaired glucose tolerance and recent-onset diabetes in the Diabetes Prevention Program. Diabet Med. 2007;24(2):137–44.

Diabetic Retinopathy Clinical Research Network (DRCR. net), A randomized trial comparing intravitreal triamcinolone acetonide and focal/grid photocoagulation for diabetic macular edema. Ophthalmology. 2008; 115(9):1447–9.

Diabetic Retinopathy Study (DRS) Group. Preliminary report on effects of photocoagulation therapy. Am J Ophthalmol. 1976;81(4):383–96.

DRS Group. Photocoagulation treatment of proliferative diabetic retinopathy. Clinical application of Diabetic Retinopathy Study (DRS) findings, DRS Report Number 8. Ophthalmology. 1981a;88(7):583–600.

DRS Group. Report Number 6. Design, methods, and baseline results. Report Number 7. A modification of the Airlie House classification of diabetic retinopathy. Prepared by the Diabetic Retinopathy. Invest Ophthalmol Vis Sci. 1981b;21(1 Pt 2):1–226.

Ding J, Wong TY. Current epidemiology of diabetic retinopathy and diabetic macular edema. Curr Diab Rep. 2012;12(4):346–54.

Dmuchowska DA, Krasnicki P, Mariak Z. Can optical coherence tomography replace fluorescein angiography in detection of ischemic diabetic maculopathy? Graefes Arch Clin Exp Ophthalmol. 2014;252(5): 731–8.

Do YK, Eggleston KN. Educational disparities in quality of diabetes care in a universal health insurance system: evidence from the 2005 Korea National Health and Nutrition Examination Survey. Int J Qual Health Care. 2011;23(4):397–404.

Do DV, Wang X, Vedula SS, et al. Blood pressure control for diabetic retinopathy. Cochrane Database Syst Rev. 2015;1:CD006127.

Doft BH, Blankenship G. Retinopathy risk factor regression after laser panretinal photocoagulation for proliferative diabetic retinopathy. Ophthalmology. 1984;91(12):1453–7.

Douvali M, Chatziralli IP, Theodossiadis PG, et al. Effect of macular ischemia on intravitreal ranibizumab treatment for diabetic macular edema. Ophthalmologica. 2014;232(3):136–43.

Dubow M, Pinhas A, Shah N, et al. Classification of human retinal microaneurysms using adaptive optics scanning light ophthalmoscope fluorescein angiography. Invest Ophthalmol Vis Sci. 2014;55(3):1299–309.

Dziuba J, Alperin P, Racketa J, et al. Modeling effects of SGLT-2 inhibitor dapagliflozin treatment versus standard diabetes therapy on cardiovascular and microvascular outcomes. Diabetes Obes Metab. 2014; 16(7):628–35.

Edwards MS, Wilson DB, Craven TE, et al. Associations between retinal microvascular abnormalities and declining renal function in the elderly population: the Cardiovascular Health Study. Am J Kidney Dis. 2005;46(2):214–24.

Ejaz S, Chekarova I, Ejaz A, et al. Importance of pericytes and mechanisms of pericyte loss during diabetes retinopathy. Diabetes Obes Metab. 2008;10(1):53–63.

Elman MJ, Aiello LP, Beck RW, et al. Randomized trial evaluating ranibizumab plus prompt or deferred laser or triamcinolone plus prompt laser for diabetic macular edema. Ophthalmology. 2010;117(6):1064–77.

Elman MJ, Bressler NM, Qin H, et al. Expanded 2-year follow-up of ranibizumab plus prompt or deferred laser or triamcinolone plus prompt laser for diabetic macular edema. Ophthalmology. 2011;118(4):609–14.

Elman MJ, Ayala A, Bressler NM, et al. Intravitreal Ranibizumab for diabetic macular edema with prompt versus deferred laser treatment: 5-year randomized trial results. Ophthalmology. 2015;122(2):375–81.

Escobar-Barranco JJ, Pina-Marin B, Fernandez-Bonet M. Dexamethasone implants in patients with naive or refractory diffuse diabetic macular edema. Ophthalmologica. 2015;233:176–85.

Early Treatment Diabetic Retinopathy Study (ETDRS) Research Group. Photocoagulation for diabetic macular edema. Early Treatment Diabetic Retinopathy Study report number 1. Arch Ophthalmol. 1985; 103(12):1796–806.

ETDRS Research Group. Grading diabetic retinopathy from stereoscopic color fundus photographs—an extension of the modified Airlie House classification ETDRS report number 10. Ophthalmology. 1991a;98(5 Suppl):786–806.

ETDRS Research Group. Classification of diabetic retinopathy from fluorescein angiograms. ETDRS report number 11. Ophthalmology. 1991b;98(5 Suppl):807–22.

ETDRS Research Group. Effects of aspirin treatment on diabetic retinopathy. ETDRS report number 8. Ophthalmology. 1991c;98(5 Suppl):757–65.

ETDRS Research Group . Fundus photographic risk factors for progression of diabetic retinopathy. ETDRS report number 12. Ophthalmology. 1991;98(5 Suppl):823–33.

ETDRS Research Group. Focal photocoagulation treatment of diabetic macular edema. Relationship of treatment effect to fluorescein angiographic and other retinal characteristics at baseline: ETDRS report no. 19. Arch Ophthalmol. 1995;113(9):1144–55.

Evans JR, Michelessi M, Virgili G. Laser photocoagulation for proliferative diabetic retinopathy. Cochrane Database Syst Rev. 2014;11:CD011234.

Ferrannini E, Cushman WC. Diabetes and hypertension: the bad companions. Lancet. 2012;380(9841):601–10.

Ferris III FL. How effective are treatments for diabetic retinopathy? JAMA. 1993;269(10):1290–1.

Ferris F. Early photocoagulation in patients with either type I or type II diabetes. Trans Am Ophthalmol Soc. 1996;94:505–37.

Fialho SL, Rego MB, Siqueira RC, et al. Safety and pharmacokinetics of an intravitreal biodegradable implant of dexamethasone acetate in rabbit eyes. Curr Eye Res. 2006;31(6):525–34.

Figueira J, Khan J, Nunes S, et al. Prospective randomised controlled trial comparing sub-threshold micropulse diode laser photocoagulation and conventional green laser for clinically significant diabetic macular oedema. Br J Ophthalmol. 2009;93(10): 1341–4.

Finger RP, Fimmers R, Holz FG, et al. Incidence of blindness and severe visual impairment in Germany: pro-

jections for 2030. Invest Ophthalmol Vis Sci. 2011;52(7):4381–9.

Fiore T, Androudi S, Iaccheri B, et al. Repeatability and reproducibility of retinal thickness measurements in diabetic patients with spectral domain optical coherence tomography. Curr Eye Res. 2013;38(6): 674–9.

Flaxel CJ, Edwards AR, Aiello LP, et al. Factors associated with visual acuity outcomes after vitrectomy for diabetic macular edema: diabetic retinopathy clinical research network. Retina. 2010;30(9):1488–95.

Fonda SJ, Bursell SE, Lewis DG, et al. The relationship of a diabetes telehealth eye care program to standard eye care and change in diabetes health outcomes. Telemed JE Health. 2007;13(6):635–44.

Fong DS, Ferris III FL, Davis MD, et al. Causes of severe visual loss in the early treatment diabetic retinopathy study: ETDRS report no. 24. Early Treatment Diabetic Retinopathy Study Research Group. Am J Ophthalmol. 1999;127(2):137–41.

Fong DS, Gottlieb J, Ferris III FL, et al. Understanding the value of diabetic retinopathy screening. Arch Ophthalmol. 2001;119(5):758–60.

Fong DS, Strauber SF, Aiello LP, et al. Comparison of the modified Early Treatment Diabetic Retinopathy Study and mild macular grid laser photocoagulation strategies for diabetic macular edema. Arch Ophthalmol. 2007;125(4):469–80.

Fortun JA, Hubbard III GB. New viscodissection instrument for use with microincisional vitrectomy in the treatment of diabetic tractional retinal detachments. Arch Ophthalmol. 2011;129(3):352–5.

Framme C, Walter A, Prahs P, et al. Structural changes of the retina after conventional laser photocoagulation and selective retina treatment (SRT) in spectral domain OCT. Curr Eye Res. 2009;34(7):568–79.

Frank RN. Systemic therapies for diabetic retinopathy: the accord eye study. Ophthalmology. 2014;121(12): 2295–6.

Friberg TR, Karatza EC. The treatment of macular disease using a micropulsed and continuous wave 810-nm diode laser. Ophthalmology. 1997;104(12):2030–8.

Frier BM. Hypoglycaemia in diabetes mellitus: epidemiology and clinical implications. Nat Rev Endocrinol. 2014;10(12):711–22.

Fullerton B, Jeitler K, Seitz M, et al. Intensive glucose control versus conventional glucose control for type 1 diabetes mellitus. Cochrane Database Syst Rev. 2014;2:CD009122.

Funatsu H, Noma H, Mimura T, et al. Association of vitreous inflammatory factors with diabetic macular edema. Ophthalmology. 2009;116(1):73–9.

Garay-Sevilla ME, Porras JS, Malacara JM. Coping strategies and adherence to treatment in patients with type 2 diabetes mellitus. Rev Invest Clin. 2011;63(2): 155–61.

Gardner TW, Antonetti DA, Barber AJ, et al. Diabetic retinopathy: more than meets the eye. Surv Ophthalmol. 2002;47 Suppl 2:S253–62.

Ghazi NG, Ciralsky JB, Shah SM, et al. Optical coherence tomography findings in persistent diabetic macular edema: the vitreomacular interface. Am J Ophthalmol. 2007;144(5):747–54.

Gillies MC, Lim LL, Campain A, et al. A randomized clinical trial of intravitreal bevacizumab versus intravitreal dexamethasone for diabetic macular edema: the BEVORDEX study. Ophthalmology. 2014;121(12):2473–81.

Giovannini A, Amato GP, Mariotti C, et al. Diabetic maculopathy induced by vitreo-macular traction: evaluation by optical coherence tomography (OCT). Doc Ophthalmol. 1999;97(3–4):361–6.

Goatman KA, Cree MJ, Olson JA, et al. Automated measurement of microaneurysm turnover. Invest Ophthalmol Vis Sci. 2003;44(12):5335–41.

Grassi MA, Tikhomirov A, Ramalingam S, et al. Replication analysis for severe diabetic retinopathy. Invest Ophthalmol Vis Sci. 2012;53(4):2377–81.

Grunwald JE, Pistilli M, Ying GS, et al. Retinopathy and progression of CKD: The CRIC study. Clin J Am Soc Nephrol. 2014;9(7):1217–24.

Gu K, Cowie CC, Harris MI. Mortality in adults with and without diabetes in a national cohort of the U.S. population, 1971–1993. Diabetes Care. 1998;21(7):1138–45.

Guigou S, Hajjar C, Parrat E, et al. Multicenter Ozurdex(R) assessment for diabetic macular edema: MOZART study. J Fr Ophtalmol. 2014;37(6):480–5.

Gulliford MC, Dodhia H, Chamley M, et al. Socioeconomic and ethnic inequalities in diabetes retinal screening. Diabet Med. 2010;27(3):282–8.

Gunderson EP, Lewis CE, Tsai AL, et al. A 20-year prospective study of childbearing and incidence of diabetes in young women, controlling for glycemia before conception: the Coronary Artery Risk Development in Young Adults (CARDIA) Study. Diabetes. 2007;56(12):2990–6.

Gunduz K, Bakri SJ. Management of proliferative diabetic retinopathy. Compr Ophthalmol Update. 2007;8(5):245–56.

Gupta B, Sivaprasad S, Wong R, et al. Visual and anatomical outcomes following vitrectomy for complications of diabetic retinopathy: the DRIVE UK study. Eye (Lond). 2012;26(4):510–6.

Haller JA, Qin H, Apte RS, et al. Vitrectomy outcomes in eyes with diabetic macular edema and vitreomacular traction. Ophthalmology. 2010;117(6):1087–93.

Hammes HP, Feng Y, Pfister F, et al. Diabetic retinopathy: targeting vasoregression. Diabetes. 2011a;60(1): 9–16.

Hammes HP, Kerner W, Hofer S, et al. Diabetic retinopathy in type 1 diabetes-a contemporary analysis of 8,784 patients. Diabetologia. 2011b;54(8):1977–84.

Hayes AJ, Leal J, Gray AM, et al. UKPDS outcomes model 2: a new version of a model to simulate lifetime health outcomes of patients with type 2 diabetes mellitus using data from the 30 year United Kingdom Prospective Diabetes Study: UKPDS 82. Diabetologia. 2013;56(9):1925–33.

Hayreh SS. Neovascular glaucoma. Prog Retin Eye Res. 2007;26(5):470–85.

Heintz E, Wirehn AB, Peebo BB, et al. Prevalence and healthcare costs of diabetic retinopathy: a population-based register study in Sweden. Diabetologia. 2010;53(10):2147–54.

Helbig H. Surgery for diabetic retinopathy. Ophthalmologica. 2007;221(2):103–11.

Hellstedt T, Vesti E, Immonen I. Identification of individual microaneurysms: a comparison between fluorescein angiograms and red-free and colour photographs. Graefes Arch Clin Exp Ophthalmol. 1996;234 Suppl 1:S13–7.

Hellstedt T, Kaaja R, Teramo K, et al. The effect of pregnancy on mild diabetic retinopathy. Graefes Arch Clin Exp Ophthalmol. 1997;235(7):437–41.

Hemmingsen B, Lund SS, Gluud C, et al. Intensive glycaemic control for patients with type 2 diabetes: systematic review with meta-analysis and trial sequential analysis of randomised clinical trials. BMJ. 2011;343:d6898.

Hietala K, Harjutsalo V, Forsblom C, et al. Age at onset and the risk of proliferative retinopathy in type 1 diabetes. Diabetes Care. 2010;33(6):1315–9.

Huang OS, Tay WT, Tai ES, et al. Lack of awareness amongst community patients with diabetes and diabetic retinopathy: the Singapore Malay eye study. Ann Acad Med Singapore. 2009;38(12):1048–55.

Hugenschmidt CE, Lovato JF, Ambrosius WT, et al. The cross-sectional and longitudinal associations of diabetic retinopathy with cognitive function and brain MRI findings: the Action to Control Cardiovascular Risk in Diabetes (ACCORD) trial. Diabetes Care. 2014;37(12):3244–52.

Hutchins E, Coppell KJ, Morris A, et al. Diabetic retinopathy screening in New Zealand requires improvement: results from a multi-centre audit. Aust N Z J Public Health. 2012;36(3):257–62.

Imai M, Iijima H, Hanada N. Optical coherence tomography of tractional macular elevations in eyes with proliferative diabetic retinopathy. Am J Ophthalmol. 2001;132(3):458–61.

Inchiostro S, Candido R, Cavalot F. How can we monitor glycaemic variability in the clinical setting? Diabetes Obes Metab. 2013;15 Suppl 2:13–6.

Ip MS, Domalpally A, Sun JK, et al. Long-term effects of therapy with ranibizumab on diabetic retinopathy severity and baseline risk factors for worsening retinopathy. Ophthalmology. 2015;122(2):367–74.

Ishibashi T, Li X, Koh A, et al. The REVEAL Study: ranibizumab monotherapy or combined with laser versus laser monotherapy in Asian patients with diabetic macular edema. Ophthalmology. 2015;122:1402–15.

Ishida S, Usui T, Yamashiro K, et al. VEGF164 is proinflammatory in the diabetic retina. Invest Ophthalmol Vis Sci. 2003;44(5):2155–62.

Ito H, Horii T, Nishijima K, et al. Association between fluorescein leakage and optical coherence tomographic characteristics of microaneurysms in diabetic retinopathy. Retina. 2013;33(4):732–9.

Jackson TL, Nicod E, Angelis A, et al. Vitreous attachment in age-related macular degeneration, diabetic macular edema, and retinal vein occlusion: a systematic review and metaanalysis. Retina. 2013; 33(6):1099–108.

Jacobson DR, Murphy RP, Rosenthal AR. The treatment of angle neovascularization with panretinal photocoagulation. Ophthalmology. 1979;86(7):1270–7.

Jaissle GB, Szurman P, Bartz-Schmidt KU. Ocular side effects and complications of intravitreal triamcinolone acetonide injection. Ophthalmologe. 2004;101(2): 121–8.

Jalli PY, Hellstedt TJ, Immonen IJ. Early versus late staining of microaneurysms in fluorescein angiography. Retina. 1997;17(3):211–5.

Javitt JC, Aiello LP. Cost-effectiveness of detecting and treating diabetic retinopathy. Ann Intern Med. 1996;124(1 Pt 2):164–9.

Kahn HA, Hiller R. Blindness caused by diabetic retinopathy. Am J Ophthalmol. 1974;78(1):58–67.

Kamoi K, Takeda K, Hashimoto K, et al. Identifying risk factors for clinically significant diabetic macula edema in patients with type 2 diabetes mellitus. Curr Diabetes Rev. 2013;9(3):209–17.

Kampik A, Kenyon KR, Michels RG, et al. Epiretinal and vitreous membranes. Comparative study of 56 cases. Arch Ophthalmol. 1981;99(8):1445–54.

Kandarakis SA, Piperi C, Topouzis F, et al. Emerging role of advanced glycation-end products (AGEs) in the pathobiology of eye diseases. Prog Retin Eye Res. 2014;42:85–102.

Kane FE, Burdan J, Cutino A, et al. Iluvien: a new sustained delivery technology for posterior eye disease. Expert Opin Drug Deliv. 2008;5(9):1039–46.

Kang H, Su L, Zhang H, et al. Early histological alteration of the retina following photocoagulation treatment in diabetic retinopathy as measured by spectral domain optical coherence tomography. Graefes Arch Clin Exp Ophthalmol. 2010;248(12):1705–11.

Karam JG, McFarlane SI. Update on the prevention of type 2 diabetes. Curr Diab Rep. 2011;11(1):56–63.

Kaul K, Hodgkinson A, Tarr JM, et al. Is inflammation a common retinal-renal-nerve pathogenic link in diabetes? Curr Diabetes Rev. 2010;6(5):294–303.

Keech AC, Mitchell P, Summanen PA, et al. Effect of fenofibrate on the need for laser treatment for diabetic retinopathy (FIELD study): a randomised controlled trial. Lancet. 2007;370(9600):1687–97.

Kempen JH, O'Colmain BJ, Leske MC, et al. The prevalence of diabetic retinopathy among adults in the United States. Arch Ophthalmol. 2004;122(4):552–63.

Kern TS. Contributions of inflammatory processes to the development of the early stages of diabetic retinopathy. Exp Diabetes Res. 2007;2007:95103.

Kern TS, Engerman RL. A mouse model of diabetic retinopathy. Arch Ophthalmol. 1996;114(8):986–90.

Khalaf SS, Al-Bdour MD, Al-Till MI. Clinical biomicroscopy versus fluorescein angiography: effectiveness and sensitivity in detecting diabetic retinopathy. Eur J Ophthalmol. 2007;17(1):84–8.

Khan MA, Haller JA. Clinical management of vitreomacular traction. Curr Opin Ophthalmol. 2015;26(3): 143–8.

Kiddee W, Trope GE, Sheng L, et al. Intraocular pressure monitoring post intravitreal steroids: a systematic review. Surv Ophthalmol. 2013;58(4):291–310.

Kiire CA, Porta M, Chong V. Medical management for the prevention and treatment of diabetic macular edema. Surv Ophthalmol. 2013;58(5):459–65.

Klaassen I, Van Noorden CJ, Schlingemann RO. Molecular basis of the inner blood-retinal barrier and its breakdown in diabetic macular edema and other pathological conditions. Prog Retin Eye Res. 2013;34:19–48.

Klein R. Screening interval for retinopathy in type 2 diabetes. Lancet. 2003;361(9353):190–1.

Klein R, Klein BE, Moss SE, et al. The Wisconsin epidemiologic study of diabetic retinopathy. II. Prevalence and risk of diabetic retinopathy when age at diagnosis is less than 30 years. Arch Ophthalmol. 1984;102(4): 520–6.

Klein BE, Moss SE, Klein R. Effect of pregnancy on progression of diabetic retinopathy. Diabetes Care. 1990;13(1):34–40.

Klein R, Klein BE, Moss SE. Epidemiology of proliferative diabetic retinopathy. Diabetes Care. 1992;15(12): 1875–91.

Klein BE, Klein R, Lee KE. Components of the metabolic syndrome and risk of cardiovascular disease and diabetes in Beaver Dam. Diabetes Care. 2002;25(10): 1790–4.

Klein R, Knudtson MD, Lee KE, et al. The Wisconsin Epidemiologic Study of Diabetic Retinopathy XXIII: the twenty-five-year incidence of macular edema in persons with type 1 diabetes. Ophthalmology. 2009;116(3):497–503.

Klein R, Lee KE, Gangnon RE, et al. Relation of smoking, drinking, and physical activity to changes in vision over a 20-year period: the Beaver Dam Eye Study. Ophthalmology. 2014;121(6):1220–8.

Klein BE, Myers CE, Howard KP, et al. Serum lipids and proliferative diabetic retinopathy and macular edema in persons with long-term type 1 diabetes mellitus: the Wisconsin Epidemiologic Study of Diabetic Retinopathy. JAMA Ophthalmol. 2015;133:503–10.

Klonoff DC, Schwartz DM. An economic analysis of interventions for diabetes. Diabetes Care. 2000;23(3): 390–404.

Kohner EM, Henkind P. Correlation of fluorescein angiogram and retinal digest in diabetic retinopathy. Am J Ophthalmol. 1970;69(3):403–14.

Kohner EM, Stratton IM, Aldington SJ, et al. Relationship between the severity of retinopathy and progression to photocoagulation in patients with type 2 diabetes mellitus in the UKPDS (UKPDS 52). Diabet Med. 2001;18(3):178–84.

Korobelnik JF, Do DV, Schmidt-Erfurth U, et al. Intravitreal aflibercept for diabetic macular edema. Ophthalmology. 2014;121(11):2247–54.

Kozak I, Oster SF, Cortes MA, et al. Clinical evaluation and treatment accuracy in diabetic macular edema using navigated laser photocoagulator NAVILAS. Ophthalmology. 2011;118(6):1119–24.

Kozak I, El-Emam SY, Cheng L, et al. Fluorescein angiography versus optical coherence tomography-guided planning for macular laser photocoagulation in diabetic macular edema. Retina. 2014;34(8): 1600–5.

Kristinsson JK, Gudmundsson JR, Stefansson E, et al. Screening for diabetic retinopathy. Initiation and frequency. Acta Ophthalmol Scand. 1995;73(6):525–8.

Kumagai K, Furukawa M, Ogino N, et al. Long-term follow-up of vitrectomy for diffuse nontractional diabetic macular edema. Retina. 2009;29(4):464–72.

Kumar A, Duraipandi K, Gogia V, et al. Comparative evaluation of 23- and 25-gauge microincision vitrectomy surgery in management of diabetic macular traction retinal detachment. Eur J Ophthalmol. 2014; 24(1):107–13.

Kuppermann BD, Blumenkranz MS, Haller JA, et al. Randomized controlled study of an intravitreous dexamethasone drug delivery system in patients with persistent macular edema. Arch Ophthalmol. 2007;125(3):309–17.

Laidlaw DA. Vitrectomy for diabetic macular oedema. Eye (Lond). 2008;22(10):1337–41.

Lang GE. Diabetic macular edema. Ophthalmologica. 2012;227 Suppl 1:21–9.

Lang GE. Mechanisms of retinal neurodegeneration as a result of diabetes mellitus. Klin Monbl Augenheilkd. 2013;230(9):929–31.

Lauszus FF, Klebe JG, Bek T, et al. Increased serum IGF-I during pregnancy is associated with progression of diabetic retinopathy. Diabetes. 2003;52(3):852–6.

LeCaire TJ, Palta M, Klein R, et al. Assessing progress in retinopathy outcomes in type 1 diabetes: comparing findings from the Wisconsin Diabetes Registry Study and the Wisconsin Epidemiologic Study of Diabetic Retinopathy. Diabetes Care. 2013;36(3):631–7.

Lee CM, Olk RJ. Modified grid laser photocoagulation for diffuse diabetic macular edema. Long-term visual results. Ophthalmology. 1991;98(10):1594–602.

Lee WJ, Sobrin L, Kang MH, et al. Ischemic diabetic retinopathy as a possible prognostic factor for chronic kidney disease progression. Eye (Lond). 2014;28(9):1119–25.

Leicht SF, Kernt M, Neubauer A, et al. Microaneurysm turnover in diabetic retinopathy assessed by automated RetmarkerDR image analysis—potential role as biomarker of response to ranibizumab treatment. Ophthalmologica. 2014;231(4):198–203.

Li CS, Neu MB, Shaw LC, et al. EPCs and pathological angiogenesis: when good cells go bad. Microvasc Res. 2010;79(3):207–16.

Li LX, Li MF, Lu JX, et al. Retinal microvascular abnormalities are associated with early carotid atherosclerotic lesions in hospitalized Chinese patients with type 2 diabetes mellitus. J Diabetes Complications. 2014;28(3):378–85.

Liegl R, Langer J, Seidensticker F, et al. Comparative evaluation of combined navigated laser photocoagulation and intravitreal ranibizumab in the treatment of diabetic macular edema. PLoS One. 2014;9(12): e113981.

Lim LS, Cheung CM, Mitchell P, et al. Emerging evidence concerning systemic safety of anti-VEGF agents—should ophthalmologists be concerned? Am J Ophthalmol. 2011;152(3):329–31.

Liu L, Wu X, Liu L, et al. Prevalence of diabetic retinopathy in mainland China: a meta-analysis. PLoS One. 2012;7(9):e45264.

Liu H, Zhang W, Xu Z, et al. Hyperoxia causes regression of vitreous neovascularization by downregulating VEGF/VEGFR2 pathway. Invest Ophthalmol Vis Sci. 2013;54(2):918–31.

Lombardo M, Parravano M, Serrao S, et al. Analysis of retinal capillaries in patients with type 1 diabetes and nonproliferative diabetic retinopathy using adaptive optics imaging. Retina. 2013;33(8):1630–9.

Looker HC, Nyangoma SO, Cromie DT, et al. Rates of referable eye disease in the Scottish National Diabetic Retinopathy Screening Programme. Br J Ophthalmol. 2014;98(6):790–5.

Loprinzi PD, Brodowicz GR, Sengupta S, et al. Accelerometer-assessed physical activity and diabetic retinopathy in the United States. JAMA Ophthalmol. 2014;132(8):1017–9.

Loukovaara S, Harju M, Kaaja R, et al. Retinal capillary blood flow in diabetic and nondiabetic women during pregnancy and postpartum period. Invest Ophthalmol Vis Sci. 2003;44(4):1486–91.

Lovestam-Adrian M, Agardh E. Photocoagulation of diabetic macular oedema—complications and visual outcome. Acta Ophthalmol Scand. 2000;78(6): 667–71.

Luke J, Nassar K, Luke M, et al. Ranibizumab as adjuvant in the treatment of rubeosis iridis and neovascular glaucoma—results from a prospective interventional case series. Graefes Arch Clin Exp Ophthalmol. 2013;251(10):2403–13.

Lung JC, Swann PG, Chan HH. Early local functional changes in the human diabetic retina: a global flash multifocal electroretinogram study. Graefes Arch Clin Exp Ophthalmol. 2012;250(12):1745–54.

Luo D, Zheng Z, Xu X, et al. Systematic review of various laser intervention strategies for proliferative diabetic retinopathy. Expert Rev Med Devices. 2015;12(1): 83–91.

Lutty GA. Effects of diabetes on the eye. Invest Ophthalmol Vis Sci. 2013;54(14):ORSF81–7.

Ly A, Scheerer MF, Zukunft S, et al. Retinal proteome alterations in a mouse model of type 2 diabetes. Diabetologia. 2014;57(1):192–203.

Maberley DA, Koushik A, Cruess AF. Factors associated with missed eye examinations in a cohort with diabetes. Can J Public Health. 2002;93(3):229–32.

Maclennan PA, McGwin Jr G, Heckemeyer C, et al. Eye care use among a high-risk diabetic population seen in a public hospital's clinics. JAMA Ophthalmol. 2014;132(2):162–7.

Madsen-Bouterse SA, Kowluru RA. Oxidative stress and diabetic retinopathy: pathophysiological mechanisms and treatment perspectives. Rev Endocr Metab Disord. 2008;9(4):315–27.

Maeshima K, Utsugi-Sutoh N, Otani T, et al. Progressive enlargement of scattered photocoagulation scars in diabetic retinopathy. Retina. 2004;24(4):507–11.

Maheshwary AS, Oster SF, Yuson RM, et al. The association between percent disruption of the photoreceptor inner segment-outer segment junction and visual acuity in diabetic macular edema. Am J Ophthalmol. 2010;150(1):63–7.

Marticorena J, Romano V, Gomez-Ulla F. Sterile endophthalmitis after intravitreal injections. Mediators Inflamm. 2012;2012:928123.

Martinez-Zapata MJ, Marti-Carvajal AJ, Sola I, et al. Anti-vascular endothelial growth factor for proliferative diabetic retinopathy. Cochrane Database Syst Rev. 2014;11:CD008721.

Massin P, Peto T, Ansquer JC, et al. Effects of fenofibric acid on diabetic macular edema: the MacuFen study. Ophthalmic Epidemiol. 2014;21(5):307–17.

Matsuda S, Tam T, Singh RP, et al. Impact of insulin treatment in diabetic macular edema therapy in type 2 diabetes. Can J Diabetes. 2015;39(1):73–7.

Matsuo T. Disappearance of diabetic macular hard exudates after hemodialysis introduction. Acta Med Okayama. 2006;60(3):201–5.

Matsuoka M, Ogata N, Minamino K, et al. Leukostasis and pigment epithelium-derived factor in rat models of diabetic retinopathy. Mol Vis. 2007;13:1058–65.

Mazhar K, Varma R, Choudhury F, et al. Severity of diabetic retinopathy and health-related quality of life: the Los Angeles Latino Eye Study. Ophthalmology. 2011;118(4):649–55.

Mehlsen J, Erlandsen M, Poulsen PL, et al. Individualized optimization of the screening interval for diabetic retinopathy: a new model. Acta Ophthalmol. 2012;90(2):109–14.

Messenger WB, Beardsley RM, Flaxel CJ. Fluocinolone acetonide intravitreal implant for the treatment of diabetic macular edema. Drug Des Devel Ther. 2013;7:425–34.

Meyer-Schwickerath G. Historical perspective of photocoagulation (in retinal vascular diseases). Doc Ophthalmol. 1977;44(1):77–9.

Miller JW, Le CJ, Strauss EC, et al. Vascular endothelial growth factor a in intraocular vascular disease. Ophthalmology. 2013;120(1):106–14.

Misra A, Bachmann MO, Greenwood RH, et al. Trends in yield and effects of screening intervals during 17 years of a large UK community-based diabetic retinopathy screening programme. Diabet Med. 2009;26(10): 1040–7.

Mitchell P, Bandello F, Schmidt-Erfurth U, et al. The RESTORE study: ranibizumab monotherapy or combined with laser versus laser monotherapy for diabetic macular edema. Ophthalmology. 2011;118(4): 615–25.

Moss SE, Klein R, Klein BE. Ten-year incidence of visual loss in a diabetic population. Ophthalmology. 1994;101(6):1061–70.

Murakami T, Uji A, Ogino K, et al. Association between perifoveal hyperfluorescence and serous retinal detachment in diabetic macular edema. Ophthalmology. 2013;120(12):2596–603.

Nam S, Chesla C, Stotts NA, et al. Barriers to diabetes management: patient and provider factors. Diabetes Res Clin Pract. 2011;93(1):1–9.

Narayan KM, Boyle JP, Thompson TJ, et al. Lifetime risk for diabetes mellitus in the United States. JAMA. 2003;290(14):1884–90.

Narayan KM, Boyle JP, Thompson TJ, et al. Effect of BMI on lifetime risk for diabetes in the U.S. Diabetes Care. 2007;30(6):1562–6.

Navarro A, Pournaras JA, Hoffart L, et al. Vitrectomy may prevent the occurrence of diabetic macular oedema. Acta Ophthalmol. 2010;88(4):483–5.

Nawaz MI, Van RK, Mohammad G, et al. Autocrine CCL2, CXCL4, CXCL9 and CXCL10 signal in retinal endothelial cells and are enhanced in diabetic retinopathy. Exp Eye Res. 2013;109:67–76.

Nehme A, Edelman J. Dexamethasone inhibits high glucose-, TNF-alpha-, and IL-1beta-induced secretion of inflammatory and angiogenic mediators from retinal microvascular pericytes. Invest Ophthalmol Vis Sci. 2008;49(5):2030–8.

Neubauer AS, Langer J, Liegl R, et al. Navigated macular laser decreases retreatment rate for diabetic macular edema: a comparison with conventional macular laser. Clin Ophthalmol. 2013;7:121–8.

Nguyen QD, Brown DM, Marcus DM, et al. Ranibizumab for diabetic macular edema: results from 2 phase III randomized trials: RISE and RIDE. Ophthalmology. 2012;119(4):789–801.

Nguyen-Khoa BA, Goehring EL, Werther W, et al. Hospitalized cardiovascular events in patients with diabetic macular edema. BMC Ophthalmol. 2012;12:11.

Nielsen LR, Pedersen-Bjergaard U, Thorsteinsson B, et al. Hypoglycemia in pregnant women with type 1 diabetes: predictors and role of metabolic control. Diabetes Care. 2008;31(1):9–14.

Nisic F, Turkovic S, Mavija M, et al. Correlation between the findings of optical coherent retinal tomography (OCT), stereo biomicroscopic images from fundus of an eye and values from visual acuity of diabetic macular edema. Acta Inform Med. 2014;22(4):232–6.

Nunes S, Pires I, Rosa A, et al. Microaneurysm turnover is a biomarker for diabetic retinopathy progression to clinically significant macular edema: findings for type 2 diabetics with nonproliferative retinopathy. Ophthalmologica. 2009;223(5):292–7.

Ogata N, Tombran-Tink J, Jo N, et al. Upregulation of pigment epithelium-derived factor after laser photocoagulation. Am J Ophthalmol. 2001;132(3):427–9.

Ola MS, Nawaz MI, Siddiquei MM, et al. Recent advances in understanding the biochemical and molecular mechanism of diabetic retinopathy. J Diabetes Complications. 2012;26(1):56–64.

Olsen TW, Adelman RA, Flaxel CJ, et al. Preferred practice pattern diabetic retinopathy. Am Acad Ophthalmol. 2014.

Ophir A. Full-field 3-D optical coherence tomography imaging and treatment decision in diffuse diabetic macular edema. Invest Ophthalmol Vis Sci. 2014;55(5):3052–3.

Ophir A, Trevino A, Fatum S. Extrafoveal vitreous traction associated with diabetic diffuse macular oedema. Eye (Lond). 2010;24(2):347–53.

Ostri C, Lux A, Lund-Andersen H, et al. Long-term results, prognostic factors and cataract surgery after diabetic vitrectomy: a 10-year follow-up study. Acta Ophthalmol. 2014;92(6):571–6.

Palermo A, Maggi D, Maurizi AR, et al. Prevention of type 2 diabetes mellitus: is it feasible? Diabetes Metab Res Rev. 2014;30 Suppl 1:4–12.

Panozzo G, Parolini B, Gusson E, et al. Diabetic macular edema: an OCT-based classification. Semin Ophthalmol. 2004;19(1–2):13–20.

Park JH, Woo SJ, Ha YJ, et al. Effect of vitrectomy on macular microcirculation in patients with diffuse diabetic macular edema. Graefes Arch Clin Exp Ophthalmol. 2009;247(8):1009–17.

Park YG, Kim EY, Roh YJ. Laser-based strategies to treat diabetic macular edema: history and new promising therapies. J Ophthalmol. 2014;2014:769213.

Parravano M, Menchini F, Virgili G. Antiangiogenic therapy with anti-vascular endothelial growth factor modalities for diabetic macular oedema. Cochrane Database Syst Rev. 2009;4:CD007419.

Patel JI, Hykin PG, Schadt M, et al. Pars plana vitrectomy with and without peeling of the inner limiting membrane for diabetic macular edema. Retina. 2006; 26(1):5–13.

Paz SH, Varma R, Klein R, et al. Noncompliance with vision care guidelines in Latinos with type 2 diabetes mellitus: the Los Angeles Latino Eye Study. Ophthalmology. 2006;113(8):1372–7.

Pearce E, Sivaprasad S, Chong NV. Factors affecting reading speed in patients with diabetic macular edema treated with laser photocoagulation. PLoS One. 2014; 9(9):e105696.

Pearson PA, Comstock TL, Ip M, et al. Fluocinolone acetonide intravitreal implant for diabetic macular edema: a 3-year multicenter, randomized, controlled clinical trial. Ophthalmology. 2011;118(8):1580–7.

Pei-Pei W, Shi-Zhou H, Zhen T, et al. Randomised clinical trial evaluating best-corrected visual acuity and central macular thickness after 532-nm subthreshold laser grid photocoagulation treatment in diabetic macular oedema. Eye (Lond). 2015;29(3):313–22.

Pelletier EM, Shim B, Ben-Joseph R, et al. Economic outcomes associated with microvascular complications of type 2 diabetes mellitus: results from a US claims data analysis. Pharmacoeconomics. 2009;27(6):479–90.

Perreault L, Pan Q, Mather KJ, et al. Effect of regression from prediabetes to normal glucose regulation on long-term reduction in diabetes risk: results from the Diabetes Prevention Program Outcomes Study. Lancet. 2012;379(9833):2243–51.

Pershing S, Enns EA, Matesic B, et al. Cost-effectiveness of treatment of diabetic macular edema. Ann Intern Med. 2014;160(1):18–29.

Pfeiffer A, Spranger J, Meyer-Schwickerath R, et al. Growth factor alterations in advanced diabetic retinopathy: a possible role of blood retina barrier breakdown. Diabetes. 1997;46 Suppl 2:S26–30.

Phelps RL, Sakol P, Metzger BE, et al. Changes in diabetic retinopathy during pregnancy. Correlations with regulation of hyperglycemia. Arch Ophthalmol. 1986;104(12):1806–10.

Pires I, Santos AR, Nunes S, et al. Subclinical macular edema as a predictor of progression to clinically significant macular edema in type 2 diabetes. Ophthalmologica. 2013;230(4):201–6.

Pokroy R, Desai UR, Du E, et al. Bevacizumab prior to vitrectomy for diabetic traction retinal detachment. Eye (Lond). 2011;25(8):989–97.

Qi HP, Bi S, Wei SQ, et al. Intravitreal versus subtenon triamcinolone acetonide injection for diabetic macular edema: a systematic review and meta-analysis. Curr Eye Res. 2012;37(12):1136–47.

Qiao Q, Keinanen-Kiukaanniemi S, Laara E. The relationship between hemoglobin levels and diabetic retinopathy. J Clin Epidemiol. 1997;50(2):153–8.

Rahman W, Rahman FZ, Yassin S, et al. Progression of retinopathy during pregnancy in type 1 diabetes mellitus. Clin Experiment Ophthalmol. 2007;35(3):231–6.

Rajendram R, Fraser-Bell S, Kaines A, et al. A 2-year prospective randomized controlled trial of intravitreal bevacizumab or laser therapy (BOLT) in the management of diabetic macular edema: 24-month data: report 3. Arch Ophthalmol. 2012;130(8):972–9.

Rangasamy S, McGuire PG, Franco NC, et al. Chemokine mediated monocyte trafficking into the retina: role of inflammation in alteration of the blood-retinal barrier in diabetic retinopathy. PLoS One. 2014;9(10): e108508.

Rasmussen KL, Laugesen CS, Ringholm L, et al. Progression of diabetic retinopathy during pregnancy in women with type 2 diabetes. Diabetologia. 2010;53(6):1076–83.

Raum P, Peto T, Pfeiffer N, Wild P, Hoehn R, Ponto K, Schneider A, Schulz A, Lamparter J, Mirshahi A. Prevalence and cardiovascular risk factors of diabetic retinopathy: results from the Gutenberg Health Study. Invest Ophthalmol Vis Sci. 2014;55:5339 (Abstract).

Regnier S, Malcolm W, Allen F, et al. Efficacy of anti-VEGF and laser photocoagulation in the treatment of visual impairment due to diabetic macular edema: a systematic review and network meta-analysis. PLoS One. 2014;9(7):e102309.

Ringholm L, Mathiesen ER, Kelstrup L, et al. Managing type 1 diabetes mellitus in pregnancy—from planning to breastfeeding. Nat Rev Endocrinol. 2012;8(11): 659–67.

Robinson R, Barathi VA, Chaurasia SS, et al. Update on animal models of diabetic retinopathy: from molecular approaches to mice and higher mammals. Dis Model Mech. 2012;5(4):444–56.

Rodrigues M, Xin X, Jee K, et al. VEGF secreted by hypoxic Muller cells induces MMP-2 expression and activity in endothelial cells to promote retinal neovascularization in proliferative diabetic retinopathy. Diabetes. 2013;62(11):3863–73.

Roider J, Brinkmann R, Wirbelauer C, et al. Subthreshold (retinal pigment epithelium) photocoagulation in macular diseases: a pilot study. Br J Ophthalmol. 2000; 84(1):40–7.

Roider J, Liew SH, Klatt C, et al. Selective retina therapy (SRT) for clinically significant diabetic macular edema. Graefes Arch Clin Exp Ophthalmol. 2010; 248(9):1263–72.

Romano MR, Gibran SK, Marticorena J, et al. Can a preoperative bevacizumab injection prevent recurrent postvitrectomy diabetic vitreous haemorrhage? Eye (Lond). 2009;23(8):1698–701.

Romero-Aroca P, Sagarra-Alamo R, Basora-Gallisa J, et al. Prospective comparison of two methods of screening for diabetic retinopathy by nonmydriatic fundus camera. Clin Ophthalmol. 2010;4:1481–8.

Rosberger DF. Diabetic retinopathy: current concepts and emerging therapy. Endocrinol Metab Clin North Am. 2013;42(4):721–45.

Roy MS, Klein R. Macular edema and retinal hard exudates in African Americans with type 1 diabetes: the New Jersey 725. Arch Ophthalmol. 2001;119(2):251–9.

Russo A, Morescalchi F, Costagliola C, et al. Comparison of smartphone ophthalmoscopy with slit-lamp biomicroscopy for grading diabetic retinopathy. Am J Ophthalmol. 2015;159(2):360–4.

Sacu S, Pemp B, Weigert G, et al. Response of retinal vessels and retrobulbar hemodynamics to intravitreal anti-VEGF treatment in eyes with branch retinal vein occlusion. Invest Ophthalmol Vis Sci. 2011;52(6):3046–50.

Sander B, Larsen M, Engler C, et al. Early changes in diabetic retinopathy: capillary loss and blood-retina barrier permeability in relation to metabolic control. Acta Ophthalmol (Copenh). 1994;72(5):553–9.

Sander B, Best J, Johansen S, et al. Fluorescein transport through the blood-aqueous and blood-retinal barriers in diabetic macular edema. Curr Eye Res. 2003;27(4):247–52.

Santos JM, Mohammad G, Zhong Q, et al. Diabetic retinopathy, superoxide damage and antioxidants. Curr Pharm Biotechnol. 2011;12(3):352–61.

Scanlon PH, Aldington SJ, Stratton IM. Epidemiological issues in diabetic retinopathy. Middle East Afr J Ophthalmol. 2013;20(4):293–300.

Scaramuzzi M, Querques G, Spina C, et al. Repeated intravitreal dexamethasone implant for diabetic macular edema. Retina. 2015;35:1216–22.

Schiffman RM, Jacobsen G, Nussbaum JJ, et al. Comparison of a digital retinal imaging system and seven-field stereo color fundus photography to detect diabetic retinopathy in the primary care environment. Ophthalmic Surg Lasers Imaging. 2005;36(1):46–56.

Schmidt-Erfurth U, Lang GE, Holz FG, et al. Three-year outcomes of individualized ranibizumab treatment in patients with diabetic macular edema: the RESTORE extension study. Ophthalmology. 2014;121(5): 1045–53.

Schultz KL, Birnbaum AD, Goldstein DA. Ocular disease in pregnancy. Curr Opin Ophthalmol. 2005;16(5): 308–14.

Schwartz SG, Brantley Jr MA, Flynn Jr HW. Genetics and diabetic retinopathy. Curr Diabetes Rev. 2013;9(1):86–92.

Schwartz SG, Flynn Jr HW, Scott IU. Emerging drugs for diabetic macular edema. Expert Opin Emerg Drugs. 2014;19(3):397–405.

Sebag J. Abnormalities of human vitreous structure in diabetes. Graefes Arch Clin Exp Ophthalmol. 1993;231(5):257–60.

Shah SM, Nguyen QD, Mir HS, et al. A randomized, double-masked controlled clinical trial of Sandostatin long-acting release depot in patients with postsurgical cystoid macular edema. Retina. 2010;30(1):160–6.

Sheetz MJ, Aiello LP, Davis MD, et al. The effect of the oral PKC beta inhibitor ruboxistaurin on vision loss in two phase 3 studies. Invest Ophthalmol Vis Sci. 2013;54(3):1750–7.

Shin HJ, Shin KC, Chung H, et al. Change of retinal nerve fiber layer thickness in various retinal diseases treated with multiple intravitreal antivascular endothelial growth factor. Invest Ophthalmol Vis Sci. 2014; 55(4):2403–11.

Shorb SR. Anemia and diabetic retinopathy. Am J Ophthalmol. 1985;100(3):434–6.

Silva KC, Pinto CC, Biswas SK, et al. Hypertension increases retinal inflammation in experimental diabetes: a possible mechanism for aggravation of diabetic retinopathy by hypertension. Curr Eye Res. 2007;32(6):533–41.

Silva PS, Sun JK, Al-Latayfeh MM, Sanchez CR, Walia S, Tolson AM, Cavallerano JD, Aiello LP. Unawareness of vision threatening diabetic retinopathy and appropriate followup in a tertiary telemedicine eye care program. Invest Ophthalmol Vis Sci. 2010;51:5059 (Abstract).

Silva PS, Cavallerano JD, Haddad NM, et al. Peripheral lesions identified on ultrawide field imaging predict increased risk of diabetic retinopathy progression over 4 years. Ophthalmology. 2015;122(5):949–56.

Sim DA, Keane PA, Zarranz-Ventura J, et al. Predictive factors for the progression of diabetic macular ischemia. Am J Ophthalmol. 2013a;156(4):684–92.

Sim DA, Keane PA, Zarranz-Ventura J, et al. The effects of macular ischemia on visual acuity in diabetic retinopathy. Invest Ophthalmol Vis Sci. 2013b;54(3): 2353–60.

Sim DA, Keane PA, Fung S, et al. Quantitative analysis of diabetic macular ischemia using optical coherence tomography. Invest Ophthalmol Vis Sci. 2014; 55(1):417–23.

Simha A, Braganza A, Abraham L, et al. Anti-vascular endothelial growth factor for neovascular glaucoma. Cochrane Database Syst Rev. 2013;10:CD007920.

Simo R, Roy S, Behar-Cohen F, et al. Fenofibrate: a new treatment for diabetic retinopathy. Molecular mechanisms and future perspectives. Curr Med Chem. 2013;20(26):3258–66.

Simunovic MP, Hunyor AP, Ho IV. Vitrectomy for diabetic macular edema: a systematic review and meta-analysis. Can J Ophthalmol. 2014;49(2):188–95.

Sivak-Callcott JA, O'Day DM, Gass JD, et al. Evidence-based recommendations for the diagnosis and treatment of neovascular glaucoma. Ophthalmology. 2001;108(10): 1767–76.

Snead DR, James S, Snead MP. Pathological changes in the vitreoretinal junction 1: epiretinal membrane formation. Eye (Lond). 2008;22(10):1310–7.

Snow V, Weiss KB, Mottur-Pilson C. The evidence base for tight blood pressure control in the management of type 2 diabetes mellitus. Ann Intern Med. 2003;138(7):587–92.

Sohn EH, He S, Kim LA, et al. Angiofibrotic response to vascular endothelial growth factor inhibition in diabetic retinal detachment: report no. 1. Arch Ophthalmol. 2012;130(9):1127–34.

Sonoda S, Sakamoto T, Shirasawa M, et al. Correlation between reflectivity of subretinal fluid in OCT images and concentration of intravitreal VEGF in eyes with diabetic macular edema. Invest Ophthalmol Vis Sci. 2013;54(8):5367–74.

Sophie R, Lu N, Campochiaro PA. Predictors of functional and anatomic outcomes in patients with diabetic macular edema treated with Ranibizumab. Ophthalmology. 2015;122:1395–401.

Stamler J, Vaccaro O, Neaton JD, et al. Diabetes, other risk factors, and 12-yr cardiovascular mortality for men screened in the multiple risk factor intervention trial. Diabetes Care. 1993;16(2):434–44.

Stefansson E. Ocular oxygenation and the treatment of diabetic retinopathy. Surv Ophthalmol. 2006;51(4): 364–80.

Stewart MW. Anti-VEGF therapy for diabetic macular edema. Curr Diab Rep. 2014;14(8):510.

Stitt AW. AGEs and diabetic retinopathy. Invest Ophthalmol Vis Sci. 2010;51(10):4867–74.

Su CC, Yang CH, Yeh PT, et al. Macular tractional retinoschisis in proliferative diabetic retinopathy: clinical characteristics and surgical outcome. Ophthalmologica. 2014;231(1):23–30.

Tahrani AA, Bailey CJ, Del PS, et al. Management of type 2 diabetes: new and future developments in treatment. Lancet. 2011;378(9786):182–97.

Tamborlane WV, Beck RW, Bode BW, et al. Continuous glucose monitoring and intensive treatment of type 1 diabetes. N Engl J Med. 2008;359(14):1464–76.

Tang J, Kern TS. Inflammation in diabetic retinopathy. Prog Retin Eye Res. 2011;30(5):343–58.

Tarr JM, Kaul K, Chopra M, et al. Pathophysiology of diabetic retinopathy. ISRN Ophthalmol. 2013;2013: 343560.

Taylor E, Dobree JH. Proliferative diabetic retinopathy. Site and size of initial lesions. Br J Ophthalmol. 1970;54(1):11–8.

The Diabetes Control and Complications Trial/Epidemiology of Diabetes Interventions and Complications Research Group. Retinopathy and nephropathy in patients with type 1 diabetes four years after a trial of intensive therapy. N Engl J Med. 2000;342(6):381–9.

The Royal College of Ophthalmologists. Diabetic Retinopathy Guidelines. London: Royal College of Ophthalmologists; 2012.

Theodossiadis PG, Theodoropoulou S, Neamonitou G, et al. Hemodialysis-induced alterations in macular thickness measured by optical coherence tomography in diabetic patients with end-stage renal disease. Ophthalmologica. 2012;227(2):90–4.

Thulliez M, Angoulvant D, Le Lez ML, et al. Cardiovascular events and bleeding risk associated with intravitreal antivascular endothelial growth factor monoclonal antibodies: systematic review and meta-analysis. JAMA Ophthalmol. 2014;132(11): 1317–26.

Tokuyama T, Ikeda T, Sato K. Effects of haemodialysis on diabetic macular leakage. Br J Ophthalmol. 2000; 84(12):1397–400.

Ugurlu N, Gerceker S, Yulek F, et al. The levels of the circulating cellular adhesion molecules ICAM-1, VCAM-1 and endothelin-1 and the flow-mediated vasodilatation values in patients with type 1 diabetes mellitus with early-stage diabetic retinopathy. Intern Med. 2013;52(19):2173–8.

UK Prospective Diabetes Study (UKPDS) Group. Tight blood pressure control and risk of macrovascular and microvascular complications in type 2 diabetes: UKPDS 38. BMJ. 1998;317(7160):703–13.

Varma R, Torres M, Pena F, et al. Prevalence of diabetic retinopathy in adult Latinos: the Los Angeles Latino eye study. Ophthalmology. 2004;111(7):1298–306.

Venkatesh P, Ramanjulu R, Azad R, et al. Subthreshold micropulse diode laser and double frequency neodymium: YAG laser in treatment of diabetic macular edema: a prospective, randomized study using multifocal electroretinography. Photomed Laser Surg. 2011;29(11):727–33.

Verma A, Raman R, Vaitheeswaran K, et al. Does neuronal damage precede vascular damage in subjects with type 2 diabetes mellitus and having no clinical diabetic retinopathy? Ophthalmic Res. 2012;47(4):202–7.

Vestgaard M, Ringholm L, Laugesen CS, et al. Pregnancy-induced sight-threatening diabetic retinopathy in women with type 1 diabetes. Diabet Med. 2010; 27(4):431–5.

Vijan S, Hofer TP, Hayward RA. Cost-utility analysis of screening intervals for diabetic retinopathy in patients with type 2 diabetes mellitus. JAMA. 2000;283(7): 889–96.

Virgili G, Parravano M, Menchini F, et al. Anti-vascular endothelial growth factor for diabetic macular oedema. Cochrane Database Syst Rev. 2014;10:CD007419.

Voykov B, Bartz-Schmidt KU. Dislocation of dexamethasone intravitreous implant. Arch Ophthalmol. 2012;130(6):706.

Vujosevic S, Bini S, Midena G, et al. Hyperreflective intraretinal spots in diabetics without and with nonproliferative diabetic retinopathy: an in vivo study using spectral domain OCT. J Diabetes Res. 2013;2013:491835.

Wang H, Chhablani J, Freeman WR, et al. Characterization of diabetic microaneurysms by simultaneous fluorescein angiography and spectral-domain optical coherence tomography. Am J Ophthalmol. 2012a; 153(5):861–7.

Wang ZY, Zhao KK, Zhao DS, et al. Dissection under perfluorocarbon liquid: a modified vitrectomy technique for diabetic tractional retinal detachment. Retina. 2012b;32(4):848–52.

Wang Y, Muqit MM, Stanga PE, et al. Spatial changes of central field loss in diabetic retinopathy after laser. Optom Vis Sci. 2014;91(1):111–20.

Wells JA, Glassman AR, Ayala AR, et al. Aflibercept, bevacizumab, or ranibizumab for diabetic macular edema. N Engl J Med. 2015;372(13):1193–203.

West SK, Klein R, Rodriguez J, et al. Diabetes and diabetic retinopathy in a Mexican-American population: Proyecto VER. Diabetes Care. 2001; 24(7):1204–9.

Wilson DJ, Finkelstein D, Quigley HA, et al. Macular grid photocoagulation. An experimental study on the primate retina. Arch Ophthalmol. 1988;106(1):100–5.

Witkin SR, Klein R. Ophthalmologic care for persons with diabetes. JAMA. 1984;251(19):2534–7.

Wong CW, Wong TY, Cheng CY, et al. Kidney and eye diseases: common risk factors, etiological mechanisms, and pathways. Kidney Int. 2014;85(6): 1290–302.

Yalvac IS, Eksioglu U, Satana B, et al. Long-term results of Ahmed glaucoma valve and Molteno implant in neovascular glaucoma. Eye (Lond). 2007;21(1): 65–70.

Yamagishi S, Ueda S, Matsui T, et al. Role of advanced glycation end products (AGEs) and oxidative stress in diabetic retinopathy. Curr Pharm Des. 2008;14(10): 962–8.

Yamamoto T, Takeuchi S, Sato Y, et al. Long-term followup results of pars plana vitrectomy for diabetic macular edema. Jpn J Ophthalmol. 2007;51(4):285–91.

Yau JW, Rogers SL, Kawasaki R, et al. Global prevalence and major risk factors of diabetic retinopathy. Diabetes Care. 2012;35(3):556–64.

Yilmaz T, Weaver CD, Gallagher MJ, et al. Intravitreal triamcinolone acetonide injection for treatment of refractory diabetic macular edema: a systematic review. Ophthalmology. 2009;116(5):902–11.

Yuen J, Clark A, Ng JQ, et al. Further survey of Australian ophthalmologist's diabetic retinopathy management: did practice adhere to National Health and Medical Research Council guidelines? Clin Exp Ophthalmol. 2010;38(6):613–9.

Zabetian A, Keli HM, Echouffo-Tcheugui JB, et al. Diabetes in the Middle East and North Africa. Diabetes Res Clin Pract. 2013;101(2):106–22.

Zandbergen AA, Vogt L, de ZD, et al. Change in albuminuria is predictive of cardiovascular outcome in normotensive patients with type 2 diabetes and microalbuminuria. Diabetes Care. 2007;30(12):3119–21.

Zechmeister-Koss I, Huic M. Vascular endothelial growth factor inhibitors (anti-VEGF) in the management of diabetic macular oedema: a systematic review. Br J Ophthalmol. 2012;96(2):167–78.

Zenoni S, Comi N, Fontana P. Individualised treatment of proliferative diabetic retinopathy: optimal surgical timing improves long-term outcomes. EPMA J. 2010;1(1):78–81.

Zhang W, Liu H, Rojas M, et al. Anti-inflammatory therapy for diabetic retinopathy. Immunotherapy. 2011;3(5):609–28.

Zhang L, Chen B, Tang L. Metabolic memory: mechanisms and implications for diabetic retinopathy. Diabetes Res Clin Pract. 2012;96(3):286–93.

Zhang X, Zhao J, Zhao T, et al. Effects of intensive glycemic control in ocular complications in patients with type 2 diabetes: a meta-analysis of randomized clinical trials. Endocrine. 2015;49:78–89.

Zheng Y, Kwong MT, Maccormick IJ, et al. A comprehensive texture segmentation framework for segmentation of capillary non-perfusion regions in fundus fluorescein angiograms. PLoS One. 2014;9(4): e93624.

Zhong Y, Li J, Chen Y, et al. Activation of endoplasmic reticulum stress by hyperglycemia is essential for Muller cell-derived inflammatory cytokine production in diabetes. Diabetes. 2012;61(2):492–504.

Zhu Y, Zhang T, Wang K, et al. Changes in choroidal thickness after panretinal photocoagulation in patients with type 2 diabetes. Retina. 2015;35(4):695–703.

Zucchiatti I, Lattanzio R, Querques G, et al. Intravitreal dexamethasone implant in patients with persistent diabetic macular edema. Ophthalmologica. 2012; 228(2):117–22.

Retinal Vein Occlusion

7

Amelie Pielen, Bernd Junker, and Nicolas Feltgen

7.1 Epidemiology and Clinical Features

Retinal vein occlusion (RVO) is the second most common vascular eye disorder after diabetic retinopathy. The prevalence of RVO is 5.2 per 1000 estimated from studies in the United States, Europe, Asia, and Australia. Branch retinal vein occlusion (BRVO) occurs more often than central retinal vein occlusion (CRVO) (4.42 versus 0.80 per 1000, respectively) (Rogers et al. 2010). The incidence rises with age and was reported to be 0.7 % under the age of 60 years compared to 4.6 % over 80 years (Rogers et al. 2010).

Clinical characteristics are dilated and engorged retinal veins, macular edema, retinal hemorrhages, retinal ischemia manifested as cotton-wool spots and peripheral ischemia visible in fluorescein angiography as capillary nonperfusion. Macular edema results in impairment of visual acuity (VA) while ischemia leads to neovascularization of the iris and of the retina. Untreated ischemic RVO may result in vitreous hemorrhage and secondary glaucoma. The longer the duration of macular edema, the more damage is done to photoreceptors and retinal pigment epithelium (Lardenoye et al. 2000). Anti-vascular endothelial growth factor (VEGF) therapy leads to prompt resolution of macular edema and early treatment may therefore result in significantly better results than delayed treatment (Pielen et al. 2013).

7.2 Pathophysiology

The exact etiology of RVO is still unknown. Patients with RVO often present with risk factors associated with arterial vascular diseases, and pathophysiology differs from systemic vein occlusions such as deep vein thrombosis (Hayreh 1994; Cugati et al. 2006). It is supposed that the process starts with a compression of the vein wall. BRVO typically occurs at arteriovenous crossings (Feltgen et al. 2010) and CRVO at the level of the lamina cribrosa (Hayreh et al. 1994). The compression causes turbulence and reduction of the venous blood flow which leads to partial thrombus formation. As a consequence, flow is further reduced, venous pressure rises and blood and plasma exudate into the surrounding tissue causing edema. In the later stages, reduced retinal perfusion causes hypoxia that triggers the

A. Pielen (✉) • B. Junker
Hannover Medical School, University Eye Hospital, Carl-Neuberg-Str.1, Hannover 30625, Germany
e-mail: Pielen.Amelie@mh-hannover.de

N. Feltgen
Universitätsmedizin Göttingen, University Eye Hospital, Robert-Koch-Str. 40, Göttingen 37075, Germany

© Springer International Publishing Switzerland 2016
A. Stahl (ed.), *Anti-Angiogenic Therapy in Ophthalmology*, Essentials in Ophthalmology, DOI 10.1007/978-3-319-24097-8_7

transcription of multiple factors, among them VEGF and inflammatory cytokines (Noma et al. 2006; Ehlken et al. 2011). VEGF further increases macular edema and contributes to the formation of neovascularization.

Risk factors for RVO are glaucoma, metabolic syndrome, and its components diabetes mellitus, arterial hypertension, hyperlipidemia, and cigarette smoke (Stem et al. 2013). A higher incidence of CRVO is found in patients with history of stroke and peripheral artery disease (Stem et al. 2013; Zhou et al. 2013). Increased levels of atherosclerotic and thrombophilic factors (factor VIII) were found to increase the risk of developing an ischemic CRVO (Sodi et al. 2011). Therapy in RVO patients should therefore not only focus on ocular treatment but also include a systematic work-up to identify any underlying systemic disease and initiate or optimize treatment of systemic risk factors.

7.3 Intravitreal Therapy

Visual impairment due to macular edema is treated with anti-inflammatory and antiangiogenic intravitreal agents targeting vascular permeability and leakage. Substances currently in clinical use are either corticosteroids or anti-VEGF.

7.3.1 Corticosteroids

Triamcinolone acetonide, dexamethasone, and fluocinolone have been investigated in eyes affected with macular edema due to RVO (Ip et al. 2009; Scott et al. 2009; Haller et al. 2010; Jain et al. 2012). Corticosteroids reduce the expression of VEGF, act as anti-inflammatory agents, inhibit vascular permeability, leakage, and the breakdown of the blood–retinal barrier (Zhang et al. 2008; Wang et al. 2008; McAllister et al. 2009; Kunikata et al. 2012). A direct neuroprotective effect was reported (Jeanneteau et al. 2008). Intravitreal treatment with corticosteroids improves VA by reducing macular edema. Main

drawbacks are cataract progression and rise in intraocular pressure (IOP).

7.3.1.1 Dexamethasone

Dexamethasone is a potent soluble corticosteroid, but half-life after intravitreal injection is very short. The development of a sustained-release biodegradable implant (Ozurdex®, Pharm Allergan GmbH) overcame this deficit. Results of the randomized controlled clinical trial (RCT) GENEVA (Global Evaluation of Implantable Dexamethasone in Retinal Vein Occlusion with Macular Edema) led to approval of Ozurdex 0.7 mg by FDA and EMA for the treatment of macular edema due to RVO (Haller et al. 2010, 2011).

Results of GENEVA: A single application of Ozurdex 0.7 mg was compared to Ozurdex 0.35 mg versus sham injection over 6 months. During the second 6 months, Ozurdex 0.7 mg was given in an open extension of the study. Ozurdex 0.7 mg reduced macular edema and led to a three-line improvement in best-corrected VA (BCVA) in 29.6 % of patients at day 60 compared to 12.5 % in the sham group ($p < 0.001$). The maximum effect as well as the maximum rise in IOP were seen at 2 months after injection and decreased thereafter. Consequently, evaluation of 12-month data showed no significant difference in BCVA (Pielen et al. 2013). Regarding adverse events, cataract progression was observed in 10.7 % of patients receiving one implant (sham/0.7 mg Ozurdex) compared to 29.8 % of patients after two Ozurdex 0.7 mg implants versus 5.7 % of sham patients (Haller et al. 2011; Pielen et al. 2013). IOP rise occurred in every third patient after Ozurdex implant at day 60 and was most often treated with local anti-glaucomatous therapy, but 1.3 % of patients underwent glaucoma surgery (versus none in sham-treated patients).

Duration of macular edema has a direct impact on the results of intravitreal treatment. In GENEVA, only 16.4 % of patients were treated after a disease duration <3 months, the majority presented with macular edema duration between 3 and 6 months (51.3 %) or longer (32.3 %). In trials investigating triamcinolone (SCORE BRVO/CRVO) and anti-VEGF agents (BRAVO, CRUISE, GALILEO, COPERNICUS) the proportion of patients with a duration of macular edema <3 months was significantly higher: SCORE BRVO > 50 %, SCORE CRVO 36 %, BRAVO 51.5–53.8 %, CRUISE 51.5–61.5 %. Secondary analysis of all trials shows that early treatment of macular edema secondary to RVO is more effective than delayed treatment (Coscas et al. 2011; Pielen et al. 2013). Therefore, intravitreal agents should be compared in head-to-head trials guaranteeing comparable baseline characteristics of patient populations and results of different RCTs should be compared with caution.

7.3.1.2 Fluocinolone

A fluocinolone implant is under investigation that showed efficacy up to 36 months after single application (Jain et al. 2012). Results in 24 eyes of 23 patients with chronic macular edema due to CRVO showed improvement of BCVA of 4.5 letters at 12 months, 8.2 at 24 months, and 3.4 at 36 months. Reduction of central retinal thickness was sustained. During the 3 years, all phakic eyes underwent cataract surgery and 5/24 eyes received glaucoma surgery. The fluocinolone implant is approved for second-line treatment in diabetic macular edema but not in RVO.

7.3.1.3 Triamcinolone Acetonide

Intravitreal injection of triamcinolone acetonide is off-label use. Triamcinolone is crystalline and is either injected in formulations with METHOCEL or as commercially available Kenalog® (Bristol-Myers Squibb) or Trivaris® (Pharm Allergan, Inc.).

The Standard Care versus Corticosteroid for Retinal Vein Occlusion (SCORE) study investigated intravitreal triamcinolone 1 mg versus 4 mg versus observation in CRVO and versus grid laser coagulation in BRVO (Ip et al. 2009; Scott et al. 2009). Retreatment could be given every 4 months. In SCORE CRVO, triamcinolone

led to a significantly higher percentage of visual gain (≥15 letters) in 26.5 % (1 mg), 25.6 % (4 mg) compared to sham treatment (6.8 %, $p = 0.001$). BCVA did not increase but was stabilized at baseline levels in triamcinolone groups, while sham patients lost BCVA. SCORE BRVO did not show a significant difference in VA gain at 12 months (26 % 1 mg, 27 % 4 mg, 29 % grid laser coagulation). Regarding adverse events, SCORE investigators found IOP rise and cataract progression as most frequent events. The adverse effects seem to be dose dependent, 20 % of patients who received 1 mg triamcinolone needed antiglaucomatous medication versus 35 % of patients in the 4 mg group (8 % observation). Glaucoma surgery was performed in 2.2 % (1 mg) and 4 % (4 mg).

7.3.2 VEGF-Inhibitors

Anti-VEGF agents act specifically: Bevacizumab (Avastin®, Roche) and ranibizumab (Lucentis®, Novartis) inhibit VEGF-A, pegaptanib sodium (Macugen®, Pfizer) binds to the isoform 165 of VEGF-A, aflibercept (Eylea®, Bayer Health Care) is a receptor fusion protein which binds all VEGF-A isoforms and placental growth factor (PlGF). The primary effect of anti-VEGF in RVO is not antiangiogenic but agents reduce vessel permeability and macular edema leading to improvement of VA.

VEGF levels are increased after CRVO and BRVO and vitreous levels of VEGF as well as interleukin-1 correlate with the amount of macular edema (Noma et al. 2005, 2006, 2008). There is evidence that different splicing variants of VEGF 165 might act controversial as either pro-angiogenic isoform (VEGF 165) or antiangiogenic isoform (VEGF 165b) (Harper and Bates 2008). In vitreous samples of RVO patients, the ratio of VEGF 165b/VEGF 165 was altered towards a pro-angiogenic shift in correlation to the severity of the occlusion (Ehlken et al. 2011). Targeting different isoforms of VEGF might be a feasible approach in the future.

7.3.2.1 Ranibizumab

Safety and efficacy of ranibizumab were investigated in the CRUISE (Ranibizumab for the Treatment of Macular Edema After Central Retinal Vein Occlusion Study) and BRAVO (Ranibizumab for the Treatment of Macular Edema Following Branch Retinal Vein Occlusion) RCTs (Brown et al. 2010; Campochiaro et al. 2010). In both pivotal trials, 6 monthly intravitreal injections of ranibizumab 0.5 mg (or 0.3 mg) were superior to sham injections and led to improvement of BCVA of +14.9 letters (CRVO 0.5 mg) and +18.3 letters (BRVO 0.5 mg) compared to sham (CRVO 0.8 letters, BRVO +7.3 letters, Table 7.1). Improvement could be stabilized over a second period of 6 months by pro re nata injections (CRVO +13.9 letters, BRVO +18.3 letters) (Brown et al. 2011; Campochiaro et al. 2011). Patients in sham groups received intravitreal ranibizumab 0.5 mg from month 6 onward. This delay in treatment of macular edema led to a significantly reduced response at month 12 (CRVO sham/ranibizumab 0.5 mg +7.3 letters, BRVO +12.1 letters sham/ranibizumab 0.5 mg) compared to 6-month data supporting the hypothesis that long-standing macular edema leads to irreversible structural damages. The rate of ocular and systemic adverse events was low, especially no signs of an increased incidence of arteriothrombotic events were noted.

Ranibizumab patients were followed up until 2 years in the HORIZON trial and showed sustained visual improvement with a relatively low mean number of ranibizumab injection in year 2 (CRVO 3.5/0.5 mg and 2.9/sham+0.5 mg; BRVO 2.1/0.5 mg and 2/sham+0.5 mg) (Heier et al. 2012). The longest follow-up currently is 48 months in the RETAIN study (Campochiaro et al. 2014). Visual improvement at 6 months could be maintained until 48 months in both CRVO (+14.0 letters) and BRVO (+20.1 letters). The percentage of patients with complete resolution of macular edema over ≥ 6 months was 50 % (BRVO) and 44 % (CRVO), of these patients, 76 % (BRVO) and 71 % (CRVO) had received their last ranibizumab injection within ≤ 2 years. The response to intravitreal ranibizumab might hint at the prognosis for VA development: Improvement of VA was significantly higher in patients presenting with completely resolved macular edema versus unresolved edema over 48 months (BRVO +25.9/+17.1 letters resolved/unresolved, CRVO +25.2/+4.3 letters, respectively). Mean number of injections was 3.2 (BRVO) and 5.9 (CRVO) in year 4.

Table 7.1 Change in best-corrected visual acuity in letters in randomized controlled trials (RCT) investigating anti-VEGF agents for macular edema secondary to central retinal vein occlusion

RCT	Agent	6 months		12 months		24 months		48 months
CRUISE (1)	Ranibizumab	+14.9		+13.9	HORIZON (2)	+12.0	RETAIN (3)	+14.0
	Sham	+0.8	Sham + Ran.	+7.3		+7.6		
Epstein (4)	Bevacizumab	+14.1		+16.0				
	Sham	−2.0	Sham + Bev.	+4.6				
COPERNICUS (5)	Aflibercept	+17.3		+16.2		+13.0		
	sham	−4.0	Sham + Afl.	+3.8		+1.5		
GALILEO (6)	Aflibercept	+18.0		+16.9		+13.1		
	Sham	+3.3		+3.8	Sham + Afl.	+6.2		

(1) Brown et al. (2010), Campochiaro et al. (2011), (2) Heier et al. (2012), (3) Campochiaro et al. (2014), (4) Epstein et al. (2012a, b), (5) Boyer et al. (2012), Brown et al. (2013), Heier et al. (2014), (6) Holz et al. (2013), Korobelnik et al. (2014), Ogura et al. (2014)

Comparison to Grid Laser Treatment in BRVO

BRAVO did not compare intravitreal ranibizumab to the gold standard of grid laser photocoagulation set forth by the Branch Vein Occlusion Study (1984). Two investigator-initiated RCTs overcame this gap of knowledge (Tan et al. 2014; Pielen et al. 2014). Tan et al. found that BCVA at 12 months was significantly higher after ranibizumab (6 monthly + PRN, +12.5 letters) compared to standard-of-care grid laser treatment (−1.6 letters). Rate of additional grid laser treatment was low in the ranibizumab group at 13 and 25 weeks (6.7 %, 8.3 % versus 68.4 %, 50 % in controls). Ranibizumab for Branch Retinal Vein Occlusion Associated Macular Edema Study (RABAMES) compared ranibizumab (3 monthly injections + observation) with grid laser (at baseline and 8 weeks optional) versus a combination (Pielen et al. 2014). Best results were found in anti-VEGF-treated patients. The combination of ranibizumab and grid laser did not lead to an additional effect and did not protect from recurrence of macular edema.

7.3.2.2 Bevacizumab

There are many publications on off-label bevacizumab in RVO indicating similar results compared to ranibizumab in RVO, but the evidence level is low due to predominantly retrospective clinical observations. There is one RCT investigating bevacizumab every 6 weeks versus sham until month 6 in macular edema due to CRVO with an open label extension until month 12 (Epstein et al. 2012a, b). BCVA significantly increased in the bevacizumab group versus sham (6 months: +14.1 versus −2.0 letters, Table 7.1) (Epstein et al. 2012b). Previously sham-treated patients did not improve as pronounced during the 6-month extension (12 months: +16.0 versus +4.6 letters), mimicking CRUISE results.

7.3.2.3 Pegaptanib

Pegaptanib sodium was investigated for macular edema secondary to CRVO and BRVO in phase II dose-ranging RCTs but was not investigated further and was not approved by FDA or EMA (Wroblewski et al. 2009, 2010). In CRVO, VA gain ≥15 letters at month 6 was not significantly higher in pegaptanib groups compared to sham (36 %/0.3 mg versus 39 %/1 mg versus 28 %/sham) (Wroblewski et al. 2009). In BRVO, pegaptanib 0.3 mg and 1 mg led to BCVA improvement of +14 letters, but the study lacked comparison to sham (Wroblewski et al. 2010).

7.3.2.4 Aflibercept

Monthly VEGF Trap-Eye (aflibercept) for macular edema secondary to CRVO was investigated over 6 months compared to sham treatment in the parallel RCTs COPERNICUS and GALILEO (Boyer et al. 2012; Holz et al. 2013). In COPERNICUS, patients from both groups received intravitreal aflibercept on PRN basis from week 24 onward with monthly (weeks 24–52) and quarterly evaluation (weeks 52–100). In GALILEO, sham patients could receive active treatment from week 52 onward, while aflibercept patients received further injections PRN from week 24 onward. Evaluation intervals were monthly (weeks 24–52) and every other month (weeks 52–76).

COPERNICUS: At 6 months, the proportion of patients with VA gain ≥15 letters was 56.1 % for aflibercept 2 mg compared to 12.3 % sham, BCVA improvement was +17.3 letters (aflibercept) versus loss of 4.0 letters (sham, Table 7.1) (Boyer et al. 2012). At 1 year, after all patients could receive intravitreal aflibercept PRN, 55.3 % of aflibercept patients and 30.1 % of sham/aflibercept showed VA gain ≥15 letters (Brown et al. 2013). Again, sham patients did not profit from delayed anti-VEGF treatment as much as patients with prompt treatment, BCVA change at month 12 was +16.2 letters (aflibercept) versus +3.8 letters (sham/aflibercept). At 2 years, VA gain was 49.1 % (aflibercept) versus 23.3 % (sham/aflibercept) and change in BCVA was +13.0 versus +1.5 letters (Heier et al. 2014). Even over the period of 18 months active aflibercept treatment, patients from the sham/aflibercept group did not catch up with those treated from baseline on.

GALILEO: At month 6, the proportion of patients gaining ≥15 letters was 60.2 % (aflibercept 2 mg monthly) versus 22.1 % (sham) (Holz et al. 2013). At month 12, the ratio was similarly pronounced (60.2 %/aflibercept versus 32.4 %/sham) because sham patients received sham injections until week 52 (Korobelnik et al. 2014). From weeks 52 to 76, patients were evaluated every 8 weeks and both groups received aflibercept 2 mg as needed (Ogura et al. 2014). After 12 months of sham treatment, the ratio of patients who gained ≥15 letters remained limited despite aflibercept treatment (29.4 %/sham+aflibercept versus 57.3 % aflibercept), while macular edema reduction was pronounced. One more clinical fact to stress the hypothesis that long-standing edema damages macular function and limits treatment outcome.

7.4 Implications for Clinical Practice

Results from RCTs demonstrate the efficacy and safety of both corticosteroids and anti-VEGF agents for macular edema secondary to RVO. Comparison of 12-month data suggests that VEGF-inhibitors might be superior to corticosteroids, but comparison of results is limited because of the lack of head-to-head trials, differences in duration of macular edema at baseline and different treatment regimens (Pielen et al. 2013). Corticosteroids, especially slow-release devices such as the dexamethasone implant allow elongated injection intervals, but they are accompanied by a relatively high rate of the ocular adverse events cataract progression and glaucoma. Intravitreal anti-VEGF agents come with little ocular and systemic events, but are accompanied by the burden of considerably higher injection frequency and the need for monthly controls in a pro re nata regimen. Long-term results, however, demonstrate that this commitment is worth the effort: the sooner the macular edema is treated, the better the structural response (resolved edema) and the longer the consequent retreatment the better is the prognosis for sustained visual acuity. Factors to predict patients'

response to treatment before the first injection remain to be determined and results of head-to-head studies may provide conclusive results for comparison of the various agents.

Compliance with Ethical Requirements

Author Amelie Pielen has received a speaker honorarium from Pharm Allergan GmbH, Novartis Pharma GmbH and Bayer Health Care. Bernd Junker has received a speaker honorarium from Novartis Pharma GmbH and Bayer Health Care. Nicolas Feltgen received a speaker honorarium from Novartis Pharma GmbH, Pharm Allergan GmbH, Bayer Health Care, and research grants from Novartis Pharma GmbH.

No human or animal studies were carried out by the authors of this chapter.

References

Boyer D, Heier J, Brown DM, et al. Vascular endothelial growth factor Trap-Eye for macular edema secondary to central retinal vein occlusion: six-month results of the phase 3 COPERNICUS study. Ophthalmology. 2012;119:1024–32. doi:10.1016/j.ophtha.2012.01.042.

Branch Vein Occlusion Study Group. Argon laser photocoagulation for macular edema in branch vein occlusion. Am J Ophthalmol. 1984;98:271–82.

Brown DM, Campochiaro PA, Singh RP, et al. Ranibizumab for macular edema following central retinal vein occlusion: six-month primary end point results of a phase III study. Ophthalmology. 2010;117:1124–33.e1. doi:10.1016/j.ophtha.2010.02.022.

Brown DM, Campochiaro PA, Bhisitkul RB, et al. Sustained benefits from ranibizumab for macular edema following branch retinal vein occlusion: 12-month outcomes of a phase III study. Ophthalmology. 2011;118:1594–602. doi:10.1016/j.ophtha.2011.02.022.

Brown DM, Heier JS, Clark WL, et al. Intravitreal aflibercept injection for macular edema secondary to central retinal vein occlusion: 1-year results from the Phase 3 COPERNICUS Study. Am J Ophthalmol. 2013;155:429–7.e7. doi:10.1016/j.ajo.2012.09.026.

Campochiaro PA, Heier JS, Feiner L, et al. Ranibizumab for macular edema following branch retinal vein occlusion: six-month primary end point results of a phase III study. Ophthalmology. 2010;117:1102–12. e1. doi:10.1016/j.ophtha.2010.02.021.

Campochiaro PA, Brown DM, Awh CC, et al. Sustained benefits from ranibizumab for macular edema following central retinal vein occlusion: twelve-month outcomes of a phase III study. Ophthalmology. 2011;118:2041–9. doi:10.1016/j.ophtha.2011.02.038.

Campochiaro PA, Sophie R, Pearlman J, et al. Long-term outcomes in patients with retinal vein occlusion treated with ranibizumab: the RETAIN study. Ophthalmology. 2014;121:209–19. doi:10.1016/j.ophtha.2013.08.038.

Coscas G, Loewenstein A, Augustin A, et al. Management of retinal vein occlusion—consensus document. Ophthalmologica. 2011;226:4–28. doi:10.1159/000327391.

Cugati S, Wang JJ, Rochtchina E, Mitchell P. Ten-year incidence of retinal vein occlusion in an older population: the Blue Mountains Eye Study. Arch Ophthalmol. 2006;124:726–32. doi:10.1001/archopht.124.5.726.

Ehlken C, Rennel ES, Michels D, et al. Levels of VEGF but not VEGF(165b) are increased in the vitreous of patients with retinal vein occlusion. Am J Ophthalmol. 2011;152:298–303.e1. doi:10.1016/j.ajo.2011.01.040.

Epstein DL, Algvere PV, von Wendt G, et al. Benefit from bevacizumab for macular edema in central retinal vein occlusion: twelve-month results of a prospective, randomized study. Ophthalmology. 2012a;119:2587–91. doi:10.1016/j.ophtha.2012.06.037.

Epstein DLJ, Algvere PV, von Wendt G, et al. Bevacizumab for macular edema in central retinal vein occlusion: a prospective, randomized, double-masked clinical study. Ophthalmology. 2012b;119:1184–9. doi:10.1016/j.ophtha.2012.01.022.

Feltgen N, Pielen A, Hansen L, et al. Intravitreal drug therapy for retinal vein occlusion—pathophysiological mechanisms and routinely used drugs. Klin Monbl Augenheilkd. 2010;227:681–93. doi:10.1055/s-0029-1245606.

Haller JA, Bandello F, Belfort Jr R, et al. Randomized, sham-controlled trial of dexamethasone intravitreal implant in patients with macular edema due to retinal vein occlusion. Ophthalmology. 2010;117:1134–46. e1. doi:10.1016/j.ophtha.2010.03.032.

Haller JA, Bandello F, Belfort Jr R, et al. Dexamethasone intravitreal implant in patients with macular edema related to branch or central retinal vein occlusion twelve-month study results. Ophthalmology. 2011;118:2453–60. doi:10.1016/j.ophtha.2011.05.014.

Harper SJ, Bates DO. VEGF-A splicing: the key to anti-angiogenic therapeutics? Nat Rev Cancer. 2008;8:880–7. doi:10.1038/nrc2505.

Hayreh SS. Retinal vein occlusion. Indian J Ophthalmol. 1994;42:109–32.

Hayreh SS, Zimmerman MB, Podhajsky P. Incidence of various types of retinal vein occlusion and their recurrence and demographic characteristics. Am J Ophthalmol. 1994;117:429–41.

Heier JS, Campochiaro PA, Yau L, et al. Ranibizumab for macular edema due to retinal vein occlusions: long-term follow-up in the HORIZON trial. Ophthalmology. 2012;119:802–9. doi:10.1016/j.ophtha.2011.12.005.

Heier JS, Clark WL, Boyer DS, et al. Intravitreal aflibercept injection for macular edema due to central retinal vein occlusion: two-year results from the COPERNICUS study. Ophthalmology. 2014;121:1414–20.e1. doi:10.1016/j.ophtha.2014.01.027.

Holz FG, Roider J, Ogura Y, et al. VEGF Trap-Eye for macular oedema secondary to central retinal vein occlusion: 6-month results of the phase III GALILEO study. Br J Ophthalmol. 2013;97:278–84. doi:10.1136/bjophthalmol-2012-301504.

Ip MS, Scott IU, VanVeldhuisen PC, et al. A randomized trial comparing the efficacy and safety of intravitreal triamcinolone with observation to treat vision loss associated with macular edema secondary to central retinal vein occlusion: the Standard Care vs Corticosteroid for Retinal Vein Occlusion (SCORE) study report 5. Arch Ophthalmol. 2009;127:1101–14. doi:10.1001/archophthalmol.2009.234.

Jain N, Stinnett SS, Jaffe GJ. Prospective study of a fluocinolone acetonide implant for chronic macular edema from central retinal vein occlusion: thirty-six-month results. Ophthalmology. 2012;119:132–7. doi:10.1016/j.ophtha.2011.06.019.

Jeanneteau F, Garabedian MJ, Chao MV. Activation of Trk neurotrophin receptors by glucocorticoids provides a neuroprotective effect. Proc Natl Acad Sci U S A. 2008;105:4862–7. doi:10.1073/pnas.0709102105.

Korobelnik J-F, Holz FG, Roider J, et al. Intravitreal aflibercept injection for macular edema resulting from central retinal vein occlusion: One-year results of the Phase 3 GALILEO study. Ophthalmology. 2014;121:202–8. doi:10.1016/j.ophtha.2013.08.012.

Kunikata H, Shimura M, Nakazawa T, et al. Chemokines in aqueous humour before and after intravitreal triamcinolone acetonide in eyes with macular oedema associated with branch retinal vein occlusion. Acta Ophthalmol. 2012;90:162–7. doi:10.1111/j.1755-3768.2010.01892.x.

Lardenoye CW, Probst K, DeLint PJ, Rothova A. Photoreceptor function in eyes with macular edema. Invest Ophthalmol Vis Sci. 2000;41:4048–53.

McAllister IL, Vijayasekaran S, Chen SD, Yu D-Y. Effect of triamcinolone acetonide on vascular endothelial growth factor and occludin levels in branch retinal vein occlusion. Am J Ophthalmol. 2009;147:838–46. e1–2. doi:10.1016/j.ajo.2008.12.006.

Noma H, Funatsu H, Yamasaki M, et al. Pathogenesis of macular edema with branch retinal vein occlusion and intraocular levels of vascular endothelial growth factor and interleukin-6. Am J Ophthalmol. 2005;140:256–61. doi:10.1016/j.ajo.2005.03.003.

Noma H, Minamoto A, Funatsu H, et al. Intravitreal levels of vascular endothelial growth factor and interleukin-6 are correlated with macular edema in branch retinal vein occlusion. Graefes Arch Clin Exp Ophthalmol. 2006;244:309–15. doi:10.1007/s00417-004-1087-4.

Noma H, Funatsu H, Mimura T, Hori S. Changes of vascular endothelial growth factor after vitrectomy for macular edema secondary to retinal vein occlusion. Eur J Ophthalmol. 2008;18:1017–9.

Ogura Y, Roider J, Korobelnik J-F, et al. Intravitreal aflibercept for macular edema secondary to central retinal vein occlusion: 18-month results of the Phase 3 GALILEO Study. Am J Ophthalmol. 2014. doi:10.1016/j.ajo.2014.07.027.

Pielen A, Feltgen N, Isserstedt C, et al. Efficacy and safety of intravitreal therapy in macular edema due to branch and central retinal vein occlusion: a systematic review. PLoS One. 2013;8, e78538. doi:10.1371/journal.pone.0078538.

Pielen A, Mirshahi A, Feltgen N, et al. Ranibizumab for Branch Retinal Vein Occlusion Associated Macular Edema Study (RABAMES): six-month results of a prospective randomized clinical trial. Acta Ophthalmol. 2014. doi:10.1111/aos.12488.

Rogers S, McIntosh RL, Cheung N, et al. The prevalence of retinal vein occlusion: pooled data from population studies from the United States, Europe, Asia, and Australia. Ophthalmology. 2010;117:313–9.e1. doi:10.1016/j.ophtha.2009.07.017.

Scott IU, Ip MS, VanVeldhuisen PC, et al. A randomized trial comparing the efficacy and safety of intravitreal triamcinolone with standard care to treat vision loss associated with macular Edema secondary to branch retinal vein occlusion: the Standard Care vs Corticosteroid for Retinal Vein Occlusion (SCORE) study report 6. Arch Ophthalmol. 2009;127:1115–28. doi:10.1001/archophthalmol.2009.233.

Sodi A, Giambene B, Marcucci R, et al. Atherosclerotic and thrombophilic risk factors in patients with ischemic central retinal vein occlusion. Retina. 2011;31:724–9. doi:10.1097/IAE.0b013e3181eef419.

Stem MS, Talwar N, Comer GM, Stein JD. A longitudinal analysis of risk factors associated with central retinal vein occlusion. Ophthalmology. 2013;120:362–70. doi:10.1016/j.ophtha.2012.07.080.

Tan MH, McAllister IL, Gillies ME, et al. Randomized controlled trial of intravitreal ranibizumab versus standard grid laser for macular edema following branch retinal vein occlusion. Am J Ophthalmol. 2014;157:237–47.e1. doi:10.1016/j.ajo.2013.08.013.

Wang K, Wang Y, Gao L, et al. Dexamethasone inhibits leukocyte accumulation and vascular permeability in retina of streptozotocin-induced diabetic rats via reducing vascular endothelial growth factor and intercellular adhesion molecule-1 expression. Biol Pharm Bull. 2008;31:1541–6.

Wroblewski JJ, Wells 3rd JA, Adamis AP, et al. Pegaptanib sodium for macular edema secondary to central retinal vein occlusion. Arch Ophthalmol. 2009;127:374–80. doi:10.1001/archophthalmol.2009.14.

Wroblewski JJ, Wells 3rd JA, Gonzales CR. Pegaptanib sodium for macular edema secondary to branch retinal vein occlusion. Am J Ophthalmol. 2010;149:147–54. doi:10.1016/j.ajo.2009.08.005.

Zhang X, Bao S, Lai D, et al. Intravitreal triamcinolone acetonide inhibits breakdown of the blood-retinal barrier through differential regulation of VEGF-A and its receptors in early diabetic rat retinas. Diabetes. 2008;57:1026–33. doi:10.2337/db07-0982.

Zhou JQ, Xu L, Wang S, et al. The 10-year incidence and risk factors of retinal vein occlusion: the Beijing eye study. Ophthalmology. 2013;120:803–8. doi:10.1016/j.ophtha.2012.09.033.

Pharmacokinetics of Intravitreally Applied VEGF Inhibitors

8

Tim U. Krohne, Frank G. Holz, and Carsten H. Meyer

8.1 Ocular Pharmacokinetics following Intravitreal Injection

The introduction of inhibitors of vascular endothelial growth factor (VEGF) in ophthalmology represents a breakthrough in the treatment of numerous retinal diseases, some of which have been untreatable before. Four medicines of this substance class have so far been used by ophthalmologists: pegaptanib (Macugen), bevacizumab (Avastin), ranibizumab (Lucentis), and aflibercept (Eylea). Although these substances are directed against the same target molecule, they

Original Publication (in German):
Tim U. Krohne, Frank G. Holz, Carsten H. Meyer. Pharmakokinetik intravitreal applizierter VEGF-Inhibitoren. Der Ophthalmologe. February 2014, Volume 111, Issue 2, pp 113-120. doi: 10.1007/s00347-013-2932-9. © Springer-Verlag Berlin Heidelberg 2013. Republication with kind permission of Springer Science+Business Media

T.U. Krohne, M.D., F.E.B.O. (✉) • F.G. Holz, M.D.
Department of Ophthalmology, University of Bonn, Ernst Abbe-Str. 2, Bonn 53127, Germany
e-mail: krohne@uni-bonn.de;
frank.holz@ukb.uni-bonn.de

C.H. Meyer, M.D.
Department of Ophthalmology, Pallas Clinics, Bahnhofplatz 4, Aarau, Aargau, Switzerland
e-mail: carsten.meyer@klinik-pallas.ch

differ considerably in terms of their molecular structure and consequently also their pharmacokinetic properties.

Pharmacokinetic studies on intravitreal VEGF inhibitors have so far been conducted primarily on rabbits and rhesus monkeys. Both animal species have a distinctly smaller ocular volume than humans so that the pharmacokinetic parameters determined usually differ considerably from those of humans. The ocular half-lives of VEGF inhibitors derived from animal experiments are usually around half of the respective human values. The pharmacokinetic values determined in animal models cannot therefore be directly transferred to humans. However, they are suitable for comparing the pharmacokinetic properties of different substances if they have been determined in the same animal model under identical conditions.

The ocular half-lives measured in rabbits and humans for the different VEGF inhibitors and other selected intravitreally administered substances are summarized in Tables 8.1 and 8.2. The ocular half-life is usually calculated directly using the values measured from aqueous humor or vitreous samples, whereby comparative measurements from animal experiments have shown that both types of sample provide virtually identical values (Bakri et al. 2007a; Gaudreault et al. 2005, 2007). Occasionally, however, the ocular half-life is also estimated using measurements from plasma samples (Basile et al. 2012; Xu et al.

Table 8.1 Ocular half-lives after intravitreal injection in rabbits (EMA, European Medicines Agency)

Molecular class	Substance (trade name)	Molecular weight (kDa)	Ocular half-life in rabbits (days)]	Reference
RNA aptamer	Pegaptanib (Macugen)	50	3.46	Eyetech Study Group (2002)
Fab fragment	Ranibizumab (Lucentis)	48	2.88	Bakri et al. (2007a)
			2.9	Gaudreault et al. (2007)
IgG antibody	Bevacizumab (Avastin)	149	4.32	Bakri et al. (2007b)
			5.95	Nomoto et al. (2009)
	Rituximab (MabThera)[a]	144	4.7	Kim et al. (2006)
	Trastuzumab (Herceptin)[b]	146	5.6	Mordenti et al. (1999)
Fc fragment fusion protein	Aflibercept (Eylea)	115	4.79	Bayer/EMA (European Medicines 2013)
	Conbercept[c]	143	4.24	Li et al. (2012)

[a]Anti-CD20 antibody
[b]Anti-HER2 antibody
[c]Fusion protein of VEGF receptor binding domains and Fc fragment, similar to aflibercept

Table 8.2 Ocular half-lives after intravitreal injection in humans

Substance (trade name)	Ocular half-life in humans (days)	Eyes examined (number)	Reference
Pegaptanib (Macugen)	8[a]	–[a]	Basile et al. (2012)
Ranibizumab (Lucentis)	7.19	18	Krohne et al. (2012)
	9[a]	–[a]	Xu et al. (2013)
Bevacizumab (Avastin)	9.82	30	Krohne et al. (2008)
	10	18	Csaky et al. (2007)
	6.7	11	Zhu et al. (2008)
Aflibercept (Eylea)	No published data		

[a]Values estimated using plasma concentration measurements

2013) provided that the examined substance is not intraocularly broken down but is eliminated from the eye by release into the systemic circulation, and that the systemic half-life can be assumed to be negligible compared to the ocular half-life. Under these conditions, the time of elimination from the bloodstream essentially corresponds to that of ocular elimination, as is the case for ranibizumab and pegaptanib for example.

For better comparability of the results, we measured the ocular half-lives of bevacizumab and ranibizumab in humans using identical methods. We determined a value of 9.82 days for the IgG antibody bevacizumab (149 kDa) and a value of 7.19 days for the Fab fragment ranibizumab (48 kDa), corresponding to a 1.4 times longer half-life of bevacizumab compared to ranibizumab (Krohne et al. 2008, 2012). This is in line with the results of a clinical trial in which a 1.4 times longer period of action of bevacizumab compared with ranibizumab was measured in patients with age-related macular degeneration (AMD) based on the retinal thickness analysis by optical coherence tomography (OCT) (Shah and Del Priore 2009). The value furthermore agrees with animal studies which describe a 1.5 times longer half-life of bevacizumab compared to ranibizumab (Bakri et al. 2007a, b). Since the molecular weight of a substance and the associated diffusion speed through the vitreous usually constitutes a main factor of the ocular elimination speed (Durairaj et al. 2009), it is notable that bevacizumab and other IgG antibodies have around three times the molecular weight compared to ranibizumab and the RNA aptamer pegaptanib (50 kDa), but only a slightly higher ocular half-life by comparison. A possible explanation for this discrepancy is the activity of the neonatal Fc receptor, as will be explained in the following section.

The VEGF inhibitor aflibercept (115 kDa), which is a fusion protein from the binding domains of VEGF receptors 1 and 2 and an Fc antibody fragment, as well as the similarly structured VEGF inhibitor conbercept (Li et al. 2012) both show ocular half-lives in rabbits which are within the range of bevacizumab and other IgG antibodies. This could indicate that the ocular half-life of aflibercept is similar to the known half-life of bevacizumab also in humans. Human data for aflibercept, however, are not available to date.

8.2 Pharmacokinetic Significance of the Neonatal Fc Receptor

The neonatal Fc receptor (FcRn) can bind IgG antibodies in order to transport them unidirectionally through various body barriers. This is important, for example, for the transportation of maternal antibodies via the placental barrier to the bloodstream of the unborn child. In the blood–brain barrier, the FcRn transports antibodies from cerebral tissues into the bloodstream and therefore possibly plays a role in the containment of intracerebral inflammatory reactions. An expression of FcRn has also been detected in the inner and outer blood–retina barrier (van Bilsen et al. 2011; Kim et al. 2008) so that here too an FcRn-mediated outward transportation of antibodies from the retina to the bloodstream is assumed (Fig. 8.1).

In addition to its transport function, the FcRn is also expressed in numerous other tissues where it prevents the degradation or elimination of IgG antibodies. For example, the antibodies absorbed by vascular endothelial cells are transported back into the blood via the FcRn so that they are not broken down intracellularly by lysosomes like other serum proteins. This recycling function of the FcRn means that antibodies have a much higher half-life in the systemic circulation than other comparable serum proteins and can therefore satisfy their immunological function for longer.

IgG antibodies are bound to the FcRn via their Fc fragment. Therefore, only complete antibodies such as bevacizumab are bound by the receptor while Fab fragments such as ranibizumab are not bound in the absence of the Fc fragment. An active FcRn-mediated outward transportation of bevacizumab but not of ranibizumab from the eye could therefore explain why bevacizumab has only a slightly higher ocular half-life than ranibizumab despite a molecular weight that is three times higher. The recycling function of the FcRn with respect to complete antibodies may also lead to the plasma half-life of bevacizumab of 20 days being distinctly extended compared to 2 h for ranibizumab (Lu et al. 2008; Xu et al. 2013). As an aptamer, pegaptanib is not bound by the FcRn, while aflibercept as a fusion protein with Fc fragment is assumed to bind to the FcRn in a similar way as IgG antibodies.

8.3 Clinical Relevance of Ocular Pharmacokinetics

The ocular elimination rate is an important factor for the effect duration of intravitreal active pharmaceutical compounds and therefore co-determines reinjection intervals and frequency. It was originally assumed that substances such as bevacizumab with a higher molecular weight compared to ranibizumab would demonstrate a longer effect and therefore a lower re-treatment frequency. However, as already explained, bevacizumab and ranibizumab have only comparatively little diverging ocular half-lives so that little differences in terms of their reinjection frequency are to be expected. The injection numbers per year for different VEGF inhibitors determined in clinical studies for pro re nata treatment regimens are summarized in Table 8.3. In agreement with the pharmacokinetic data, essentially equal injection frequencies for bevacizumab and ranibizumab were found. For aflibercept, data is so far only available from the marketing authorization studies which currently

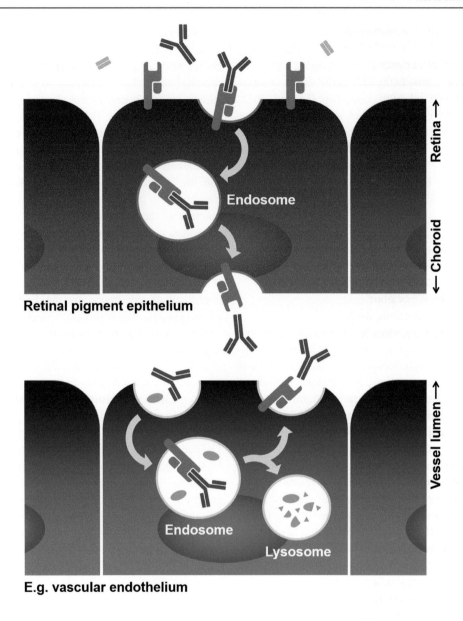

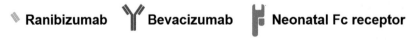

Ranibizumab   **Bevacizumab**   **Neonatal Fc receptor**

Fig. 8.1 Possible role of the neonatal Fc receptor (FcRn) in the transportation of bevacizumab (Avastin) and ranibizumab (Lucentis). Bevacizumab, but not ranibizumab, binds to the FcRn via the Fc fragment. The FcRn acceler-ates elimination from the eye by outward transportation via the blood–retina barrier (*top*) and increases the duration of retention in the systemic circulation through protection from lysosomal breakdown (*bottom*)

Table 8.3 Average number of injections per year with a treatment regimen including an initial fixed upload phase and subsequent monthly treatments as needed (pro re nata, PRN) in neovascular age-related macular degeneration

Substance (trade name)	Study	Injections in first year	Injections in second year
Pegaptanib (Macugen)	No published data		
Bevacizumab (Avastin)	CATT	7.7	6.4
Ranibizumab (Lucentis)	CATT	6.9	5.7
	SUSTAIN	5.7	No second year
	HARBOR	7.7	5.6
	PrONTO	5.6	4.2
	VIEW 1/2	No PRN arm	5.6[a]
Aflibercept (Eylea)	VIEW 1/2	No PRN arm	4.8[b]
	CLEAR-IT 2	5.6[c]	No second year

[a]Corresponds to 4.7 injections in 44 study weeks with capped PRN treatment regimen
[b]Corresponds to 4.1 injections in 44 study weeks in 2q4 study arm with "capped PRN" treatment regimen
[c]In "2q4" study arm including initial fixed upload phase of 4 monthly injections

do not allow any conclusion as to whether the number of injections differs significantly from other VEGF inhibitors in a pro re nata treatment regimen.

8.4 Systemic Pharmacokinetics following Intravitreal Injection

VEGF inhibitors are eliminated from the eye not through intraocular breakdown but by release into the systemic circulation so that following intravitreal administration a suppression of systemic VEGF activity with potentially systemic adverse events is possible. The systemic exposure depends on the systemic half-lives of the substances. Data is available on the systemic half-lives particularly for bevacizumab and aflibercept used systemically for cancer treatment, and also for other VEGF inhibitors. An overview of the values in humans is summarized in Table 8.4. A distinct difference is shown here between substances with and without Fc fragment which is most likely attributable to the above described different binding to the neonatal Fc receptor and the associated protection from a rapid systemic breakdown of the substances.

Using the ocular and systemic half-lives measured, the systemic level of active substances following intravitreal administration can be modelled using the Bateman function (Fig. 8.2). The model indicates a distinctly higher systemic exposure to bevacizumab compared to ranibizumab so that a stronger effect of bevacizumab on the systemic VEGF activity would be expected. Indeed, clinical studies on patients with AMD, diabetic macular edema, and retinopathy of prematurity indicate that intravitreally injected bevacizumab can lead to suppression of systemic VEGF activity over a period of several weeks after injection (Carneiro et al. 2012; Matsuyama et al. 2010; Sato et al. 2011; Zehetner et al. 2013). In agreement with the pharmacokinetic data, two comparative investigations into bevacizumab and other VEGF inhibitors could not detect such a systemic effect for ranibizumab and pegaptanib (Carneiro et al. 2012; Zehetner et al. 2013). Therefore, the pharmacokinetic properties of ranibizumab would appear more advantageous compared to bevacizumab for areas of application which are particularly sensitive in terms of a systemic VEGF suppression, such as the treatment of retinopathy of prematurity (Krohne et al. 2012). An effect on the untreated fellow eye was also determined in a study on diabetic macular edema only after the injection of bevacizumab, but not of ranibizumab (Bakbak et al. 2013). However, other studies were unable to detect either a measurable substance level of bevacizumab or a reduction in the VEGF activity in the untreated fellow eye (Meyer et al. 2012; Sawada et al. 2008). So far, there is no published data on the effect of aflibercept on the systemic VEGF level or contralateral eye exposure.

In cancer treatment, VEGF inhibitors such as bevacizumab are used in distinctly higher dosages and can lead to known adverse events such as bleeding, neutropenia, and intestinal perforations. By comparison, the serum levels achieved after intravitreal treatment are about 100 times lower. In all larger ophthalmological studies on

anti-VEGF treatment including VISION, ANCHOR/MARINA, CATT, IVAN, and VIEW 1/2, the rates of systemic serious adverse events (SAE) were low in all study groups. Moreover, SAE rates in studies such as VISION and MARINA were not significantly different in treatment groups compared with the untreated control groups. Even the fixed monthly administration of ranibizumab with four times the usual dose over a period of 12 months as part of the HABOR study did not lead to a significant rise in the SAE rate (Busbee et al. 2013). However, with the low SAE incidence, patient numbers in all studies have so far been insufficient for a statistically relevant statement to be made on systemic safety. A current meta-analysis of several clinical studies and an analysis of the data from the CATT and IVAN studies both come to the conclusion that there are indications of an increased general SAE rate under bevacizumab compared with ranibizumab, without it being possible, however, to determine higher incidences in a specific organ system (Chakravarthy et al. 2013; Schmucker et al. 2012). These results on the SAE rate correlate with the stated pharmacokinetic differences of the VEGF inhibitors with respect to their systemic exposure.

Table 8.4 Systemic half-lives in humans (EMA, European Medicines Agency)

Substance (trade name)	Systemic half-life in humans (days)	Reference
Pegaptanib (Macugen)	No published human data; 0.4[a] in monkey	(Tucker et al. 1999)
Ranibizumab (Lucentis)	0.08[b]	Xu et al. (2013)
Bevacizumab (Avastin)	20	Lu et al. (2008)
Aflibercept (Eylea)	2–6	Bayer/EMA (2013)

[a]Corresponds to 9.3 h
[b]Corresponds to 2 h

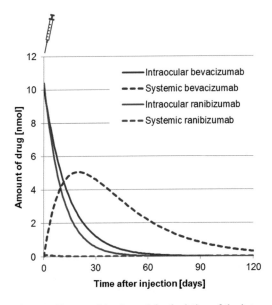 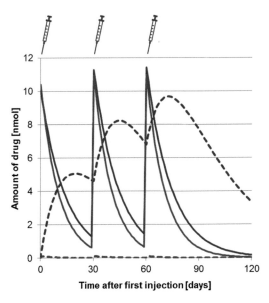

Fig. 8.2 Pharmacokinetic model calculation of the intraocular and systemic substance levels after a single (*left*) and three consecutive monthly (right) intravitreal injections of 1.5 mg bevacizumab (Avastin) or 0.5 mg ranibizumab (Lucentis) using the ocular and systemic half-lives measured in humans

8.5 Refraction and Ocular Pharmacokinetics

Refraction differences may be accompanied by significant axial length differences and therefore a different ocular distribution volume for intravitreally injected medicines. If by way of simplification the eye is viewed as a sphere, then arithmetically one eye with an axial length of 27 mm, for example, will have around double the volume of an eye with an axial length of 22 mm. The standard dosage of an intravitreal medicine in such an eye would therefore achieve only half the substance concentration, and the duration of action of the medicine would arithmetically be reduced by 1 half-life (in the case of bevacizumab, for example, around 10 days). This effect may possibly be enhanced by a faster elimination of the active substance from larger eyes as a result of the larger retinal surface. Even if in reality the myopic eye in particular can deviate substantially from the spherical shape so that the true differences in volumes will probably be smaller, this arithmetical example does show the pronounced effects that axial length differences may possibly have on the pharmacokinetics of intravitreal medicine. Although the arithmetical effect of ocular volume on intraocular drug concentration and duration of action could not yet be confirmed in experimental studies (Krohne et al. 2015), individual authors recommend to adjust the dosage of intravitreal medicines in eyes with axial lengths which differ extremely from the norm (Teichmann 2002). Another possibility would be to reduce the control and reinjection intervals of anti-VEGF treatment for highly myopic eyes, particularly if an inadequate therapeutic effect is observed. However, no studies have so far investigated the effect of axial length on duration and extent of the clinical effect.

8.6 Effects of Vitreous Liquefaction, Vitrectomy, and Silicone Oil Endotamponade

The liquefaction of the vitreous which increases with age causes the viscosity of the vitreous to decrease so that a faster diffusion and therefore altered pharmacokinetics of intravitreal substances are to be assumed. Experimental studies on animals have actually detected a significantly accelerated elimination of intravitreally injected substances from the vitreous after enzymatic liquefaction of the vitreous (Tan et al. 2011; Wu et al. 2011). However, to what extent the duration of effect of VEGF inhibitors in humans decreases with increasing age and degree of vitreous liquefaction and whether this influences the therapeutic effect in a clinically relevant manner has not so far been examined.

Following a vitrectomy, the vitreous is replaced by the distinctly less viscous aqueous humor. Data from animal experiments provide evidence of an accelerated elimination from the vitrectomized eye for different intravitreal substances (Chin et al. 2005; Doft et al. 1985; Jarus et al. 1985). The molecular weight of many of the active substances investigated in these studies such as triamcinolone (0.4 kDa), amphotericin B (0.9 kDa), and 5-fluorouracil (0.1 kDa) is, however, considerably lower than that of VEGF inhibitors such as bevacizumab (149 kDa) so that the pharmacokinetic results may possibly be transferred to the VEGF inhibitors only to a limited extent. Due to the anatomical features of the animal models used here, the vitrectomy was also combined with a lensectomy in many studies which results in the absence of a barrier to the anterior chamber with possibly easier diffusion of the substances from the vitreous, therefore making comparability with the situation in the vitrectomized but phakic/pseudophakic human eye difficult.

So far, only very restricted data on the pharmacokinetics in the vitrectomized eye exist for VEGF inhibitors. A retrospective case series on 11 vitrectomized eyes which were treated with bevacizumab for diabetic macular edema reports on the absence of a clinical effect on retinal thickness and vision, possibly due to an accelerated ocular elimination of the substance (Yanyali et al. 2007). Contrary to this, another retrospective study on diabetic macular edema describes an effect of bevacizumab in vitrectomized eyes which, however, is smaller than in non-vitrectomized eyes (Mehta et al. 2010). In monkeys, a 54 % lower ocular half-life of bevacizumab was measured after combined lensectomy and vitrectomy (Kakinoki et al. 2012). In rabbits, a 46

% reduction was demonstrated for bevacizumab and a 24 % decrease for ranibizumab following vitrectomy alone, while the reduction after lensectomy alone was even more pronounced (Christoforidis et al. 2013). By contrast, a different study on rabbits came to the conclusion that vitrectomy alone has no influence on ocular half-life (Ahn et al. 2013). The data on the effect of VEGF inhibitors in vitrectomized eyes is therefore not uniform so far. Even after vitrectomy, an intravitreal anti-VEGF treatment may be effective. However, in view of the possibly faster elimination of the active pharmaceutical ingredients from the eye, it may be expedient to shorten the standard check-up and reinjection intervals.

The injection into silicone oil-filled eyes is a rather rare application of VEGF inhibitors. Experimental animal studies, however, exist and show that the transition from the vitreous to the retinal tissue and into the anterior chamber in silicone oil-filled eyes is delayed, but that the subsequent elimination rate in retinal tissue and anterior chamber does not differ from that of non-vitrectomized eyes (Xu et al. 2012). This indicates that a treatment with intravitreal VEGF inhibitors could be effective also in silicone oil-filled eyes. Clinical data on the treatment of retinal diseases are not available, however. Only for diabetic rubeosis iridis is a decline of the disease following intravitreal injection of bevacizumab in silicone oil-filled eyes reported in a case series of five patients (Falavarjani et al. 2010).

8.7 Outlook on Future Developments

In order to reduce the necessity of intravitreal injections and therefore the burden on patients as well as the endophthalmitis risk, new forms of administration such as topical VEGF inhibitors and sustained release drug carriers are desirable. Topical administration could be achieved by a lower molecular weight and improved corneal penetrability. VEGF inhibitors from new substance classes such as single-chain antibody fragments (ESBA1008, MW 26 kDa) and DARPins (AGN-150998, MW 34 kDa) could possess properties of this nature and are already undergoing clinical testing, but still as intravitreal injection for the time being. Sustained release drug carriers are already being used with steroids (e.g., Ozurdex, Iluvien, Retisert) and antiviral drugs (e.g., Vitrasert) for ophthalmic treatment. They are able to evenly release the active substance contained in them over months or years after intravitreal implantation. Therefore with these devices, it is less the pharmacokinetic properties of the active substances but more the release characteristics of the carrier that determines ocular substance levels. The use of sustained release drug technology with proteins such as the currently available VEGF inhibitors is proving to be difficult, however, due to the lower stability of these substances compared to, for example, steroids. Sustained release drug carriers charged with VEGF inhibitors are therefore currently only being investigated at a preclinical level.

8.8 Conclusions for Clinicians

- The ocular and systemic pharmacokinetics of intravitreally injected substances determine the ocular effect duration and the systemic exposure and are therefore of clinical relevance with respect to reinjection frequency and systemic safety.
- Despite distinct differences in molecular weight, the currently available VEGF inhibitors show only comparatively small differences in terms of ocular half-lives (Tables 8.1 and 8.2), possibly because the slower diffusion of larger, Fc fragment-containing substances from the eye is compensated by an active outward transportation via the neonatal Fc receptor.
- VEGF inhibitors containing an Fc fragment can have a distinctly longer systemic half-life compared with Fc-free substances (Table 8.4) because binding to the neonatal Fc receptor on extraocular cells such as vascular endothelial cells may slow its systemic breakdown.
- The pharmacokinetics of intravitreal VEGF inhibitors can also be influenced by properties of the individual patient or eye, such as refraction (ocular volume), age (vitreous liquefaction), and previous surgeries (vitrectomy).

Compliance with Ethical Requirements
T.U. Krohne—support of research projects and clinical studies: Alcon, Novartis; consultancy honoraria, lecture fees, travel expenses: Bayer, Heidelberg Engineering, Novartis. F.G. Holz—support of research projects and clinical studies: Acucela, Alcon, Allergan, Bayer, Carl Zeiss Meditec, Genentech, Heidelberg Engineering, Novartis, Optos; consultancy honoraria, lecture fees, travel expenses: Acucela, Alcon, Allergan, Bayer, Genentech, Heidelberg Engineering, Novartis, Roche. C.H. Meyer—support of research projects and clinical studies: Novartis, Allergan; consultancy honoraria, lecture fees, travel expenses: Bayer, GSK, Novartis.

No human or animal studies were carried out by the authors for this chapter.

References

Ahn J, Kim H, Woo SJ, et al. Pharmacokinetics of intravitreally injected bevacizumab in vitrectomized eyes. J Ocul Pharmacol Ther. 2013;29(7):612–8.

Bakbak B, Ozturk BT, Gonul S, et al. Comparison of the effect of unilateral intravitreal bevacizumab and ranibizumab injection on diabetic macular edema of the fellow eye. J Ocul Pharmacol Ther. 2013;29(8): 728–32.

Bakri SJ, Snyder MR, Reid JM, et al. Pharmacokinetics of intravitreal ranibizumab (Lucentis). Ophthalmology. 2007a;114:2179–82.

Bakri SJ, Snyder MR, Reid JM, et al. Pharmacokinetics of intravitreal ranibizumab (Lucentis). Ophthalmology. 2007b;114:2179–82.

Basile AS, Hutmacher M, Nickens D, et al. Population pharmacokinetics of pegaptanib in patients with neovascular, age-related macular degeneration. J Clin Pharmacol. 2012;52:1186–99.

Busbee BG, Ho AC, Brown DM, et al. Twelve-month efficacy and safety of 0.5 mg or 2.0 mg ranibizumab in patients with subfoveal neovascular age-related macular degeneration. Ophthalmology. 2013;120:1046–56.

Carneiro AM, Costa R, Falcao MS, et al. Vascular endothelial growth factor plasma levels before and after treatment of neovascular age-related macular degeneration with bevacizumab or ranibizumab. Acta Ophthalmol. 2012;90:e25–30.

Chakravarthy U, Harding SP, Rogers CA, et al. Alternative treatments to inhibit VEGF in age-related choroidal neovascularisation: 2-year findings of the IVAN randomised controlled trial. Lancet. 2013;382(9900): 1258–67.

Chin HS, Park TS, Moon YS, et al. Difference in clearance of intravitreal triamcinolone acetonide between vitrectomized and nonvitrectomized eyes. Retina. 2005;25:556–60.

Christoforidis JB, Williams MM, Wang J, et al. Anatomic and pharmacokinetic properties of intravitreal bevacizumab and ranibizumab after vitrectomy and lensectomy. Retina. 2013;33:946–52.

Csaky KG, Gordiyenko N, Rabena MG et al. Pharmacokinetics of intravitreal bevacizumab in humans. Invest Ophthalmol Vis Sci 2007;48: E-Abstract 4936.

Doft BH, Weiskopf J, Nilsson-Ehle I, et al. Amphotericin clearance in vitrectomized versus nonvitrectomized eyes. Ophthalmology. 1985;92:1601–5.

Durairaj C, Shah JC, Senapati S, et al. Prediction of vitreal half-life based on drug physicochemical properties: quantitative structure-pharmacokinetic relationships (QSPKR). Pharm Res. 2009;26:1236–60.

European Medicines Agency. Eylea: EPAR—European public assessment report (September 20, 2012). http://www.ema.europa.eu/docs/en_GB/document_library/EPAR_-_Public_assessment_report/human/002392/WC500135744.pdf. 2013. Accessed: January 23, 2015.

Eyetech Study Group. Preclinical and phase 1A clinical evaluation of an anti-VEGF pegylated aptamer (EYE001) for the treatment of exudative age-related macular degeneration. Retina. 2002;22:143–52.

Falavarjani KG, Modarres M, Nazari H. Therapeutic effect of bevacizumab injected into the silicone oil in eyes with neovascular glaucoma after vitrectomy for advanced diabetic retinopathy. Eye (Lond). 2010; 24:717–9.

Gaudreault J, Fei D, Rusit J, et al. Preclinical pharmacokinetics of Ranibizumab (rhuFabV2) after a single intravitreal administration. Invest Ophthalmol Vis Sci. 2005;46:726–33.

Gaudreault J, Fei D, Beyer JC, et al. Pharmacokinetics and retinal distribution of ranibizumab, a humanized antibody fragment directed against VEGF-A, following intravitreal administration in rabbits. Retina. 2007;27:1260–6.

Jarus G, Blumenkranz M, Hernandez E, et al. Clearance of intravitreal fluorouracil. Normal and aphakic vitrectomized eyes. Ophthalmology. 1985;92:91–6.

Kakinoki M, Sawada O, Sawada T, et al. Effect of vitrectomy on aqueous VEGF concentration and pharmacokinetics of bevacizumab in macaque monkeys. Invest Ophthalmol Vis Sci. 2012;53:5877–80.

Kim H, Csaky KG, Chan CC, et al. The pharmacokinetics of rituximab following an intravitreal injection. Exp Eye Res. 2006;82:760–6.

Kim H, Fariss RN, Zhang C, et al. Mapping of the neonatal Fc receptor in the rodent eye. Invest Ophthalmol Vis Sci. 2008;49:2025–9.

Krohne TU, Eter N, Holz FG, et al. Intraocular pharmacokinetics of bevacizumab after a single intravitreal injection in humans. Am J Ophthalmol. 2008;146:508–12.

Krohne TU, Aisenbrey S, Holz FG. Current therapeutic options in retinopathy of prematurity. Ophthalmologe. 2012a;109:1189–97.

Krohne TU, Liu Z, Holz FG, et al. Intraocular pharmacokinetics of ranibizumab following a single intravitreal injection in humans. Am J Ophthalmol. 2012b; 154(682-686), e682.

Krohne TU, Muether PS, Stratmann NK, et al. Influence of ocular volume and lens status on pharmacokinetics and duration of action of intravitreal vascular endothelial growth factor inhibitors. Retina. 2015;35(1): 69–74.

Li H, Lei N, Zhang M, et al. Pharmacokinetics of a long-lasting anti-VEGF fusion protein in rabbit. Exp Eye Res. 2012;97:154–9.

Lu JF, Bruno R, Eppler S, et al. Clinical pharmacokinetics of bevacizumab in patients with solid tumors. Cancer Chemother Pharmacol. 2008;62:779–86.

Matsuyama K, Ogata N, Matsuoka M, et al. Plasma levels of vascular endothelial growth factor and pigment epithelium-derived factor before and after intravitreal injection of bevacizumab. Br J Ophthalmol. 2010;94: 1215–8.

Mehta S, Blinder KJ, Shah GK, et al. Intravitreal bevacizumab for the treatment of refractory diabetic macular edema. Ophthalmic Surg Lasers Imaging. 2010;41:323–9.

Meyer CH, Krohne TU, Holz FG. Concentrations of unbound bevacizumab in the aqueous of untreated fellow eyes after a single intravitreal injection in humans. Acta Ophthalmol. 2012;90:68–70.

Mordenti J, Cuthbertson RA, Ferrara N, et al. Comparisons of the intraocular tissue distribution, pharmacokinetics, and safety of 125I-labeled full-length and Fab antibodies in rhesus monkeys following intravitreal administration. Toxicol Pathol. 1999;27:536–44.

Nomoto H, Shiraga F, Kuno N, et al. Pharmacokinetics of bevacizumab after topical, subconjunctival, and intravitreal administration in rabbits. Invest Ophthalmol Vis Sci. 2009;50:4807–13.

Sato T, Wada K, Arahori H, et al. Serum concentrations of bevacizumab (Avastin) and vascular endothelial growth factor in infants with retinopathy of prematurity. Am J Ophthalmol. 2011;153(2):327–33.e1.

Sawada O, Kawamura H, Kakinoki M, et al. Vascular endothelial growth factor in fellow eyes of eyes injected with intravitreal bevacizumab. Graefes Arch Clin Exp Ophthalmol. 2008;246:1379–81.

Schmucker C, Ehlken C, Agostini HT, et al. A safety review and meta-analyses of bevacizumab and ranibizumab: off-label versus gold standard. PLoS One. 2012;7, e42701.

Shah AR, Del Priore LV. Duration of action of intravitreal ranibizumab and bevacizumab in exudative AMD eyes based on macular volume measurements. Br J Ophthalmol. 2009;93:1027–32.

Tan LE, Orilla W, Hughes PM, et al. Effects of vitreous liquefaction on the intravitreal distribution of sodium fluorescein, fluorescein dextran, and fluorescent microparticles. Invest Ophthalmol Vis Sci. 2011;52: 1111–8.

Teichmann KD. Intravitreal injections: does globe size matter? J Cataract Refract Surg. 2002;28:1886–9.

Tucker CE, Chen LS, Judkins MB, et al. Detection and plasma pharmacokinetics of an anti-vascular endothelial growth factor oligonucleotide-aptamer (NX1838) in rhesus monkeys. J Chromatogr B Biomed Sci Appl. 1999;732:203–12.

van Bilsen K, van Hagen PM, Bastiaans J, et al. The neonatal Fc receptor is expressed by human retinal pigment epithelial cells and is downregulated by tumour necrosis factor-alpha. Br J Ophthalmol. 2011;95: 864–8.

Wu WC, Chen CC, Liu CH, et al. Plasmin treatment accelerates vascular endothelial growth factor clearance from rabbit eyes. Invest Ophthalmol Vis Sci. 2011;52:6162–7.

Xu Y, You Y, Du W, et al. Ocular pharmacokinetics of bevacizumab in vitrectomized eyes with silicone oil tamponade. Invest Ophthalmol Vis Sci. 2012;53: 5221–6.

Xu L, Lu T, Tuomi L, et al. Pharmacokinetics of ranibizumab in patients with neovascular age-related macular degeneration: a population approach. Invest Ophthalmol Vis Sci. 2013;54:1616–24.

Yanyali A, Aytug B, Horozoglu F, et al. Bevacizumab (Avastin) for diabetic macular edema in previously vitrectomized eyes. Am J Ophthalmol. 2007;144: 124–6.

Zehetner C, Kirchmair R, Huber S, et al. Plasma levels of vascular endothelial growth factor before and after intravitreal injection of bevacizumab, ranibizumab and pegaptanib in patients with age-related macular degeneration, and in patients with diabetic macular oedema. Br J Ophthalmol. 2013;97:454–9.

Zhu Q, Ziemssen F, Henke-Fahle S et al. Vitreous levels of bevacizumab and vascular endothelial growth factor-A in patients with choroidal neovascularization. Ophthalmology. 2008;115:1750–5, 1755e1751.

Neovascular Glaucoma

9

Julia Lüke, Matthias Lüke, and Salvatore Grisanti

9.1 Pathogenesis of Neovascular Glaucoma

Ischemic retinopathies and the concomitant increased level of vascular endothelial growth factor (VEGF) are the leading causes of neovascularization of the iris surface. In progressive stages, fibrovascular membranes occlude the anterior chamber angle and inhibit aqueous outflow resulting in elevated intraocular pressure (IOP). This is often difficult to control and frequently results in loss of vision. Rubeosis iridis was initially described by Coats in 1906. Since his original description, neovascularization of the iris and anterior chamber angle has been described in many diseases, 97 % of which are associated with retinal ischemia (Brown et al. 1984). The most common conditions are diabetes mellitus, central retinal vein occlusion (CRVO), and ocular ischemic syndrome. Diseases associated with rubeosis and neovascular glaucoma (NVG) are listed in Table 9.1. The reason for this process is elevated intraocular VEGF levels.

Similarly, intravitreal injections of recombinant human VEGF in amounts comparable to those measured in eyes with active neovascularization induce noninflammatory iris neovascularization in nonhuman primates. Prolonged exposure to VEGF can therefore produce neovascular glaucoma (Tolentino et al. 1996).

9.2 Conventional Therapeutic Approach in Neovascular Glaucoma

There are two key aspects to the management of neovascular glaucoma: treatment of the underlying angiogenic disease process and treatment of the increased IOP. Previous treatment modalities include (a) panretinal photocoagulation (PRP) or cryocoagulation to ablate the source of VEGF and (b) cyclodestructive or drainage procedures to counteract the angular obstruction and to reduce IOP.

PRP is considered the standard treatment of ischemic retinal diseases. Ohnishi and colleagues documented regression of rubeosis in 68 % of patients and normalization of IOP in 42 % of patients treated with PRP. The efficacy of PRP has been studied in specific disease processes, including diabetic retinopathy, CRVO, radiation retinopathy following plaque treatment, and central retinal artery occlusion (Wand et al. 1978). PRP results in new vessel regression in all of

J. Lüke, M.D., P.D. (✉) • M. Lüke, M.D., P.D.
S. Grisanti, M.D.
Department of Ophthalmology, University of Lübeck, Ratzeburger Allee 160, Lübeck, Schleswig-Holstein 23538, Germany
e-mail: julia.lueke@uksh.de;
Matthias.lueke@uksh.de; Salvatore.grisanti@uksh.de

© Springer International Publishing Switzerland 2016
A. Stahl (ed.), *Anti-Angiogenic Therapy in Ophthalmology*,
Essentials in Ophthalmology, DOI 10.1007/978-3-319-24097-8_9

Table 9.1 Disease in which rubeosis iridis has been reported (Sivak-Callcott et al. 2001)

Retinal ischemic diseases
Diabetic retinopathy
Central retinal vein occlusion
Ocular ischemic syndrome/carotid occlusive disease
Central retinal artery occlusion
Retinal detachment
Leber's congenital amaurosis
Coat's disease
Eales disease
Sickle cell retinopathy
Retinal hemangioma
Persistent hyperplastic primary vitreous
Norrie's disease
Wyburn Mason
Carotid-cavernous fistula
Dural shunt
Stickler's syndrome
X-linked retinoschisis
Takayasu's aortitis
Juxtafoveal telangiectasis
Surgically induced
Carotid endarterectomy
Cataract extraction
Pars plana vitrectomy/lensectomy
Silicone oil
Scleral buckle
Neodymium-doped yttrium aluminium garnet capsulotomy
Laser coreoplasty
Tumors
Iris: melanoma, hemangioma, metastatic lesion
Ciliary body: ring melanoma
Retina: retinoblastoma, large cell lymphoma
Choroid: melanoma
Conjunctiva: squamous cell melanoma
Radiation
External beam
Charged particle: proton, helium
Plaques
Photoradiation
Inflammatory diseases
Uveitis: chronic iridocyclitis, Behcet's disease
Vogt–Koyanagi–Harada syndrome
Syphilitic retinitis
Sympathetic ophthalmia
Endophthalmitis
Miscellaneous
Vitreous wick syndrome
Interferon alpha

these conditions. Extensive cryotherapy of the anterior retina has been shown to be effective in causing regression of rubeosis. Fernandez-Vigo et al. did not find any difference in the regression of rubeosis with cryotherapy when compared with PRP (Fernández-Vigo et al. 1997).

Medical management of neovascular glaucoma is based on IOP-lowering agents, including topical beta-adrenergic antagonists, alpha-2 agonists, and topical and oral carbonic anhydrase inhibitors. Partial destruction of the ciliary body lowers aqueous humor production and therefore reduces IOP. Although diode laser cyclodestruction seems to show promise for successful IOP control in patients with neovascular glaucoma, its long-term success rate has not been well described. Moreover, standardization of a formal treatment protocol is required. Although cryotherapy of the ciliary body may be highly effective in lowering IOP, its rate of complications including progression to phthisis seems to be higher than that associated with cyclophotocoagulation. In 1972, Feibl and Bigger reported a 50 % reduction in IOP treated with cyclocryotherapy (Feibel and Bigger 1972). Despite adequate IOP control, up to 70 % of patients treated with cyclocryotherapy for refractory neovascular glaucoma have been reported to lose vision (Caprioli et al. 1985). Although laser cyclophotocoagulation seems to have a lower complication rate, the percentage of patients with neovascular glaucoma who lose vision with this modality remains high, with long-term vision loss of 46.6 % reported by Shields and Shields (1994).

Filtering surgery for neovascular glaucoma is initially effective but often unsuccessful at the end due to the wound-healing process. Many modifications have been tried to improve the outcome of these procedures (Brouillette and Chebil 1987; Kahook et al. 2006b; L'Esperance et al. 1983; Tripathi et al. 1998). A different approach of aqueous drainage has been described by Kirchhof (1994). He performed pars plana vitrectomy, lensectomy, and retinectomy to re-route aqueous drainage through the choroidal circulation in nine eyes with neovascular glaucoma. An average decrease of 20–50 mmHg in IOP was noted. Phthisis occurred in two eyes, hypotony in three eyes, and a retinal detachment in one eye. This treatment, however, was often associated with cyclophotocoagulation ab interno. The IOP-lowering effect could therefore not be clearly associated with the retinectomy alone.

Aqueous tube shunts have reported success rates of 22 % up to 97 % for patients with neovascular glaucoma (Assaad et al. 1999). However, the authors cautioned that the visual prognosis might still be poor because of the severe underlying disease process and postoperative complications.

9.3 Anti-VEGF Drugs in Neovascular Glaucoma

In 2006, the first short-term case reports described the effects of intravitreal bevacizumab on the regression of anterior segment neovascularization (Avery 2006; Davidorf et al. 2006). At the same time, we presented iris fluorescein angiography in a case series of six eyes of three patients receiving a bevacizumab injection (1.0 mg) into the anterior chamber. As early as 1 day after the

injection a reduction of leakage was observed that persisted throughout the follow-up time of 1 month (Fig. 9.1) (Grisanti et al. 2006). Three years later, a report described a decrease in aqueous VEGF concentration in NVG patients who received intracameral bevacizumab (Grover et al. 2009). Since then, multiple case series reported on the regression of neovascularization of both the iris and the angle with the use of VEGF inhibitors. In one case report, a patient with neovascular glaucoma who failed IOP control with transscleral cyclophotocoagulation and PRP, showed an immediate decrease in IOP after injection of bevacizumab (1 mg in 0.04 mL) (Kahook et al. 2006a). Six consecutive patients with NVG described by Iliev et al. showed a marked regression of anterior segment neovascularization. Half of the patients showed a significant reduction of IOP after bevacizumab, and the remaining patients were controlled after additional cyclophotocoagulation and PRP (Iliev et al. 2006). VEGF-inhibition and regression of neovascularizations may therefore have an additional IOP-lowering effect that can develop rapidly within a few days.

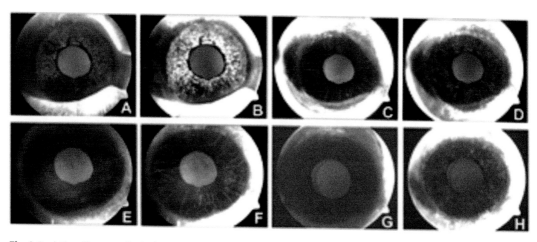

Fig. 9.1 At baseline, one day before intracameral Avastin injection (1.0 mg bevacizumab, Genentech, USA) iris fluorescein angiography revealed an advanced rubeosis (**a**: 30 s, **b**: 5 min). As early as 5 days after bevacizumab injection a massive reduction of rubeosis was evident in iris fluorescein angiography (**c**: 30 s, **d**: 5 min). The stabile regression of rubeosis was observed 30 days (**e**: 30 s, **f**: 5 min) as well as 170 days (**g**: 30 s, **h**: 5 min) after initial bevacizumab injection

9.4   Pharmacokinetics of Anti-VEGF Drugs in NVG

The degree and duration of the antiproliferative effect induced by anti-VEGF drugs is still a matter of debate. Both depend on the area of ischemic retina and the associated intravitreal VEGF level. Tripathi et al. demonstrated significantly increased levels of VEGF in the aqueous humor of patients with NVG that were 40- and 113-fold higher than in patients with primary open angle glaucoma or cataract, respectively (Tripathi et al. 1998). Comparable findings were reported for ischemic retinal disease such as diabetic retinopathy and central retinal vein occlusion (Shinoda et al. 2000). A direct blockade of VEGF by, e.g., bevacizumab interrupts this signaling cascade. The clinical effect can be observed as early as 1 day after injection (Grisanti et al. 2006). Therefore, the application of anti-VEGF drugs in patients with NVG allows a rapid control of the neovascularizations. In a rabbit model, the vitreous half-life of bevacizumab (1.25 mg) was shown to be 4.32 days. Small amounts of bevacizumab were also found in the serum and in the fellow uninjected eye (Bakri et al. 2007).

Gheith et al. analyzed the length of the therapeutic benefit of bevacizumab in a case series of 6 patients with an average follow-up of 9.7 months. They applied 1.25 mg/0.05 mL of bevacizumab intravitreally followed by PRP 1 week later which led to a complete regression of iris and angle neovascularizations in all patients. After 3 and 5 months, respectively, 2 patients had recurrence of rubeosis but displayed regression after another injection of bevacizumab (Gheith et al. 2007). Based on the pathomechanisms, a recurrence of iris neovascularizations must be expected if the underlying ischemic disease is not sufficiently treated. The date of recurrence varied depending on the amount of untreated retina. In our own series of 20 eyes (of 18 patients) with neovascular glaucoma. 14 (70 %) received additional to a mean of 2.75 bevacizumab injections (1.25/0.05 mL) an ablation of the ischemic retina (laser photoablation: $n = 13$, cryoablation: $n = 6$) during a follow-up of 1 year (Beutel et al. 2010).

Clinical studies addressed the question if the injection of anti-VEGF drugs should be applied in the vitreous or in the anterior chamber. Osamu et al. found that the VEGF concentration in the aqueous humor averaged 326 ± 125 pg/mL before intravitreal injection of bevacizumab and decreased to less than 31 pg/mL in all eyes 1 week after injection (Sawada et al. 2007). Lim et al. reported on the VEGF levels after intracameral bevacizumab injection. In this case series of 5 NVG patients, the intracameral VEGF levels were remarkably lowered from 1181.8 ± 1248.3 pg/mL to 33.2 pg/mL, which was much higher than that seen after intravitreal injection (Lim et al. 2009). The application of anti-VEFG in the anterior chamber may approach the anterior segment pathology more directly, but the injection of anti-VEGF in the vitreous seems to achieve a comparable clinical regression of NVI and may have even a longer lasting effect in view of the depot effect of the vitreous.

9.5   Treatment Regime in NVG Patients

Treatment of neovascular glaucoma needs a comprehensive approach. In view of the heterogeneity of the underlying diseases, the varying degree of ischemia and differences in anterior chamber angle involvement, the selection of therapeutic instruments must be carefully and individually assessed for every patient. First of all, the involvement of the anterior chamber angle has to be considered for treatment planning. The study group of Whakayabashi et al. analyzed NVG patients divided into different subgroups depending on the degree of involvement of the anterior chamber angle. In patients with NVG and an open angle, intravitreal bevacizumab injection (IVB) seems to be effective in stabilizing the IOP. In these cases, the aqueous outflow is not inhibited by neovascular membranes and one injection of IVB reduced the elevated IOP into the normal range in approximately 70 % of the study eyes. Rubeosis, however, recurred in 44 % by 6 months of follow-up. In contrast, the recurrence rate in the NVG group with a closed anterior chamber angle was even higher (71 %), indicating that the burden of VEGF in this advanced stage is more prominent. Nevertheless, the IOP decreased rapidly to a near-normal level by IVB monotherapy or IVB with topical antiglaucoma medication in 9 eyes (53 %). Therefore, IVB seems to be effective at least in selected cases also in this group. Nevertheless, a high proportion of patients (41 %) needed surgical intervention. This indicates that established fibrous membranes in the anterior chamber angle that are not sensitive to VEGF-inhibition were present. The increased IOP was controlled successfully by filtering surgery after repeated IVB without perioperative bleedings. In the last group with synechiae and closure of the anterior chamber angle, the efficacy of bevacizumab for achieving rapid and marked regression of iris and angle neovascularization in patients was similar to that in the other groups. Nevertheless, IVB was not able to reduce the elevated IOP in the majority of patients in this group with closed anterior chamber angle and progressive synechiae. Within 1 week after the initial IVB injection, 11 eyes (73 %) required

early surgical intervention. In total, 14 eyes (93 %) underwent surgery to stabilize the markedly elevated IOP by the first 2 months of follow-up. In these advanced stages of NVG, the role of anti-VEGF drugs is limited to halting the neovascular activities (Wakabayashi et al. 2008). However, this adjuvant allows reducing the risk of bleeding and inflammation which are well-known risks of trabeculectomy or shunt-tube drainage procedures for NVG independent of the degree of anterior chamber angle involvement (Elgin et al. 2006; Parrish and Herschler 1983; Tsai et al. 1995).

Therefore, a situation with early neovascularization and an open anterior chamber angle requires a less aggressive treatment to lower the IOP than a situation with an advanced involvement and closure of the anterior chamber angle.

Regarding the combination with other treatment modalities different therapeutic options are available (see Fig. 9.2). Treatment of the

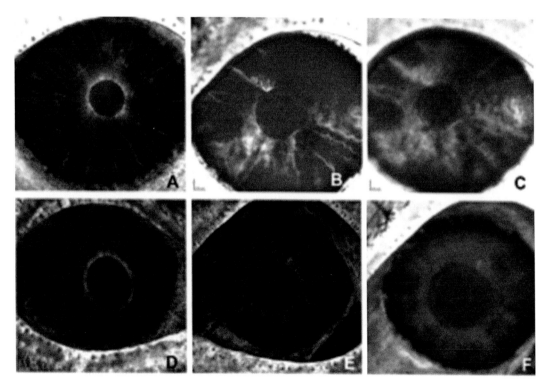

Fig. 9.2 A 84-year-female patient with a rubeotic secondary glaucoma based on a central retinal vein occlusion presented initially with an intraocular pressure of 48 mmHg. The iris fluorescein angiography (early phase, **a**; 60 s, **b**; 3 min, **c**) revealed a stage 4 rubeosis. After 3 days of intravitreal injection of ranibizumab, a rapid regression of rubeosis occurred (early phase, **d**; 60 s, **e**; 3 min, **f**) as well as a reduction of intraocular pressure (11 mmHg)

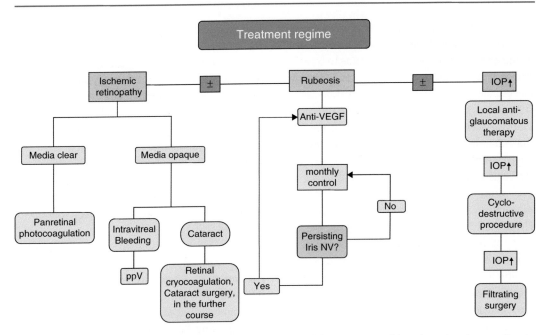

Fig. 9.3 Flow-chart demonstrating the different interventions chosen depending on the stage of ischemic retinopathy and the intraocular pressure. Anti-VEGF should be injected in every case with active rubeosis according to this treatment regime (Lüke et al. 2013)

underlying ischemic disease remains fundamental in all cases. PRP is the treatment of choice in case of clear optical media. Ehlers et al. compared the effect of PRP monotherapy with a combined approach of PRP and IVB. In this retrospective comparative analysis, the patients that received adjuvant bevacizumab injection had neovascular regression, while only 17 % of patients who underwent PRP monotherapy had regression. The high response rate in the combination treatment group supports the critical role that VEGF plays in anterior segment neovascularization (Ehlers et al. 2008). In a prospective series of 10 patients with NVG and 10 patients with rubeosis of the iris, all patients presented with a rapid regression of rubeosis (see Fig. 9.2) and a fast and a significant reduction of IOP in the NVG group. All patients required treatment of the underlying ischemic disease (Lüke et al. 2013). In one case, a vitrectomy was performed combined with PRP in one case. In three patients, cataract surgery was necessary to allow further laser coagulation of the retina. In the NVG group, the vast majority (90 %) received an IOP-lowering operative procedure. Based on these findings, we recommend a treatment

regime which is based on the IOP level, the degree of untreated retinal ischemia, the status of the optical media, and the involvement of the anterior chamber angle (see Fig. 9.3).

So far ranibizumab (Lüke et al. 2013, Fig. 9.2) and bevacizumab (Fig. 9.1) have been tested successfully for this indication. A study comparing the effect of different VEGF inhibitors has not been performed yet. In view of the off-label character of all anti-VEGF drugs for NVG, the choice will depend on underlying disease and comorbidities.

In terms of safety, concerns may arise regarding the VEGF-inhibition of all VEGF isoforms possibly leading to side effects in normal retinal tissues and circulation (Inan et al. 2007; Ishida et al. 2003). In our case series of severe ischemic retinal diseases, no increase of retinal ischemia was observed during a follow-up of 12 month after repeated ranibizumab injection for rubeosis and NVG. Additionally, no severe systemic side effects were observed. Nevertheless, 2 out of 18 patients (11 %) had a Serious Adverse Event per FDA definition that is in the range of previous ranibizumab studies especially of those with a comparable patients' selection (Massin et al.

2010). In view of the results of the CATT 2 study, which reported on higher rates of serious adverse events with bevacizumab, ranibizumab should be preferentially selected in those patients with cardiovascular risk factors (Martin et al. 2012). Additionally, it has to be considered that only ranibizumab is an approved therapy for CRVO or diabetic macular edema which can be coexistent in rubeotic secondary glaucoma (Massin et al. 2010; Mitchell et al. 2011).

9.6 Adjuvant Treatment in Filtering Surgery for Neovascular Glaucoma

Angiogenesis is part of the wound-healing process that may lead to scar formation after glaucoma filtration surgery. The risk for this unwanted side effect is augmented in neovascular glaucoma patients. VEGF promotes the early phase of angiogenesis especially endothelial cell migration and proliferation. The strongest stimulus for VEGF secretion is hypoxia. But also other paracrine acting factors such as TGF-ß1, EGF, TGF-α, bFGF, PDGF-BB, and IL-1b stimulate VEGF-expression (Barrientos et al. 2008).

The inhibition of VEGF to prevent angiogenesis during wound healing on the one hand and the reduction of fibroblast proliferation on the other hand by influencing the supply of FGF are synergistic effects of VEGF blockade and inhibit therefore both wound healing and angiogenesis (Corral et al. 1999; Jonas et al. 2007; Seghezzi et al. 1998). Preclinical studies, which compared anti-VEGF (bevacizumab) with 5-FU or BSS in a rabbit model revealed a significant delayed scarring after bevacizumab injection (Memarzadeh et al. 2009). Several case reports describe a positive effect of anti-VEGF as adjuvant in glaucoma filtration surgery in neovascular glaucoma patients (Katz et al. 1995; Kahook et al. 2006a; Kitnarong et al. 2008). A positive effect was reported after intravitreal injection (Jonas et al. 2007; Kitnarong et al. 2008) and after subconjunctival injection during (Caprioli et al. 1985; Gheith et al. 2007) or after glaucoma filtration surgery (Kahook et al. 2006a). The preoperative

intravitreal application may additionally prevent intraoperative bleedings (Cornish et al. 2009; Li et al. 2009). The subconjunctival injection in contrast may have a better local antifibrotic effect (Grewal et al. 2008).

9.7 Summary

Neovascular glaucoma may be the cause of severe loss in visual function and has mainly a bad prognosis as it is highly resistant to different treatment modalities. In this severe disease, adjuvant application of anti-VEGF drugs allows a rapid regression of rubeosis. Dependent on the stage of the disease, a fast IOP reduction will help to improve prognosis. Anti-VEGF treatment is meaningful for short-term control, but it achieves also a long-term effect by inhibiting the progression and establishment of angle obstruction, which is a severe complication of rubeosis. In the treatment of NVG, conventional therapeutic procedures addressing the retinal ischemia and the source of the angiogenic stimulus should always be performed, but the adjuvant application of anti-VEGF therapy is a necessary instrument in a modern treatment approach in patients with rubeosis and neovascular glaucoma. The need for continued monitoring of NVI has to be considered in this complex disease.

Compliance with Ethical Requirements Compliance with Ethical Requirements: Julia Lüke, Matthias Lüke, and Salvatore Grisanti declare that they have no conflict of interest. All procedures followed were in accordance with the ethical standards of the responsible committee on human experimentation (institutional and national) and with the Helsinki Declaration of 1975, as revised in 2000. Informed consent was obtained from all patients for being included in the study.

The authors were supported by Novartis Pharma to perform an IIT.

References

Assaad MH, Baerveldt G, Rockwood EJ. Glaucoma drainage devices: pros and cons. Curr Opin Ophthalmol. 1999;10:147–53.

Avery RL. Regression of retinal and iris neovascularization after intravitreal bevacizumab (Avastin) treatment. Retina. 2006;26:352–4.

Bakri SJ, Snyder MR, Reid JM, Pulido JS, Singh RJ. Pharmacokinetics of intravitreal bevacizumab (Avastin). Ophthalmology. 2007;114:855–9.

Barrientos S, Stojadinovic O, Golinko MS, Brem H, Tomic-Canic M. Growth factors and cytokines in wound healing. Wound Repair Regen. 2008;16:585–601.

Beutel J, Peters S, Lüke M, Aisenbrey S, Szurman P, Spitzer MS, Yoeruek E, Bevacizumab Study Group, Grisanti S. Bevacizumab as adjuvant for neovascular glaucoma. Acta Ophthalmol. 2010;88:103–9.

Brouillette G, Chebil A. Long-term results of modified trabeculectomy with supramid implant for neovascular glaucoma. Can J Ophthalmol. 1987;22:254–6.

Brown GC, Magargal LE, Schachat A, Shah H. Neovascular glaucoma. Etiologic considerations. Ophthalmology. 1984;91:315–20.

Caprioli J, Strang SL, Spaeth GL, Poryzees EH. Cyclocryotherapy in the treatment of advanced glaucoma. Ophthalmology. 1985;92:947–54.

Cornish KS, Ramamurthi S, Saidkasimova S, Ramaesh K. Intravitreal bevacizumab and augmented trabeculectomy for neovascular glaucoma in young diabetic patients. Eye (Lond). 2009;23:979–81.

Corral CJ, Siddiqui A, Wu L, Farrell CL, Lyons D, Mustoe TA. Vascular endothelial growth factor is more important than basic fibroblastic growth factor during ischemic wound healing. Arch Surg. 1999;134:200–5.

Davidorf FH, Mouser JG, Derick RJ. Rapid improvement of rubeosis iridis from a single bevacizumab (Avastin) injection. Retina. 2006;26:354–6.

Ehlers JP, Spirn MJ, Lam A, Sivalingam A, Samuel MA, Tasman W. Combination intravitreal bevacizumab/panretinal photocoagulation versus panretinal photocoagulation alone in the treatment of neovascular glaucoma. Retina. 2008;28:696–702.

Elgin U, Berker N, Batman A, Simsek T, Cankaya B. Trabeculectomy with mitomycin C combined with direct cauterization of peripheral iris in the management of neovascular glaucoma. J Glaucoma. 2006;15:466–70.

Feibel RM, Bigger JF. Rubeosis iridis and neovascular glaucoma. Evaluation of cyclocryotherapy. Am J Ophthalmol. 1972;74:862–7.

Fernández-Vigo J, Castro J, Macarro A. Diabetic iris neovascularization. Natural history and treatment. Acta Ophthalmol Scand. 1997;75:89–93.

Gheith ME, Siam GA, de Barros DS, Garg SJ, Moster MR. Role of intravitreal bevacizumab in neovascular glaucoma. J Ocul Pharmacol Ther. 2007;23:487–91.

Grewal DS, Jain R, Kumar H, Grewal SP. Evaluation of subconjunctival bevacizumab as an adjunct to trabeculectomy a pilot study. Ophthalmology. 2008; 115:2141–5.

Grisanti S, Biester S, Peters S, Tatar O, Ziemssen F, Bartz-Schmidt KU, Tuebingen Bevacizumab Study Group. Intracameral bevacizumab for iris rubeosis. Am J Ophthalmol. 2006;142:158–60.

Grover S, Gupta S, Sharma R, Brar VS, Chalam KV. Intracameral bevacizumab effectively reduces aqueous vascular endothelial growth factor concentrations in neovascular glaucoma. Br J Ophthalmol. 2009;93:273–4.

Iliev ME, Domig D, Wolf-Schnurrbursch U, Wolf S, Sarra GM. Intravitreal bevacizumab (Avastin) in the treatment of neovascular glaucoma. Am J Ophthalmol. 2006;142:1054–6.

Inan UU, Avci B, Kusbeci T, Kaderli B, Avci R, Temel SG. Preclinical evaluation of intravitreal injection of full-length humanized vascular endothelial growth factor antibody in rabbit eyes. Invest Ophthalmol Vis Sci. 2007;48:1773–81.

Ishida S, Usui T, Yamashiro K, Kaji Y, Amano S, Ogura Y, Hida T, Oguchi Y, Ambati J, Miller JW, Gragoudas ES, Ng YS, D'Amore PA, Shima DT, Adamis AP. VEGF164-mediated inflammation is required for pathological, but not physiological, ischemia-induced retinal neovascularization. J Exp Med. 2003;198:483–9.

Jonas JB, Spandau UH, Schlichtenbrede F. Intravitreal bevacizumab for filtering surgery. Ophthalmic Res. 2007;39:121–2.

Kahook MY, Schuman JS, Noecker RJ. Intravitreal bevacizumab in a patient with neovascular glaucoma. Ophthalmic Surg Lasers Imaging. 2006a;37:144–6.

Kahook MY, Schuman JS, Noecker RJ. Needle bleb revision of encapsulated filtering bleb with bevacizumab. Ophthalmic Surg Lasers Imaging. 2006b;37:148–50.

Katz GJ, Higginbotham EJ, Lichter PR, Skuta GL, Musch DC, Bergstrom TJ, Johnson AT. Mitomycin C versus 5-fluorouracil in high-risk glaucoma filtering surgery. Extended follow-up. Ophthalmology. 1995;102: 1263–9.

Kirchhof B. Retinectomy lowers intraocular pressure in otherwise intractable glaucoma: preliminary results. Ophthalmic Surg. 1994;25:262–7.

Kitnarong N, Chindasub P, Metheetrairut A. Surgical outcome of intravitreal bevacizumab and filtration surgery in neovascular glaucoma. Adv Ther. 2008;25: 438–43.

L'Esperance Jr FA, Mittl RN, James Jr WA. Carbon dioxide laser trabeculostomy for the treatment of neovascular glaucoma. Ophthalmology. 1983;90:821–9.

Li D, Zhang C, Song F, Lubenec I, Tian Y, Song QH. VEGF regulates FGF-2 and TGF-beta1 expression in injury endothelial cells and mediates smooth muscle cells proliferation and migration. VEGF regulates FGF-2 and TGF-beta1 expression in injury endothelial cells and mediates smooth muscle cells proliferation and migration. Microvasc Res. 2009;77:134–42.

Lim TH, Bae SH, Cho YJ, Lee JH, Kim HK, Sohn YH. Concentration of vascular endothelial growth factor after intracameral bevacizumab injection in eyes with neovascular glaucoma. Korean J Ophthalmol. 2009;23(3):188–92.

Lüke J, Nassar K, Lüke M, Grisanti S. Ranibizumab as adjuvant in the treatment of rubeosis iridis and neovascular glaucoma—results from a prospective interventional case series. Graefes Arch Clin Exp Ophthalmol. 2013;251:2403–13.

Martin DF, Maguire MG, Fine SL, Fine SL, Ying GS, Jaffe GJ, Grunwald JE, Toth C, Redford M, Ferris 3rd FL. Comparison of Age-related Macular Degeneration Treatments Trials (CATT) Research Group Writing Committee: Ranibizumab and Bevacizumab for treatment of neovascular age-related macular degeneration: two-year results. Ophthalmology. 2012;119: 1388–98.

Massin P, Bandello F, Garweg JG, Hansen LL, Harding SP, Larsen M, Mitchell P, Sharp D, Wolf-Schnurrbusch UE, Gekkieva M, Weichselberger A, Wolf S. Safety and efficacy of ranibizumab in diabetic macular edema (RESOLVE Study): a 12-month, randomized, controlled, double-masked, multicenter phase II study. Diabetes Care. 2010;33:2399–405.

Memarzadeh F, Varma R, Lin LT, Parikh JG, Dustin L, Alcaraz A, Eliott D. Postoperative use of bevacizumab as an antifibrotic agent in glaucoma filtration surgery in the rabbit. Invest Ophthalmol Vis Sci. 2009;50:3233–7.

Mitchell P, Bandello F, Schmidt-Erfurth U, Lang GE, Massin P, Schlingemann RO, Sutter F, Simader C, Burian G, Gerstner O, Weichselberger A, RESTORE Study Group. The RESTORE study: ranibizumab monotherapy or combined with laser versus laser monotherapy for diabetic macular edema. Ophthalmology. 2011;118:615–62.

Parrish R, Herschler J. Eyes with end-stage neovascular glaucoma: natural history following successful modified filtering operation. Arch Ophthalmol. 1983; 101:745–6.

Sawada O, Kawamura H, Kakinoki M, Sawada T, Ohji M. Vascular endothelial growth factor in aqueous humor before and after intravitreal injection of Bevacizumab in eyes with diabetic retinopathy. Arch Ophthalmol. 2007;125:1363–6.

Seghezzi G, Patel S, Ren CJ, Gualandris A, Pintucci G, Robbins ES, Shapiro RL, Galloway AC, Rifkin DB, Mignatti P. Fibroblast growth factor-2 (FGF-2) induces vascular endothelial growth factor (VEGF) expression in the endothelial cells of forming capillaries: an autocrine mechanism contributing to angiogenesis. J Cell Biol. 1998;141(7):1659–73.

Shields MB, Shields SE. Noncontact transscleral Nd:YAG cyclophotocoagulation: a long-term follow-up of 500 patients. Trans Am Ophthalmol Soc. 1994;92:271–83. discussion 283-287.

Shinoda K, Ishida S, Kawashima S, Wakabayashi T, Uchita M, Matsuzaki T, Takayama M, Shinmura K, Yamada M. Clinical factors related to the aqueous levels of vascular endothelial growth factor and hepatocyte growth factor in proliferative diabetic retinopathy. Curr Eye Res. 2000;21:655–61.

Sivak-Callcott JA, O'Day DM, Gass JDM, Tsai JC. Evidence-based recommendations for the diagnosis and treatment of neovascular glaucoma. Ophthalmology. 2001;108:1767–78.

Tolentino MJ, Miller JW, Gragoudas ES, Chatzistefanou K, Ferrara N, Adamis AP. Vascular endothelial growth factor is sufficient to produce iris neovascularization and neovascular glaucoma in a nonhuman primate. Arch Ophthalmol. 1996;114(8):964–70.

Tripathi RC, Li J, Tripathi BJ, Chalam KV, Adamis AP. Increased level of vascular endothelial growth factor in aqueous humor of patients with neovascular glaucoma. Ophthalmology. 1998;105:232–7.

Tsai JC, Feuer WJ, Parrish 2nd RK, Grajewski AL. 5-Fluorouracil filtering surgery and neovascular glaucoma. Long-term follow-up of the original pilot study. Ophthalmology. 1995;102:887–92.

Wakabayashi T, Oshima Y, Sakaguchi H, Ikuno Y, Miki A, Gomi F, Otori Y, Kamei M, Kusaka S, Tano Y. Intravitreal bevacizumab to treat iris neovascularization and neovascular glaucoma secondary to ischemic retinal diseases in 41 consecutive cases. Ophthalmology. 2008;115:1571–80.

Wand M, Dueker DK, Aiello LM, Grant WM. Effects of panretinal photocoagulation on rubeosis iridis, angle neovascularization, and neovascular glaucoma. Am J Ophthalmol. 1978;86:332–9.

Corneal Neovascular Diseases

10

Deniz Hos, Felix Bock, Björn Bachmann,
and Claus Cursiefen

10.1 Introduction

The healthy cornea is one of the very few avascular tissues of the body that contains no blood and lymphatic vessels. This avascularity, which is also termed the corneal "(lymph)angiogenic privilege", is evolutionary highly conserved and is essential for corneal transparency and proper vision (Cursiefen 2007). Thus, minor inflammatory and angiogenic stimuli, to which the cornea is constantly exposed due to its anatomical position, generally do not result in corneal neovascularization, as the cornea expresses potent antiangiogenic molecules to actively maintain its avascular state (Albuquerque et al. 2009; Ambati et al. 2006; Cursiefen et al. 2006, 2011; Singh et al. 2013). However, severe corneal damage can overcome this corneal angiogenic privilege and lead to the pathological ingrowths of blood as well as lymphatic vessels from the limbus into the cornea (corneal neovascularization) (Cursiefen 2007). This corneal neovascularization (1) results in reduced corneal transparency and visual acuity; (2) is the most important risk factor for graft rejection after keratoplasty; and (3) has recently been shown to contribute to the development of several corneal pathologies such as dry eye disease (Bock et al. 2013; Hos and Cursiefen 2014; Hos et al. 2014; Goyal et al. 2010). The inhibition of corneal neovascularization as a therapeutic approach has recently been translated into the clinic and shows promising results (Bock et al. 2013).

This review will recapitulate recent findings in the field of corneal neovascular disease. We will first give an overview of recently discovered mechanisms that contribute to the corneal angiogenic privilege. Second, we will present diseases that are associated with corneal neovascularization and review the impact of corneal neovascularization on visual acuity and on corneal graft survival after transplantation. Third, we will present how corneal neovessels can be morphometrically analyzed. Finally, we will specify current clinically applied antiangiogenic treatment strategies against corneal neovascularization. As was declared by a recent consensus meeting, there is a huge unmet need for topical inhibitors of angiogenesis at the ocular surface (Cursiefen et al. 2012).

D. Hos, M.D. • F. Bock, Ph.D.
B. Bachmann, M.D. (✉) • C. Cursiefen M.D.
Department of Ophthalmology, University
of Cologne, Kerpener Strasse 62, 50924
Cologne, Germany
e-mail: deniz.hos@uk-koeln.de; felix.bock@
uk-koeln.de; bjoern.bachmann@uk-koeln.de;
claus.cursiefen@uk-koeln.de

© Springer International Publishing Switzerland 2016
A. Stahl (ed.), *Anti-Angiogenic Therapy in Ophthalmology*,
Essentials in Ophthalmology, DOI 10.1007/978-3-319-24097-8_10

10.2 Corneal (Lymph)angiogenic Privilege

Recently, several molecular mechanisms that contribute to the corneal angiogenic privilege could be identified. In this context, especially the corneal epithelium seems to be crucial for the maintenance of corneal avascularity, as it expresses several potent antiangiogenic factors such as endostatin, angiostatin, thrombospondin-1, thrombospondin-2, pigment epithelium-derived factor, and others (Armstrong and Bornstein 2003; Cursiefen et al. 2004c, 2011; Lin et al. 2001). These molecules are able to directly inhibit vascular endothelial cell proliferation and migration, and it has also been shown that these factors can interfere with growth factor mobilization and binding. Additionally, the corneal epithelium expresses soluble VEGF receptor-1 (sVEGFR-1), soluble VEGFR-2 (sVEGFR-2), and soluble VEGFR-3 (sVEGFR-3) which all act as decoy receptors and sequester (lymph)angiogenic VEGFs (Albuquerque et al. 2009; Ambati et al. 2006; Singh et al. 2013). In addition, we could previously demonstrate that the corneal epithelium also ectopically expresses membrane bound VEGFR-3, which is able to bind angiogenic ligands and therefore reduce binding of these to VEGFR-3 expressed on lymphatic vascular endothelial cells (Cursiefen et al. 2006). Furthermore, the cornea is also able to actively suppress neovascularization under hypoxic conditions by the expression of inhibitory PAS domain protein (IPAS), which negatively regulates hypoxia-induced upregulation of VEGF (Makino et al. 2001).

Due to these antiangiogenic mechanisms, corneal neovascularization usually does not occur as the cornea is able to buffer most minor angiogenic stimuli. However, severe and eye-threatening inflammation can overcome the corneal antiangiogenic mechanisms and result in the pathological ingrowths of blood and clinically invisible lymphatic vessels from the limbus into the cornea (Fig. 10.1) (Cursiefen 2007).

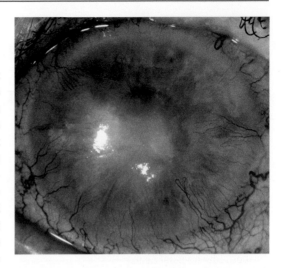

Fig. 10.1 Corneal neovascularization in a patient with recurrent herpetic ulcerative keratitis. Blood vessels originate from the limbus and grow towards the center of the cornea. Note secondary central corneal scar

10.3 Corneal Neovascular Disease

10.3.1 Corneal Diseases Resulting in Corneal Neovascularization

As mentioned in the previous chapter, severe pathological processes can lead to a breakdown of the corneal angiogenic privilege and result in secondary ingrowths of blood and lymphatic vessels from the limbus into the cornea. These processes include inflammatory (e.g., ocular pemphigoid, Lyell-syndrome, Stevens–Johnson syndrome, graft-versus-host disease, corneal graft rejection, dry eye disease), infectious (e.g., viral, bacterial, or fungal dermatitis), degenerative (e.g., Terrien marginal degeneration, pterygium), hypoxic (e.g., extended contact lens wear), and traumatic diseases (e.g., chemical burns). Ocular pathologies that lead to a loss of limbal barrier function (e.g., limbal stem cell deficiency) are also frequently accompanied by corneal neovessels. In this context, corneal inflammation and ulceration accompanied by corneal neovascularization are amongst the leading causes of severe vision loss worldwide (Whither et al. 2002).

10.3.2 Reduction of Visual Acuity and Promotion of Immune Responses by Corneal Blood and Lymphatic Vessels

Independent of the underlying disease, corneal blood vessels can lead to corneal scarring and significantly impair corneal transparency and vision. Visual acuity can become directly impaired by the ingrowths of corneal blood vessels into the optical zone leading to light scattering or obscuration. Also secondary effects such as corneal edema, lipid deposition, and hemorrhage through immature and leaky capillaries can further reduce visual acuity. In addition, immune effector cells such as macrophages and T lymphocytes can easily reach the cornea via pathological blood vessels and can damage the structural integrity of the cornea.

Clinically, improvements in visual acuity frequently occur when central corneal neovascularization or central lipid keratopathy decrease (Fig. 10.2). However, peripheral corneal edema or corneal obscuration outside the optic zone might still allow for good visual function. In contrast to the clinical experience, only little evidence in the literature suggests a positive effect of the reduction of corneal neovascularization on visual acuity (Bachmann et al. 2013). So far, studies are missing that investigate the space-resolved change of corneal neovascularization and its influence on visual acuity. However, the localization of corneal neovascularization is decisive whether a successful antiangiogenic treatment results in improved visual acuity. Future studies are needed that correlate the regression of centrally located corneal vessels with visual acuity.

Unlike blood vessels, clinically invisible lymphatic vessels do not lead to a significant reduction of corneal transparency per se, but have been shown to substantially contribute to several corneal pathologies such as corneal transplant rejection, dry eye disease, and ocular allergy (Lee et al. 2015 Bock et al. 2013; Dietrich et al. 2010; Goyal et al. 2010; Hos and Cursiefen 2014). Here, corneal lymphatic vessels seem to

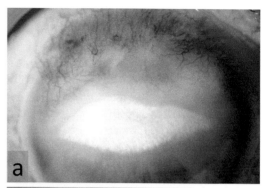

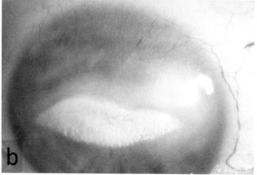

Fig. 10.2 (**a**) Dense corneal neovascularization associated with secondary lipid keratopathy. The patient was only able to see hand movements. (**b**) Improvement of corneal neovascularization and lipid keratopathy 1 month after fine needle diathermy of corneal vessels combined with topical application of Bevacizumab. Visual acuity also increased to 20/100. The aim of this measure was to improve graft survival after subsequent penetrating keratoplasty

serve as conduits that enable accelerated migration of antigen-presenting cells from the ocular surface to the lymph nodes and contribute to—as in the case of these diseases—undesired immune responses (Hos et al. 2014).

10.3.3 Corneal Neovascularization as a Risk Factor for Corneal Transplant Rejection

Corneal neovascularization has long been accepted as a risk factor for graft rejection and graft failure after perforating corneal transplantation (Dana and Streilein 1996; Sano et al. 1995). The cornea is considered to be an immune privileged anatomical structure not only due to its angiogenic privilege but also because of the absence of MHCII positive antigen-presenting cells in the central part of the cornea and the expression of Fas ligand on corneal endothelial cells which induces apoptosis in immune competent cells expressing the Fas receptor (Niederkorn 1999, 2010). Moreover, certain neuropeptides secreted by sensory corneal nerves seem to contribute to the corneal immune privilege (Niederkorn 2010). Thus, graft rejection after keratoplasty performed in avascular normal-risk corneas occurs in less than 20 % within 5 years after transplantation even without systemic immunosuppressive therapy (Williams et al. 2012). However, in prevascularized, high-risk corneas the rejection rate is higher than 50 %, even with systemic immunosuppressive therapy.

The definition of high-risk corneal transplantation is primarily based on the degree of corneal neovessels in the host's cornea. Corneas are thought to be on a higher risk for graft rejection, which is the most frequent reason for graft failure, when the host's deep corneal stoma is vascularized in a minimum of two quadrants. Compared with avascular recipients the relative risk for graft rejection is 2.67 if more than two quadrants are vascularized (Bachmann et al. 2010). Based on these findings, the concept of preconditioning high-risk grafts aims on a reduction of the preoperative corneal vessel load by adopting different antiangiogenic therapies (see Sect. 10.5).

In contrast to many clinical studies evaluating the effect of preexisting corneal neovessels before corneal transplantation so far only limited study evidence describes the influence of postoperative corneal neovascularization on graft rejection or graft failure (Altenburger et al. 2012; Lam et al. 2006; Cursiefen et al. 2001b, 2002a; Jonas et al. 2002). In fact, about ¾ of patients undergoing penetrating keratoplasty develop post-keratoplasty corneal neovascularization (Altenburger et al. 2012; Cursiefen et al. 2001b, 2002a; Jonas et al. 2002; Lam et al. 2006). In about 10 %, these new vessels even reach the host–graft interface (Altenburger et al. 2012; Cursiefen et al. 2001b; Lam et al. 2006). This post-keratoplasty neovascularization also seems to increase the risk for subsequent immune reactions (Jonas et al. 2002).

After corneal grafting, preexisting corneal vessels can further increase. Whether this affects graft rejection has so far only been evaluated experimentally. In mice, the additional ingrowths of blood and lymphatic vessels after corneal transplantation leads to higher rejection rates not only in normal corneas, but also in high-risk corneas (Bachmann et al. 2008, 2009; Cursiefen et al. 2004a). This suggests that the inhibition of corneal neovascularization after keratoplasty might also have a protective effect against graft rejection in humans (Fig. 10.3).

10.3.4 Corneal Lymphangiogenesis in Dry Eye Disease and Ocular Allergy

Studies analyzing the time course of pathologic corneal hem- and lymphangiogenesis during corneal inflammation have revealed that blood and lymphatic vessels usually grow in parallel into the cornea (Cursiefen et al. 2004b, 2006b). Furthermore, it is known that after brief inflammation corneal lymphatic vessels regress earlier and more completely in comparison to corneal blood vessels (Cursiefen et al. 2002b, 2006b). Accordingly, vascularized corneas may contain only blood but no more lymphatic vessels, when inflammation is no longer present and had occurred more than 6 months ago. However, several experimental studies could demonstrate that there are also diseases of the ocular surface that result in selective corneal lymphangiogenesis without hemangiogenesis, namely dry eye and ocular allergy.

It is widely accepted that dry eye is not only a condition with alterations in tear quantity and composition, but a complex disease, where chronic inflammation is maintained by adaptive immune responses (Niederkorn et al. 2006; Schaumburg et al. 2011). Recently, our group showed that in thrombospondin-1 deficient mice, which develop dry eye similar to Sjogren's syndrome, an isolated growth of corneal lymphatic

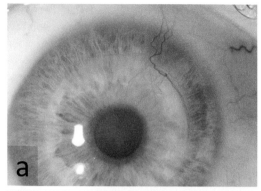

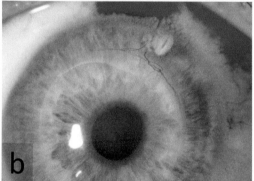

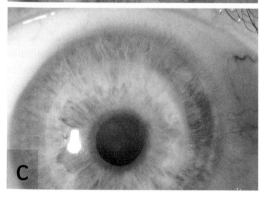

Fig. 10.3 (**a**) Corneal blood vessels reaching the graft–host interface after perforating keratoplasty. (**b**) One day after fine needle diathermy combined with topical application of Bevacizumab the site of coagulation is visible. (**c**) Two months after fine needle diathermy, no blood vessels are visible in the graft or in the host's cornea. This shall reduce the risk of graft rejection after keratoplasty

vessels occurs (Cursiefen et al. 2011). Furthermore, mice that are exposed to desiccating stress with high air flow and low humidity also develop corneal inflammation accompanied by lymphangiogenesis without concurrent

hemangiogenesis (Goyal et al. 2010). These corneal lymphatics seem to facilitate trafficking of antigen-presenting cells from the ocular surface to the lymph nodes, where accelerated autosensitization occurs. Importantly, selective inhibition of lymphangiogenesis can significantly improve the clinical course of dry eye disease, at least in the experimental setting (Goyal et al. 2012).

Very recently, the contribution of lymphangiogenesis to ocular allergy has also been determined. It was shown that mice with severe forms of experimentally induced ocular allergy develop corneal lymphatic, but not blood vessels (Lee et al. 2015). Further analysis of allergic mice revealed that these pathologic lymphatic vessels enable egress of activated antigen-presenting cells from the cornea to the regional lymph nodes and contribute to Th-2 responses. Notably, inhibition of corneal lymphangiogenesis in these mice reduced allergy-associated Th-2 responses and significantly ameliorated clinical disease (Lee et al. 2015).

Taken together, corneal lymphangiogenesis seems to play an essential role in the development of dry eye disease and ocular allergy. This offers an exciting and promising therapeutic target to treat these very frequently occurring diseases.

10.4 Morphological Characterization and Quantification of Corneal Neovascularization

As described in the above chapters, blood and lymphatic vessels play a crucial role in several corneal diseases. To analyze the morphology of corneal blood and lymphatic vessels, the cornea provides unique properties in several ways: the cornea is physiologically transparent and is also easily accessible for in vivo imaging. This chapter will summarize current imaging and quantification methods to characterize corneal hem- and lymphangiogenesis.

10.4.1 Morphology of Corneal Vessels

In 1998, Cursiefen et al. performed a histopathological study to analyze the incidence and localization of vessels in diseased corneas. Within over 1200 corneal buttons obtained by keratoplasty, the group detected corneal neovascularization in about 20 % of the buttons with different disease associations. The occurrence of vessels was accompanied by corneal edema and an inflammatory cell infiltrate. Most of the vessels were located in the upper and middle third of the corneal stroma, whereas only few vessels were located in the deep stromal layers (Cursiefen et al. 1998). Within the vascularized corneas in this study, 87 % of the vessels were covered by pericytes, which support the long-term, growth factor independent survival of vascular endothelial cells. The coverage of corneal blood vessels by pericytes starts early and increases with the duration of neovascularization, until almost all vessels have recruited pericytes (Cursiefen et al. 2003).

By ultrastructural analysis it was shown that, in addition to corneal blood vessels, thin-walled, erythrocyte-free lymphatic vessels could be found in human corneal buttons obtained from keratoplasty. These lymphatics can be stained with the lymphatic markers LYVE-1 and podoplanin and represented about 8 % of all vessels. Lymphatic vessels were mainly present in the early phase of corneal neovascularization and were always accompanied by blood vessels as well as by stromal inflammatory cells (Cursiefen et al. 2002b).

10.4.2 Quantification of Corneal Blood and Lymphatic Vessels

As described in the previous chapters, corneal neovascularization serves as an indicator of corneal inflammation and is a major risk factor for corneal graft rejection (Bachmann et al. 2010). Therefore, the quantification of the corneal vessel load is an important tool to monitor the course of ongoing inflammatory processes at the cornea as well as for the follow-up of antiangiogenic therapies.

The most common method to quantify corneal neovascularization is the assessment of numbers of corneal quadrants which show vascularization (Bachmann et al. 2010; Niederkorn 2003). A more sophisticated method is the digital image analysis. This method was first used in our laboratories for the quantification of blood and lymphatic vessels in a murine model of corneal neovascularization, where the vascularized corneas were stained immunohistochemically with CD31 as blood endothelial marker and LYVE-1 as lymph endothelial marker (Bock et al. 2008b). The morphometry of corneal hem- and lymphangiogenesis is afterwards performed semiautomatically on digital images using image analysis software. The semiautomatic method is mainly based on a threshold analysis. After the use of different digital filters, the blood and lymphatic vessels appear bright and are represented by gray values which are very well distinguishable from the background gray values (Fig. 10.4). We could show that the semiautomatic quantification of corneal neovascularization is very valid in measuring the area covered by blood or lymphatic vessels and has a good reproducibility with respect to both vessel types. This new semiautomatic morphometry method based on threshold analysis therefore provides a high accuracy. Using this method, we analyzed experimental corneal hem- and lymphangiogenesis in various scenarios and were able to even detect small differences within the analyzed groups (Bock et al. 2007, 2008a; Bucher et al. 2012; Dietrich et al. 2007; Hos et al. 2008a, b, 2011a, b, 2013; Regenfuss et al. 2010; Lipp et al. 2014). Based on this method, further characteristics of the vessel network like vessel endpoints, branching points, vessel length, or vessel diameter can now be assessed (Blacher et al. 2009).

The method of semiautomatic quantification of corneal vessels is also already transferred into clinical studies (Cursiefen et al. 2009, 2014). In this context, we performed a multicenter, randomized, double-blind study in which we analyzed the area covered by vessels in a three-month follow-up time period (Fig. 10.5) (Cursiefen et al. 2009). The extent of corneal neovascularization was determined by repeatedly performed

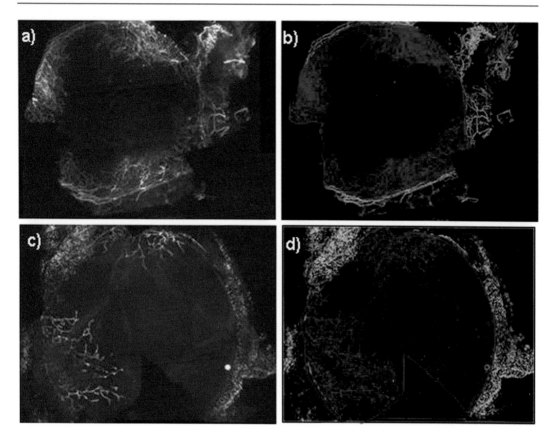

Fig. 10.4 Digital quantification of corneal blood and lymphatic vessels in a mouse model of corneal vascularization. (**a**) Original flat mount specifically stained for blood vessels (CD31); (**b**) modified image of (**a**) with detected blood vessels in *red*; (**c**) original flat mount specifically stained for lymphatic vessels (LYVE-1); (**d**) modified image of (**c**) with detected lymphatic vessels in *red*. Modified from Bock et al. 2008b, with permission of Elsevier

standardized digital slit-lamp photographs, which then were analyzed morphometrically using the image analysis software based on gray filter sampling. The method made it possible to detect significant changes of neovascularization in a range of 2 % of the total corneal area.

10.5   Therapeutic Inhibition of Corneal Neovascularization

Numerous potential antiangiogenic treatment strategies for corneal neovascular diseases have already been tested in preclinical models with promising results. However, only few have so far reached the way into clinical trials or are used off-label to treat patients with corneal neovascularization. Although several specific angiogenesis inhibitors such as Ranibizumab, Aflibercept, and Pegaptanib have been approved by the US Food and Drug Administration for the treatment of pathologic neovascularization at the posterior pole of the eye, no specific angiogenesis inhibitor against corneal neovascularization has been approved so far. This part of the review will focus on antiangiogenic therapies at the cornea with already existing clinical experience.

10.5.1   Corticosteroids

Corticosteroids are potent anti-inflammatory drugs which are still the clinical standard of antiangiogenic therapy at the cornea (Bock et al. 2013; Hos et al. 2011b). These drugs are known

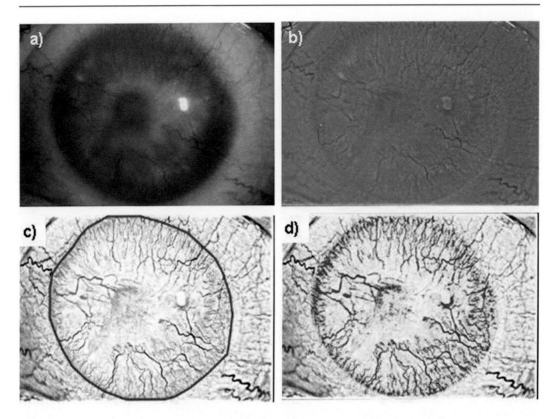

Fig. 10.5 Digital quantification of corneal blood vessels in the clinical setting. (**a**) Original image of a vascularized cornea; (**b**) shading correction of (a); (**c**) gray value image of (**b**) with defined region of interest; (**d**) detection of blood vessels (red) in the modified corneal image. Modified from Cursiefen et al. 2009, with permission of Elsevier

to reduce corneal hemangiogenesis and, as recently demonstrated, also corneal lymphangiogenesis (Hos et al. 2011b). The antiangiogenic effect of corticosteroids is mainly indirect due to the reduction of inflammation in the cornea. In addition, corticosteroids also show direct inhibitory effects on vascular endothelial cells (Hos et al. 2011b). The anti(lymph)angiogenic potency of corticosteroids varies with prednisolone having the strongest effects. Nonetheless, although corticosteroids are effective antiangiogenic agents, the prolonged use of these drugs may cause several side effects such as delayed epithelial wound healing, elevated intraocular pressure, or cataract. Furthermore, although corticosteroids suppress the formation of new vessels in progressive corneal neovascular diseases, they are less effective in regressing already present, mature vessels. Furthermore, especially in highly

inflamed settings such as after penetrating keratoplasty, steroids even at high dosage are not sufficient to block corneal neovascularization (Cursiefen et al. 2001a).

10.5.2 Anti-VEGF Therapy

Preclinically, several specific antiangiogenic treatment strategies targeting VEGF have already been tested in the past. In 2004, the $VEGF_{R1R2}$ trap (Aflibercept) showed an almost complete blockade of both hem- and lymphangiogenesis in the inflamed mouse cornea (Cursiefen et al. 2004a). Further anti-VEGF therapeutic strategies that were experimentally tested so far are antibodies directed against VEGF (Bevacizumab, Ranibizumab) (Bock et al. 2007; Bucher et al. 2012), aptamers binding VEGF (Pegaptanib)

(Lipp et al. 2014), VEGF receptor blocking antibodies (anti-VEGFR3) (Bock et al. 2008a), VEGF receptor tyrosine kinases (Detry et al. 2013; Hos et al. 2008b), and several others. Despite the progress in the experimental setting, none of these specific inhibitors has an FDA approval for the use at the cornea, as already mentioned above. Nonetheless, Bevacizumab is frequently used off-label to treat patients with corneal neovascularization also in the context of corneal transplantation, and several groups have already proven the effectiveness and safety of Bevacizumab in inhibiting corneal hemangiogenesis (Koenig et al. 2012). In addition, recent studies have also shown the effectiveness of Ranibizumab in inhibiting corneal neovascularization in patients (Ferrari et al. 2013). Bevacizumab and Ranibizumab can penetrate well into the cornea and reach sufficient concentrations especially in case of an absent or altered corneal epithelial barrier (as is the case in vascularized corneas). In this context, Dastjerdi et al. analyzed if Bevacizumab as a full length antibody can penetrate the cornea. They found that indeed the intact corneal epithelium almost completely avoids the penetration of this antibody. As soon as the cornea is vascularized the penetration is much better. The subconjunctival application of this antibody also resulted in strong deposition of the drug in the corneal stroma even in healthy eyes (Dastjerdi et al. 2011). Ranibizumab and Bevacizumab show comparable antiangiogenic results at the cornea although Ranibizumab seems to be slightly more effective. In addition, both have recently been shown to block also corneal lymphangiogenesis, at least in the experimental setting (Bock et al. 2007; Bucher et al. 2012).

10.5.3 GS-101: Antisense Oligonucleotide against IRS-1

Insulin receptor substrate-1 (IRS-1) has recently been shown to be an important intracellular signalling molecule in the angiogenic cascade. The main function of IRS-1 is the recruitment of cytosolic proteins to the corresponding receptors and thereby contributing to intracellular signal cascades. IRS-1 has been shown to assist in multiple growth hormone and cytokine receptor signalling pathways, including the VEGF/VEGFR pathway (White 1998). It was shown that IRS-1 is expressed in the cornea (Andrieu-Soler et al. 2005). The blockade of IRS-1 signalling inhibits corneal hemangiogenesis and, as recently shown, also lymphangiogenesis (Hos et al. 2011a). An antisense oligonucleotide against IRS-1 (GS-101, Aganirsen) has successfully been tested as eyedrops in phase II and phase III clinical trials (Cursiefen et al. 2009, 2014) (Fig. 10.6). The phase II/III data showed that Aganirsen eyedrops are safe, were well tolerated and effective in inhibiting progressive corneal neovascularization when applied twice daily (Fig. 10.6) (Cursiefen et al. 2009, 2014). Furthermore, Aganirsen eyedrops were able to reduce the need for corneal transplantation in patients with viral keratitis-associated central corneal neovascularization (Cursiefen et al. 2014). Aganirsen therefore holds great promise to be the first therapeutic that will be approved for the topical treatment of corneal neovascularization by the FDA. Since Aganirsen eyedrops in primate models also reached sufficient tissue levels at the retina, Aganirsen may be a novel topical treatment option against AMD and retinal vascular diseases without the need for intravitreal injections (Cloutier et al. 2012).

10.5.4 Fine Needle Diathermy of Corneal Vessels

In mature blood vessels, a pure pharmaceutical antiangiogenic approach is not effective in reducing the degree of corneal neovascularization, as these vessels have pericyte covered walls and are less dependent on growth levels for the maintenance of their anatomical structure. Fine needle diathermy is a method to physically occlude mature vessels by cauterization (Koenig et al. 2012; Pillai et al. 2000). This is achieved by introducing a 10-0 stainless steel side cutting needle into the lumen of a corneal vessel. Thereafter, electric current is applied to the needle by the use of a diathermy device. This approach can be

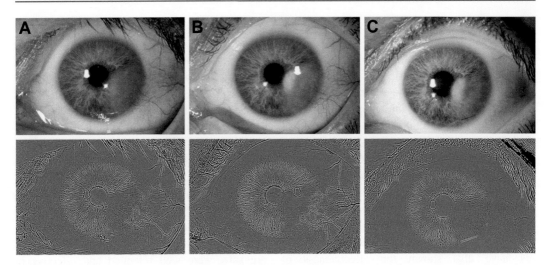

Fig. 10.6 Aganirsen antisense oligonucleotide eyedrops inhibit and regress corneal neovascularization in a patient with herpetic keratitis. *Top*: photographs before treatment (**a**), after 90 days (**b**) and 180 days (**c**) of topical Aganirsen treatment. *Bottom*: Corresponding morphometric analyses. Note the significant reduction in area covered by pathologic corneal blood vessels. Modified from Cursiefen et al. 2014, with permission of Elsevier

combined with topical adjunct anti-VEGF treatment (Koenig et al. 2009, 2012) which seems to reduce the rate of reperfusion of cauterized vessels and thereby the rate of retreatments (Koenig et al. 2012). In case of intense corneal neovascularization, repeated vessel cauterizations might be necessary (Faraj et al. 2014). Sufficient corneal vessel reduction can lead to improvements of lipid keratopathy and increase visual acuity (Wertheim et al. 2007). Moreover, improvements in corneal neovascularization are associated with a reversal of graft rejection episodes.

10.5.5 Photodynamic Therapy with Verteporfin

Verteporfin, a benzoporphyrin derivative, is a photosensitizer, which selectively binds to the endothelium of immature, actively proliferating vessels. After activation of this compound by nonthermal red light in the presence of oxygen, highly reactive short-lived singlet oxygen and other reactive oxygen radicals are produced and cause damage to the proliferating endothelium (photodynamic therapy, PDT). Verteporfin is widely used for the treatment of patients with chronic or recurrent central serous chorioretinopathy. Further indications for photodynamic therapy with Verteporfin are subfoveal choroidal neovascularization in age-related macular degeneration, pathologic myopia, choroidal hemangioma, and polypoidal choroidal vasculopathy.

Several studies have analyzed whether PDT with Verteporfin is an effective treatment for patients with corneal neovascularization and have demonstrated that corneal blood vessels can be regressed by this approach (Brooks et al. 2004; Yoon et al. 2007; Al-Abdullah and Al-Assiri 2011). This is particularly of interest, since many patients present with already mature and stable corneal vessels that are refractory to conservative treatment. These studies that aimed to regress corneal blood vessels applied Verteporfin systemically. In addition, we have previously shown that it is also possible to selectively regress corneal lymphatic vessels with PDT, when Verteporfin is applied locally by intrastromal injection. After local application, Verteporfin seems to selectively bind to the draining lymphatics, which can then be selectively regressed by PDT (Bucher et al. 2014).

10.6 Concluding Remarks

Although actively maintained by a variety of anti(lymph)angiogenic mechanisms, the (lymph)angiogenic privilege of the cornea is not invincible and can be overcome by severe diseases of the ocular surface. As corneal blood and lymphatic vessels reduce visual acuity, increase the risk for graft rejection after corneal transplantation and contribute to the development and maintenance of a variety of corneal diseases such as dry eye and ocular allergy, anti(lymph)angiogenic therapy has emerged as a novel therapeutic concept to treat patients with these diseases. Several anti(lymph)angiogenic treatment strategies have been established so far and include conservative therapy with anti-inflammatory or specific anti(lymph)angiogenic pharmaceuticals as well as invasive surgical and laser-assisted approaches. Although no specific (lymph)angiogenesis inhibitor against corneal neovascularization has been approved so far, several promising candidates have already reached the clinic, with others likely to follow.

Compliance with Ethical Requirements
Authors DH, FB, and BB declare that they have no conflict of interest.

Author CC is a consultant for Gene Signal, France

All procedures followed were in accordance with the ethical standards of the responsible committee on human experimentation (institutional and national) and with the Helsinki Declaration of 1975, as revised in 2000. Informed consent was obtained from all patients for being included in the study.

All institutional and national guidelines for the care and use of laboratory animals were followed.

Funding/Support German Research Foundation: DFG Cu 47/4-1 (CC), DFG Cu 47/6-1 (CC), DFG Forschergruppe FOR 2240 "(Lymph)Angiogenesis and Cellular Immunity in Inflammatory Diseases of the Eye" (DH, FB, CC); EU COST BM1302 (DH, FB, BB, CC); GEROK-Programme, University of Cologne (DH)

References

Al-Abdullah AA, Al-Assiri A. Resolution of bilateral corneal neovascularization and lipid keratopathy after photodynamic therapy with verteporfin. Optometry. 2011;82(4):212–4. doi:10.1016/j.optm.2010.09.012.

Albuquerque RJ, Hayashi T, Cho WG, Kleinman ME, Dridi S, Takeda A, Baffi JZ, Yamada K, Kaneko H, Green MG, Chappell J, Wilting J, Weich HA, Yamagami S, Amano S, Mizuki N, Alexander JS, Peterson ML, Brekken RA, Hirashima M, Capoor S, Usui T, Ambati BK, Ambati J. Alternatively spliced vascular endothelial growth factor receptor-2 is an essential endogenous inhibitor of lymphatic vessel growth. Nat Med. 2009;15(9):1023–30. doi:10.1038/nm.2018.

Altenburger AE, Bachmann B, Seitz B, Cursiefen C. Morphometric analysis of postoperative corneal neovascularization after high-risk keratoplasty: herpetic versus non-herpetic disease. Graefes Arch Clin Exp Ophthalmol. 2012;250(11):1663–71. doi:10.1007/s00417-012-1988-6.

Ambati BK, Nozaki M, Singh N, Takeda A, Jani PD, Suthar T, Albuquerque RJ, Richter E, Sakurai E, Newcomb MT, Kleinman ME, Caldwell RB, Lin Q, Ogura Y, Orecchia A, Samuelson DA, Agnew DW, St Leger J, Green WR, Mahasreshti PJ, Curiel DT, Kwan D, Marsh H, Ikeda S, Leiper LJ, Collinson JM, Bogdanovich S, Khurana TS, Shibuya M, Baldwin ME, Ferrara N, Gerber HP, De Falco S, Witta J, Baffi JZ, Raisler BJ, Ambati J. Corneal avascularity is due to soluble VEGF receptor-1. Nature. 2006;443(7114):993–7. doi:10.1038/nature05249.

Andrieu-Soler C, Berdugo M, Doat M, Courtois Y, BenEzra D, Behar-Cohen F. Downregulation of IRS-1 expression causes inhibition of corneal angiogenesis. Invest Ophthalmol Vis Sci. 2005;46(11):4072–8. doi:10.1167/iovs.05-0105.

Armstrong LC, Bornstein P. Thrombospondins 1 and 2 function as inhibitors of angiogenesis. Matrix Biol. 2003;22(1):63–71.

Bachmann B, Taylor RS, Cursiefen C. Corneal neovascularization as a risk factor for graft failure and rejection after keratoplasty: an evidence-based meta-analysis. Ophthalmology. 2010;117(7):1300–5. doi:10.1016/j.ophtha.2010.01.039. e1307.

Bachmann B, Taylor RS, Cursiefen C. The association between corneal neovascularization and visual acuity: a systematic review. Acta Ophthalmol. 2013;91(1):12–9. doi:10.1111/j.1755-3768.2011.02312.x.

Bachmann BO, Bock F, Wiegand SJ, Maruyama K, Dana MR, Kruse FE, Luetjen-Drecoll E, Cursiefen C. Promotion of graft survival by vascular endothelial growth factor a neutralization after high-risk corneal transplantation. Arch Ophthalmol. 2008;126(1):71–7. doi:10.1001/archopht.126.1.71.

Bachmann BO, Luetjen-Drecoll E, Bock F, Wiegand SJ, Hos D, Dana R, Kruse FE, Cursiefen C. Transient postoperative vascular endothelial growth factor (VEGF)-neutralisation improves graft survival in corneas with partly regressed inflammatory neovascularisation. Br J Ophthalmol. 2009;93(8):1075–80. doi:10.1136/bjo.2008.145128.

Blacher S, Detry B, Bruyere F, Foidart JM, Noel A. Additional parameters for the morphometry of angiogenesis and lymphangiogenesis in corneal flat mounts. Exp Eye Res. 2009;89(2):274–6. doi:10.1016/j.exer.2009.02.021.

Bock F, Maruyama K, Regenfuss B, Hos D, Steven P, Heindl LM, Cursiefen C. Novel anti(lymph)angiogenic treatment strategies for corneal and ocular surface diseases. Prog Retin Eye Res. 2013;34:89–124. doi:10.1016/j.preteyeres.2013.01.001.

Bock F, Onderka J, Dietrich T, Bachmann B, Kruse FE, Paschke M, Zahn G, Cursiefen C. Bevacizumab as a potent inhibitor of inflammatory corneal angiogenesis and lymphangiogenesis. Invest Ophthalmol Vis Sci. 2007;48(6):2545–52. doi:10.1167/iovs.06-0570.

Bock F, Onderka J, Dietrich T, Bachmann B, Pytowski B, Cursiefen C. Blockade of VEGFR3-signalling specifically inhibits lymphangiogenesis in inflammatory corneal neovascularisation. Graefes Arch Clin Exp Ophthalmol. 2008a;246(1):115–9. doi:10.1007/s00417-007-0683-5.

Bock F, Onderka J, Hos D, Horn F, Martus P, Cursiefen C. Improved semiautomatic method for morphometry of angiogenesis and lymphangiogenesis in corneal flatmounts. Exp Eye Res. 2008b;87(5):462–70. doi:10.1016/j.exer.2008.08.007.

Brooks BJ, Ambati BK, Marcus DM, Ratanasit A. Photodynamic therapy for corneal neovascularisation and lipid degeneration. Br J Ophthalmol. 2004;88(6):840.

Bucher F, Bi Y, Gehlsen U, Hos D, Cursiefen C, Bock F. Regression of mature lymphatic vessels in the cornea by photodynamic therapy. Br J Ophthalmol. 2014;98(3):391–5. doi:10.1136/bjophthalmol-2013-303887.

Bucher F, Parthasarathy A, Bergua A, Onderka J, Regenfuss B, Cursiefen C, Bock F. Topical Ranibizumab inhibits inflammatory corneal hem- and lymphangiogenesis. Acta Ophthalmol. 2012. doi:10.1111/j.1755-3768.2012.02525.x.

Cloutier F, Lawrence M, Goody R, Lamoureux S, Al-Mahmood S, Colin S, Ferry A, Conduzorgues JP,

Hadri A, Cursiefen C, Udaondo P, Viaud E, Thorin E, Chemtob S. Antiangiogenic activity of aganirsen in nonhuman primate and rodent models of retinal neovascular disease after topical administration. Invest Ophthalmol Vis Sci. 2012;53(3):1195–203. doi:10.1167/iovs.11-9064.

Cursiefen C. Immune privilege and angiogenic privilege of the cornea. Chem Immunol Allergy. 2007;92:50–7. doi:10.1159/000099253.

Cursiefen C, Bock F, Horn FK, Kruse FE, Seitz B, Borderie V, Fruh B, Thiel MA, Wilhelm F, Geudelin B, Descohand I, Steuhl KP, Hahn A, Meller D. GS-101 antisense oligonucleotide eye drops inhibit corneal neovascularization: interim results of a randomized phase II trial. Ophthalmology. 2009;116(9):1630–7. doi:10.1016/j.ophtha.2009.04.016.

Cursiefen C, Cao J, Chen L, Liu Y, Maruyama K, Jackson D, Kruse FE, Wiegand SJ, Dana MR, Sterile JW. Inhibition of hemangiogenesis and lymphangiogenesis after normal-risk corneal transplantation by neutralizing VEGF promotes graft survival. Invest Ophthalmol Vis Sci. 2004a;45(8):2666–73. doi:10.1167/iovs.03-1380.

Cursiefen C, Chen L, Borges LP, Jackson D, Cao J, Radziejewski C, D'Amore PA, Dana MR, Wiegand SJ, Sterile JW. VEGF-A stimulates lymph angiogenesis and hemangiogenesis in inflammatory neovascularization via macrophage recruitment. J Clin Invest. 2004b;113(7):1040–50. doi:10.1172/JCI20465.

Cursiefen C, Chen L, Saint-Geniez M, Hamrah P, Jin Y, Rashid S, Pytowski B, Persaud K, Wu Y, Sterile JW, Dana R. Nonvascular VEGF receptor 3 expression by corneal epithelium maintains avascularity and vision. Proc Natl Acad Sci U S A. 2006a;103(30):11405–10. doi:10.1073/pnas.0506112103.

Cursiefen C, Colin J, Dana R, Diaz-Llopis M, Faraj LA, Garcia-Delpech S, Geerling G, Price FW, Remeijer L, Rouse BT, Seitz B, Udaondo P, Meller D, Dua H. Consensus statement on indications for anti-angiogenic therapy in the management of corneal diseases associated with neovascularisation: outcome of an expert roundtable. Br J Ophthalmol. 2012;96(1):3–9. doi:10.1136/bjo.2011.204701.

Cursiefen C, Hofmann-Rummelt C, Kuchle M, Schlotzer-Schrehardt U. Pericyte recruitment in human corneal angiogenesis: an ultrastructural study with clinicopathological correlation. Br J Ophthalmol. 2003; 87(1):101–6.

Cursiefen C, Kuchle M, Naumann GO. Angiogenesis in corneal diseases: histopathologic evaluation of 254 human corneal buttons with neovascularization. Cornea. 1998;17(6):611–3.

Cursiefen C, Martus P, Nguyen NX, Langenbucher A, Seitz B, Kuchle M. Corneal neovascularization after nonmechanical versus mechanical corneal trephination for non-high-risk keratoplasty. Cornea. 2002a; 21(7):648–52.

Cursiefen C, Maruyama K, Bock F, Saban D, Sadrai Z, Lawler J, Dana R, Masli S. Thrombospondin 1 inhibits inflammatory lymph angiogenesis by CD36 ligation on monocytes. J Exp Med. 2011;208(5):1083–92. doi:10.1084/jem.20092277.

Cursiefen C, Maruyama K, Jackson DG, Sterile JW, Kruse FE. Time course of angiogenesis and lymph angiogenesis after brief corneal inflammation. Cornea. 2006b;25(4):443–7. doi:10.1097/01.ico.0000183485. 85636.ff.

Cursiefen C, Masli S, Ng TF, Dana MR, Bornstein P, Lawler J, Sterile JW. Roles of thrombospondin-1 and -2 in regulating corneal and iris angiogenesis. Invest Ophthalmol Vis Sci. 2004c;45(4):1117–24.

Cursiefen C, Schlotzer-Schrehardt U, Kuchle M, Sorokin L, Breiteneder-Geleff S, Alitalo K, Jackson D. Lymphatic vessels in vascular zed human corneas: immunohistochemical investigation using LYVE-1 and podoplanin. Invest Ophthalmol Vis Sci. 2002b;43(7):2127–35.

Cursiefen C, Viaud E, Bock F, Geudelin B, Ferry A, Kadlecova P, Levy M, Al Mahmood S, Colin S, Thorin E, Majo F, Frueh B, Wilhelm F, Meyer-Ter-Vehn T, Geerling G, Bohringer D, Reinhard T, Meller D, Pleyer U, Bachmann B, Seitz B. Aganirsen antisense oligonucleotide eye drops inhibit dermatitis-induced corneal neovascularization and reduce need for transplantation: The I-CAN Study. Ophthalmology. 2014. doi:10.1016/j.ophtha.2014.03.038.

Cursiefen C, Wenkel H, Martus P, Langenbucher A, Nguyen NX, Seitz B, Kuchle M, Naumann GO. Impact of short-term versus long-term topical steroids on corneal neovascularization after non-high-risk keratoplasty. Graefes Arch Clin Exp Ophthalmol. 2001a;239(7):514–21.

Cursiefen C, Wenkel H, Martus P, Langenbucher A, Seitz B, Kuchle M. Standardized semiquantitative analysis of corneal neovascularization using projected corneal photographs--pilot study after perforating corneal keratoplasty before immune reaction. Klin Monbl Augenheilkd. 2001b;218(7):484–91. doi:10.1055/s-2001-16291.

Dana MR, Streilein JW. Loss and restoration of immune privilege in eyes with corneal neovascularization. Invest Ophthalmol Vis Sci. 1996;37(12):2485–94.

Dastjerdi MH, Sadrai Z, Saban DR, Zhang Q, Dana R. Corneal penetration of topical and subconjunctival bevacizumab. Invest Ophthalmol Vis Sci. 2011;52(12):8718–23. doi:10.1167/iovs.11-7871.

Detry B, Blacher S, Erpicum C, Paupert J, Maertens L, Maillard C, Munaut C, Sounni NE, Lambert V, Foidart JM, Rakic JM, Cataldo D, Noel A. Sunitinib inhibits inflammatory corneal lymph angiogenesis. Invest Ophthalmol Vis Sci. 2013;54(5):3082–93. doi:10.1167/iovs.12-10856.

Dietrich T, Bock F, Yuen D, Hos D, Bachmann BO, Zahn G, Wiegand S, Chen L, Cursiefen C. Cutting edge: lymphatic vessels, not blood vessels, primarily mediate immune rejections after transplantation. J Immunol. 2010;184(2):535–9. doi:10.4049/jimmunol.0903180.

Dietrich T, Onderka J, Bock F, Kruse FE, Vossmeyer D, Stragies R, Zahn G, Cursiefen C. Inhibition of inflammatory lymphangiogenesis by integrin alpha5 blockade. Am J Pathol. 2007;171(1):361–72.

Faraj LA, Elalfy MS, Said DG, Dua HS. Fine needle diathermy occlusion of corneal vessels. Br J Ophthalmol. 2014;98(9):1287–90.doi:10.1136/bjophthalmol-2014-304891.

Ferrari G, Dastjerdi MH, Okanobo A, Cheng SF, Amparo F, Nallasamy N, Dana R. Topical Ranibizumab as a treatment of corneal neovascularization. Cornea. 2013;32(7):992–7.doi:10.1097/ICO.0b013e3182775f8d.

Goyal S, Chauhan SK, Dana R. Blockade of prolymphangiogenic vascular endothelial growth factor C in dry eye disease. Arch Ophthalmol. 2012;130(1):84–9. doi:10.1001/archophthalmol.2011.266.

Goyal S, Chauhan SK, El Annan J, Nallasamy N, Zhang Q, Dana R. Evidence of corneal lymphangiogenesis in dry eye disease: a potential link to adaptive immunity? Arch Ophthalmol. 2010;128(7):819–24. doi:10.1001/archophthalmol.2010.124.

Hos D, Bachmann B, Bock F, Onderka J, Cursiefen C. Age-related changes in murine limbal lymphatic vessels and corneal lymphangiogenesis. Exp Eye Res. 2008a;87(5):427–32. doi:10.1016/j.exer.2008.07.013.

Hos D, Bock F, Dietrich T, Onderka J, Kruse FE, Thierauch KH, Cursiefen C. Inflammatory corneal (lymph)angiogenesis is blocked by VEGFR-tyrosine kinase inhibitor ZK 261991, resulting in improved graft survival after corneal transplantation. Invest Ophthalmol Vis Sci. 2008b;49(5):1836–42. doi:10.1167/iovs.07-1314.

Hos D, Cursiefen C. Lymphatic vessels in the development of tissue and organ rejection. Adv Anat Embryol Cell Biol. 2014;214:119–41. doi:10.1007/978-3-7091-1646-3_10.

Hos D, Koch KR, Bucher F, Bock F, Cursiefen C, Heindl LM. Serum eyedrops antagonize the anti(lymph) angiogenic effects of Bevacizumab in vitro and in vivo. Invest Ophthalmol Vis Sci. 2013;54(9):6133–42. doi:10.1167/iovs.13-12460.

Hos D, Regenfuss B, Bock F, Onderka J, Cursiefen C. Blockade of insulin receptor substrate-1 inhibits corneal lymphangiogenesis. Invest Ophthalmol Vis Sci. 2011a;52(8):5778–85. doi:10.1167/iovs.10-6816.

Hos D, Saban DR, Bock F, Regenfuss B, Onderka J, Masli S, Cursiefen C. Suppression of inflammatory corneal lymphangiogenesis by application of topical corticosteroids. Arch Ophthalmol. 2011b;129(4):445–52. doi:10.1001/archophthalmol.2011.42.

Hos D, Schlereth SL, Bock F, Heindl LM, Cursiefen C. Antilymphangiogenic therapy to promote transplant survival and to reduce cancer metastasis: what can we learn from the eye? Semin Cell Dev Biol. 2014;38:117–30. doi:10.1016/j.semcdb.2014.11.003.

Jonas JB, Rank RM, Budde WM. Immunologic graft reactions after allogenic penetrating keratoplasty. Am J Ophthalmol. 2002;133(4):437–43.

Koenig Y, Bock F, Horn F, Kruse F, Straub K, Cursiefen C. Short- and long-term safety profile and efficacy of topical bevacizumab (Avastin) eyedrops against corneal neovascularization. Graefes Arch Clin Exp Ophthalmol. 2009;247(10):1375–82. doi:10.1007/s00417-009-1099-1.

Koenig Y, Bock F, Kruse FE, Stock K, Cursiefen C. Angioregressive pretreatment of mature corneal blood vessels before keratoplasty: fine-needle vessel coagulation combined with anti-VEGFs. Cornea. 2012;31(8): 887–92. doi:10.1097/ICO.0b013e31823f8f7a.

Lam VM, Nguyen NX, Martus P, Seitz B, Kruse FE, Cursiefen C. Surgery-related factors influencing corneal neovascularization after low-risk keratoplasty. Am J Ophthalmol. 2006;141(2):260–6. doi:10.1016/j.ajo.2005.08.080.

Lee HS, Hos D, Blanco T, Bock F, Reyes NJ, Mathew R, Cursiefen C, Dana R, Saban DR. Involvement of corneal lymphangiogenesis in a mouse model of allergic eye disease. Invest Ophthalmol Vis Sci. 2015;56(5):3140–8.

Lin HC, Chang JH, Jain S, Gabison EE, Kure T, Kato T, Fukai N, Azar DT. Matrilysin cleavage of corneal collagen type XVIII NC1 domain and generation of a 28-kDa fragment. Invest Ophthalmol Vis Sci. 2001;42(11):2517–24.

Lipp M, Bucher F, Parthasarathy A, Hos D, Onderka J, Cursiefen C, Bock F. Blockade of the VEGF isoforms in inflammatory corneal hemangiogenesis and lymphangiogenesis. Graefes Arch Clin Exp Ophthalmol. 2014;252(6):943–9. doi:10.1007/s00417-014-2626-2.

Makino Y, Cao R, Svensson K, Bertilsson G, Asman M, Tanaka H, Cao Y, Berkenstam A, Poellinger L. Inhibitory PAS domain protein is a negative regulator of hypoxia-inducible gene expression. Nature. 2001;414(6863):550–4. doi:10.1038/35107085.

Niederkorn JY. The immune privilege of corneal allografts. Transplantation. 1999;67(12):1503–8.

Niederkorn JY. The immune privilege of corneal grafts. J Leukoc Biol. 2003;74(2):167–71.

Niederkorn JY. High-risk corneal allografts and why they lose their immune privilege. Curr Opin Allergy Clin Immunol. 2010;10(5):493–7. doi:10.1097/ACI.0b013e32833dfa11.

Niederkorn JY, Stern ME, Pflugfelder SC, De Paiva CS, Corrales RM, Gao J, Siemasko K. Desiccating stress induces T cell-mediated Sjogren's syndrome-like lacrimal keratoconjunctivitis. J Immunol. 2006;176(7):3950–7.

Pillai CT, Dua HS, Hossain P. Fine needle diathermy occlusion of corneal vessels. Invest Ophthalmol Vis Sci. 2000;41(8):2148–53.

Regenfuss B, Onderka J, Bock F, Hos D, Maruyama K, Cursiefen C. Genetic heterogeneity of lymphangiogenesis in different mouse strains. Am J Pathol. 2010;177(1):501–10. doi:10.2353/ajpath.2010.090794.

Sano Y, Ksander BR, Streilein JW. Fate of orthotopic corneal allografts in eyes that cannot support anterior chamber-associated immune deviation induction. Invest Ophthalmol Vis Sci. 1995;36(11):2176–85.

Schaumburg CS, Siemasko KF, De Paiva CS, Wheeler LA, Niederkorn JY, Pflugfelder SC, Stern ME. Ocular surface APCs are necessary for autoreactive T cell-mediated experimental autoimmune lacrimal keratoconjunctivitis. J Immunol. 2011;187(7):3653–62. doi:10.4049/jimmunol.1101442.

Singh N, Tiem M, Watkins R, Cho YK, Wang Y, Olsen T, Uehara H, Mamalis C, Luo L, Oakey Z, Ambati BK. Soluble vascular endothelial growth factor receptor-3 is essential for corneal alymphaticity. Blood. 2013;121(20):4242–9. doi:10.1182/blood-2012-08-453043.

Wertheim MS, Cook SD, Knox-Cartwright NE, Van DL, Tole DM. Electrolysis-needle cauterization of corneal vessels in patients with lipid keratopathy. Cornea. 2007;26(2):230–1. doi:10.1097/01.ico.0000248383.09272.ee.

Whitcher JP, Srinivasan M, Upadhyay MP. Prevention of corneal ulceration in the developing world. Int Ophthalmol Clin. 2002;42(1):71–7.

White MF. The IRS-signaling system: a network of docking proteins that mediate insulin and cytokine action. Recent Prog Horm Res. 1998;53:119–38.

Williams KA, Lowe MT, Keane MC, Jones VJ, Loh RS, Coster DJ. The Australian Corneal Graft Registry 2012 Report. Adelaide, Australia: SnapPrinting; 2012, p. 235–42. Accessed 1 October 2014.

Yoon KC, You IC, Kang IS, Im SK, Ahn JK, Park YG, Ahn KY. Photodynamic therapy with verteporfin for corneal neovascularization. Am J Ophthalmol. 2007;144(3):390–5. doi:10.1016/j.ajo.2007.05.028.

Anti-Angiogenic Gene Therapy: Basic Science and Challenges for Translation into the Clinic

11

Clemens Lange and James Bainbridge

11.1 Introduction

The growth of abnormal blood vessels (neovascularisation) is a central feature of retinal disorders including retinopathy of prematurity (ROP), retinal vein occlusions (RVO), proliferative diabetic retinopathy (PDR), and neovascular age-related macular degeneration (nAMD), which are the leading causes of blindness in infants, individuals of working age and the elderly in the Western world, respectively. Although neovascularisation occurs at a relatively late stage of disease, it is nonetheless an attractive target for therapeutic intervention, since it represents a pathway common to many different diseases and typically leads directly to visual loss. Intraocular delivery of antibodies directed against VEGF has become the conventional treatment modality for neovascular AMD and increasingly for proliferative diabetic retinopathy (Rofagha et al. 2013; Salam et al. 2001). The success of this treatment, however, is limited by the relative short half-life of antibodies in the eye and depends on frequently repeated injections that pose a significant cumulative risk of local complications including intraocular infection, vitreous haemorrhage, and retinal detachment.

Ocular gene therapy is an emerging therapeutic approach that offers the potential for targeted, sustained, and regulatable delivery of angiostatic proteins to the retina after a single procedure. The eye has major advantages as a target organ for gene therapy. It is a well-confined and highly compartmentalised organ that is readily accessible for vector administration by microsurgical techniques. Vector suspensions can be delivered precisely under direct visualisation into the desired compartment, including the vitreous body and the subretinal or suprachoroidal spaces, enabling specific ocular cell targeting with minimal risk of systemic dissemination. The blood–retina barrier further limits the systemic spread of locally administered vectors and reduces the possibility of systemic adverse events and exposure to vector antigens that might cause inflammation and limit transgene expression. Because of its small size, only small volumes of vector suspensions are required to reach a significant proportion of the desired target cells. Furthermore, the eye's unique immune environment confers additional protection against

C. Lange, M.D., Ph.D.
Eye Center, University Hospital Freiburg,
Killianstrasse 5, Freiburg 79106, Germany
e-mail: Clemens.lange@uniklinik-freiburg.de

J. Bainbridge, Ph.D., F.R.C.Ophth. (✉)
Department of Genetics, UCL Institute of
Ophthalmology, 11-43 Bath Street, London
EC1V 9EL, UK

Moorfields Eye Hospital, London, UK
e-mail: j.bainbridge@ucl.ac.uk

© Springer International Publishing Switzerland 2016
A. Stahl (ed.), *Anti-Angiogenic Therapy in Ophthalmology*,
Essentials in Ophthalmology, DOI 10.1007/978-3-319-24097-8_11

immune responses to foreign antigens (Forrester and Xu 2012) that could otherwise limit long-term transgene expression (Bennett et al. 1996). Finally, therapeutic effects on structure and function can be easily observed, recorded, and quantified using a variety of in vivo techniques both experimentally and clinically. These advantages have led to numerous preclinical studies and the first clinical gene therapy trials to treat patients with Leber congenital amaurosis (Bainbridge et al. 2008; Hauswirth et al. 2008; Maguire et al. 2008) choroideremia (MacLaren et al. 2014), and exudative age-related macular degeneration (Campochiaro et al. 2006).

11.2 Concepts of Ocular Gene Therapy

The fundamental concepts of gene therapy were developed in the 1960s following the identification of nucleic acids and the discovery of viral transduction. Recombinant DNA techniques enabled the cloning of genes that could be used to correct genetic defects and disease phenotypes in mammalian cells in vitro (Friedmann 1992). Since then, significant advances in vector design and gene transfer methods have been made in the field of human gene therapy. In the eye, gene transfer strategies can be used for gene supplementation in recessive disease, gene inactivation in dominant disease, expression of neuroprotective mediators in degenerative disease, "suicide genes" for example in tumour diseases, and expression of immunomodulatory and angiostatic factors in immunological and neovascular eye disease.

Many different viral and non-viral vector systems, designed to improve the efficiency of gene delivery to target cells, have been evaluated and optimised for use in the eye (Reichel et al. 1999; Buch et al. 2008). Among these vectors, lentivirus (LV), adenovirus (AV), and adeno-associated virus (AAV) are the most frequently used viral vector systems for gene therapy. Lentiviral vectors such as HIV, SIV, or EIAV are retroviruses and able to transduce non-dividing cells. In the eye, these vector systems can induce stable, long-

term transgene expression in tissues of the anterior segment and the retinal pigment epithelium, but transduce photoreceptor cells with only low efficiency (Bainbridge et al. 2001; Balaggan et al. 2006a). Lentiviral vectors promote integration of the transferred gene into the host chromosome, posing a risk of oncogenesis as a result of insertional mutagenesis. For this reason, self-inactivating and non-integrating lentiviral vectors are being developed as potentially safer alternatives.

Adenoviral vectors are non-integrating viruses that efficiently target both dividing and non-dividing cells in the outer retina (Ali et al. 1998; Bennett et al. 1994). However, the duration of gene expression in the targeted cell is limited by a significant T-cell-mediated immune response (Reichel et al. 1998). This limitation might be overcome by the use of helper-dependent Ad vectors, which lengthen the duration of transgene expression from shorter than 3 months to up to 1 year (Lamartina et al. 2007).

Recombinant adeno-associated virus (rAAV) vectors are currently the vector of choice for ocular gene therapy. They typically do not integrate into the genome but persist mainly as extragenomic circular episomes, with only low risk of insertional oncogenesis. rAAV vectors mediate stable, long-term transgene expression in a variety of retinal cells, including photoreceptors, RPE cells, ganglion cells, and Müller cells, with minimal immune response. Most recombinant AAV vectors are composed of the genomic component of AAV serotype 2 packaged using capsids derived from other AAV serotypes. The capsid serotype determines the tropism and efficacy of the vector. Whereas AAV2/2 (i.e., the genome based on AAV-2 and packaged in AAV-2 capsid), 2/5, and 2/8 transduce the RPE and photoreceptors following subretinal delivery. AAV2/1, AAV2/6, and AAV2/4 exclusively target the RPE, and AAV2/9 efficiently transduces Müller cells (for a detailed review, see Buch et al. 2008). The AAV variant ShH10 efficiently and selectively transduces Müller cells by about 94 % following intravitreal injection (Klimczak et al. 2009), and other AAV variants have been reported to efficiently transduce human and rat astrocytes (Koerber et al. 2009). A major limitation of AAV vectors, however, is their small payload capacity, which is limited to 5 KB irrespective of the capsid type (Wu et al. 2010). Therefore, large genes or extensive promoter/regulatory elements cannot be introduced. This limitation may be addressed by a trans-splicing technique in which a large coding sequence is divided into smaller sequences for delivery, and subsequently recombined intracellularly.

11.3 Gene Therapy for Neovascular Eye Disease

The unique potential of gene therapy is that a single intraocular injection of a vector can lead to the sustained expression of an angiostatic protein to address the chronic pro-angiogenic drive in neovascular eye disease. The principle of angiostatic gene therapy has been intensively examined in various animal models of ocular neovascularisation. Ocular neovascularisation can be induced experimentally via focal laser photocoagulation of Bruch's membrane, which causes choroidal neovascularisation (CNV) to develop, or by exposing rodents to hyperoxia which causes retinal ischaemia and the development of retinal neovascularisation (RNV). Furthermore, the effect of ocular gene therapy can be assessed in various transgenic mice which develop spontaneous RNV and CNV. Although none of these models recapitulates the full spectrum of pathology of human diseases, they model some features in the development of RNV and CNV and have proven invaluable in proof-of-concept experiments for anti-angiogenic drug development.

11.3.1 Candidate Genes for Angiostatic Gene Therapy

11.3.1.1 VEGF-Inhibiting Molecules

Because of the convincing clinical success of anti-VEGF therapy in neovascular eye disease, a gene therapy approach that enables sustained long-term VEGF blockade could be highly effective. Anti-VEGF gene therapy can be achieved by inducing the expression of molecules that bind extracellular VEGF, such as the VEGF receptor sFlt1 (see Fig. 11.1) or VEGF antibodies, or by inhibiting intracellular VEGF protein expression using sh- and siRNA. Soluble fms-like tyrosine kinase-1 (sFlt1 or sVEGFR-1) is a splice variant of the VEGF receptor (Flt1) and a potent inhibitor of extracellular VEGF. Numerous reports confirm the efficiency of sFlt1 gene therapy in reducing the development of ocular neovascularisation (see Tables 11.1 and 11.2). Systemic, intravitreal or subretinal injection of Ad or AAV vectors carrying the sFlt1 gene suppress the development of retinal (Lamartina et al. 2007; Rota et al. 2004; Bainbridge et al. 2002; Lai et al. 2009) and CNV in rodents (Lai et al. 2001, 2009; Honda et al. 2000; Igarashi et al. 2010), and AAV-mediated sFlt-1 expression reduces the development of laser-induced CNV in non-human primates (Lai et al. 2005). Furthermore, the intraocular injection of AAV2 viruses encoding sFLT01, a chimeric VEGF-binding molecule consisting of domain 2 of Flt-1 linked to a human IgG1 heavy-chain fragment, suppresses RNV and CNV in mice and primates without histological evidence of toxicity for 12 months (Pechan et al. 2009; Lukason et al. 2011). Similarly, a single intravitreal administration of AAV vectors expressing the VEGF antibody bevacizumab was shown to cause long-term expression of bevacizumab in the RPE which was associated with suppression of neovascularisation in transgenic mice overexpressing human VEGF165 in photoreceptors (Mao et al. 2011). Moreover, subretinal delivery of AAV2 vectors encoding anti-VEGF siRNA and shRNA or the VEGF-binding intraceptor Flt23k reduced both VEGF protein levels and laser-induced CNV in mice (Igarashi et al. 2014; Askou et al. 2012; Zhang et al. 2015). Notably, a safety study in cynomolgus monkeys using AAV2.sFLT01 demonstrated no cell-mediated immune reaction or adverse effects on retinal vascular or electroretinal function for up to 1 year after intraocular administration (Maclachlan et al. 2011). These encouraging pre-clinical data in non-human primates led to two

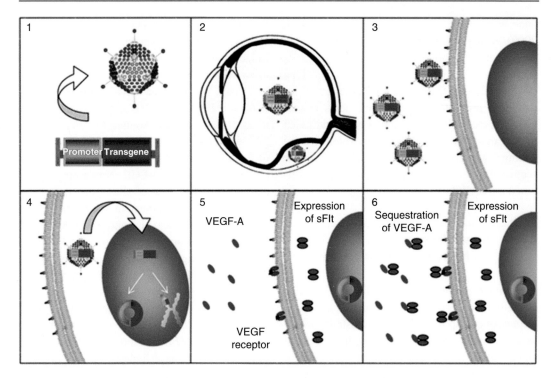

Fig. 11.1 Schematic drawing of anti-VEGF (sFLT1) angiostatic gene therapy. The angiostatic transgene (e.g. sFLT1) is introduced into viral vectors (1). Upon intravitreal or subretinal delivery of the viral vector in the eye (2) the viruses bind to cellular surface antigens (3) and enter the target cells. The transgene is then transported into the nucleus, integrates in the genome, or rests episomal depending on the virus (4) and is continuously expressed by the host cells (5). These angiostatic proteins are secreted and antagonise VEGF action (6). Illustrated by Scott Robbie, London

phase I/II clinical trials currently investigating the safety and tolerability of AAV2-SFlt01 (NCT01024998, sponsored by Genzyme) and rAAV.sFlt-1 (NCT01494805, sponsored by the Lions Eye Institute, Perth, Australia) in neovascular AMD. These studies are expected to complete in July 2018 and May 2017 respectively (see Table 11.3).

11.3.1.2 Pigment Epithelium-Derived Factor

Pigment epithelium-derived factor (PEDF) is a multifunctional secreted protein possessing both anti-angiogenic and neuroprotective properties. It is constitutively secreted by Müller and RPE cells and acts as a potent endogenous angiostatic molecule which contributes to the avascularity of the outer retina in the healthy state. Reciprocal to VEGF, PEDF levels are significantly reduced in the vitreous of eyes with PDR and nAMD compared with healthy eyes (Holekamp et al. 2002; Spranger et al. 2000). As PEDF inhibits hypoxia-induced VEGF expression at the transcriptional level, it has been postulated that the decrease in PEDF is at least partially responsible for increased VEGF levels and the associated vascular leakage and neovascularisation in neovascular eye disease (Zhang et al. 2006). Furthermore, PEDF promotes the survival of neurons in vitro and protects photoreceptors from excessive light exposure (Cao et al. 2001; Steele et al. 1993). Vector-mediated overexpression of PEDF therefore offers the attractive possibility of both countering harmful VEGF-induced angiogenesis and preventing retinal cell death in neovascular eye disease. Intravitreal or subretinal injection of adenoviruses encoding human PEDF (AdPEDF.11) suppresses the development of

Table 11.1 Summary of preclinical angiostatic gene therapy studies for retinal neovascularisation

Gene	Vector	Delivery	Experimental model	Result	Reference
Gene therapy in experimental models of ocular neovascularisation					
Retinal neovascularisation					
Angiostatin	HIV	Intravitreal	OIR mouse model	Reduced RNV in 90 % of animals	Igarashi et al. (2003)
CD59	AAV2/8	Intravitreal	Streptozotocin diabetes	Reduced leakage and non-perfusion	Adhi et al. (2013)
Endostatin	Ad-Tx	Subretinal	Transgenic mice	Reduced vasopermeability and RNV	Takahashi et al. (2003)
Endostatin	rAAV2/1	Subretinal	OIR mouse model	Reduced RNV	Auricchio et al. (2002b)
PEDF	Ad	Intravitreal	OIR mouse model	Reduced RNV	Mori et al. (2001)
PEDF	rAAV2	Intravitreal	OIR mouse model	Reduced RNV by 74 %	Raisler et al. (2002)
PEDF	AAV2	Intravitreal	Transgenic mice	Reduced RNV and capillary dropout	Haurigot et al. (2012)
TIMP3	rAAV2/1	Subretinal	OIR mouse model	Reduced RNV	Auricchio et al. (2002b)
Vasohibin	Ad	Intravitreal	OIR mouse model	Reduced RNV	Shen et al. (2006)
Vasoinhibin	AAV2	Intravitreal	VEGF-induced VP	Reduced vasopermeability	Ramírez et al. (2011)
Anti-VEGF					
Anti-VEGF shRNA	Lentivirus	Subretinal	OIR rat model	Transfected Müller cells, reduced RNV	Wang et al. (2013)
Anti-VEGF$_{164}$ shRNA	Lentivirus	Subretinal	OIR rat model	Transfection of Müller cells, reduced RNV	Jiang et al. (2014)
Bevacizumab	AAVrh.10	Intravitreal	Transgenic mice	Reduced RNV by 90 % for 168 days	Mao et al. (2011)
sFLT01	AAV2	Intravitreal	Non-human primate	Reduced CNV, transfected ganglion cells	Lukason et al. (2011)
sFLT1	HD-Ad/dox	Intravitreal	OIR rat model	transfected Müller cells reduced RNV	Lamartina et al. (2007)
sFLT1	Ad	Intravitreal	OIR rat model	Reduced RNV by 97 %	Rota et al. (2004)
sFLT1	Ad or AAV	Intravitreal	OIR mouse model	Reduced RNV by more than 50 %	Bainbridge et al. (2002)
sFLT1	rAAV	Intravitreal	Transgenic mice	Reduced RNV, leukocyte accumulation	Lai et al. (2009)
sFLT1 chimaera	AAV2	Intravitreal	OIR mouse model	Reduced RNV, no toxicity for 12 months	Pechan et al. (2009)
VEGF peptides	rAAV	Intravitreal	OIR mouse model	Reduced RNV by 71–83 %	Deng et al. (2005)

HD-Ad helper-dependent adenovirus, *dox* doxycycline-inducible, *VP* vasopermeability. Updated November 2014

RNV and CNV in mice. Interestingly, when given after neovascularisation has become established, overexpression of PEDF is associated with the apoptosis of activated, but not quiescent endothelial cells, and the regression of pathological neovascularisation (Mori et al. 2001, 2002).

Furthermore, periocular injection of the same vector results in an efficient transduction of the episclera, PEDF penetration into the choroid, and reduced laser-induced CNV in mice and pigs (Gehlbach et al. 2003; Saishin et al. 2005). Intraocular delivery of AAV-encoding PEDF

Table 11.2 Summary of preclinical angiostatic gene therapy studies for choroidal neovascularisation

Choroidal neovascularisatio					
Gene	Vector	Delivery	Experimental model	Result	Reference
Angiostatin	rAAV	Subretinal	Laser-induced CNV, rat	Reduced CNV area for >150 days	Lai et al. (2001)
Angiostatin	EIAV	Subretinal	Laser-induced CNV, mouse	Reduced CNV area by 50 %	Balaggan et al. (2006b)
CD59	Ad	Subretinal	Laser-induced CNV, mouse	Reduced MAC and CNV formation	Cashman et al. (2011)
Endostatin	EIAV	Subretinal	Laser-induced CNV, mouse	Reduce CNV area by 60 %	Balaggan et al. (2006b)
PEDF	AAV	Subretinal	Laser-induced CNV, mouse	Reduced CNV	Mori et al. (2002)
PEDF	Ad	Subretinal	Laser-induced CNV, mouse	Reduced CNV	Mori et al. (2001)
PEDF	Ad	Periocular	Laser-induced CNV, pig	Reduced CNV	Saishin et al. (2005)
PEDF	Ad	Intravitreal	Cynomolgus monkey	Dose-related inflammation	Rasmussen et al. (2001)
PEDF	Ad	Periocular	Laser-induced CNV, mouse	Increased choroidal PEDF, reduced CNV	Gehlbach et al. (2003)
TIMP3	Nonviral HVJ	Subretinal	Laser-induced CNV, rat	Reduced CNV	Takahashi et al. (2000)
Anti-VEGF					
Anti-VEGF intraceptor (Flt23k)	AAV2	Subretinal	Laser-induced CNV, mouse	Expression for >6 months, CNV reduction by 62 %, no AE observed	Zhang et al. (2015)
Anti-VEGF shRNA	AAV	Subretinal	Laser-induced CNV, mouse	Reduced CNV by 84 %	Cashman et al. (2006)
Anti-VEGF shRNA	scAAV2/8	Subretinal	Laser-induced CNV, mouse	Reduced CNV by 48 %	Askou et al. (2012)
Anti-VEGF siRNA	AAV2/8	Subretinal	Laser-induced CNV, mouse	VEGF reduced by 50 %, CNV reduced	Igarashi et al. (2014)
sFLT1	AAV8	Subretinal	Laser-induced CNV, mouse	Reduced CNV	Igarashi et al. (2010)
sFLT1	AAV	Subretinal	Laser-induced CNV, mouse and monkeys	Long-term expression of Flt1, CNV suppression in 85 %	Lai et al. (2005)
sFLT1 (3 variants)	Nonviral/EP	Ciliary muscle	Laser-induced CNV, rat	Reduced CNV, VEGF inhibition for 6M	El Sanharawi et al. (2013)
sFLT1	Ad	Systemic	Laser-induced CNV, rat	Reduced fibroblast proliferation and inflammatory cell infiltration in CNV	Honda et al. (2000)

HVJ hemagglutinating virus of Japan liposomes, *scAAV2*/8-hU6-sh9 self-complementary AAV vectors were packaged in serotype 8 capsids, Updated November 2014

leads to long-term PEDF production, suppressed retinal and choroidal NV (Mori et al. 2002; Raisler et al. 2002), and is associated with reduced RNV, normal retinal capillary density, and reduced incidence of retinal detachment in a transgenic mouse model that mimics the chronic progression of human DR (Haurigot et al. 2012). Toxicology studies performed in non-human primates demonstrate a dose-related inflammatory response which is minimal and fully reversible at doses below 1×10^9 (Rasmussen et al. 2001). These encouraging preclinical results led to a

Table 11.3 Summary of human trials of angiostatic retinal gene therapy (updated November 2014)

Ongoing human trials of retinal gene therapy for neovascular eye disease							
Neovascular AMD							
Gene	Vector	Delivery	Description	Status	Estimated completion	Country	Reference
sFLT-01	AAV2	Intravitreal	Phase I, open-label, multi-centre, dose-escalating, safety and tolerability study sponsored by Genzyme	ongoing	July 2018	USA	NCT01024998
sFLT-1	rAAV	Subretinal	Phase I/II, controlled dose-escalating trial, safety, and efficacy study	Ongoing	May 2017	Australia	NCT01494805
Endostatin/ Angiostatin	EIAV, lentivirus	Subretinal	Phase I, dose-escalating safety study sponsored by Oxford BioMedica	Ongoing	March 2015	USA	NCT01301443
PEDF	Ad	Intravitreal	Phase I, open-label, single-administration, dose-escalation study sponsored by GenVec	Completed	N/A	USA	NCT00109499 Campochiaro et al. (2006)

phase-I clinical trial of ocular gene therapy investigating the safety of subretinal delivery of adenoviruses encoding PEDF (AdPEDF) in 28 patients with neovascular AMD. Following a single intravitreal delivery of AdPEDF, no serious adverse events related to the virus occurred, nor were any dose-limiting toxicities documented. Mild, transient intraocular inflammation was evident in seven patients, and raised intraocular pressure in six patients was controlled by topical medication alone. Sputum and urine cultures were negative for replicating adenovirus, though, serum-neutralising antibodies directed against adenovirus were raised in several patients indicating a systemic response following intravitreal vector delivery. Following administration of low-dose vector, the mean CNV lesion size doubled from 6 to 12 months, whereas following administration of a higher dose the CNV size remained stable. This study demonstrated an encouraging safety profile and suggested angiostatic activity following a single intravitreal injection of AdPEDF in AMD (Campochiaro et al. 2006). Despite these findings, no phase-II trial has been reported to date.

11.3.1.3 Endostatin and Angiostatin

Endostatin is a naturally occurring protein produced by proteolytic cleavage of collagen type 18, which acts as an endogenous inhibitor of angiogenesis. The subretinal injection of lentiviral vectors encoding for Endostatin was associated with an increased expression of Endostatin in the RPE and reduced vasopermeability and RNV in transgenic mice (Takahashi et al. 2003). The intravitreal or subretinal administration of lentiviruses or AAV containing the Endostatin gene is associated with attenuation of laser-induced CNV (Mori et al. 2002; Balaggan et al. 2006b) and of RNV in the OIR mouse model (Auricchio et al. 2002a) indicating that overexpression of Endostatin restricts the development of ocular neovascularisation. Angiostatin, on the other hand, is a naturally occurring fragment of plasmin, which inhibits endothelial cell migration and induces apoptosis (O'Reilly et al. 1997). Intravitreal injection of either adeno-associated or lentiviral vectors encoding Angiostatin suppresses RNV and CNV in mice (Lai et al. 2001; Raisler et al. 2002; Balaggan et al. 2006b; Igarashi et al. 2003). Based on these preclinical data, a phase-I clinical trial is currently ongoing to determine the bioactivity and safety of subretinal delivery of EIAV lentiviral vectors encoding both Endostatin and Angiostatin in neovascular AMD (Retinostat, Oxford BioMedica UK Ltd., NCT01301443). This trial is expected to have completed by March 2015.

11.3.1.4 Miscellaneous Factors

In addition to the factors previously described, several other angiostatic and neuroprotective molecules are the subject of investigation for potential delivery in neovascular eye disease by gene therapy (see Tables 11.1 and 11.2). These factors include the Tissue Inhibitor Metalloproteinase 3 (Auricchio et al. 2002b; Takahashi et al. 2000), Vasohibin (Wakusawa et al. 2011; Shen et al. 2006; Ramírez et al. 2011), and CD59 (Adhi et al. 2013; Cashman et al. 2006). Owing to the limited data available, these factors are not discussed in detail.

11.4 Challenges for Translation into the Clinic

11.4.1 Potential Side Effects of Ocular Gene Therapy

The duration of vector-mediated transgene expression in the eye is not yet known. AAV-mediated transgene expression appears to last the entire life in rodents and for more than 2½ years in non-human primates (Lebherz et al. 2005). Although such long-term expression is an advantage from one viewpoint, it also raises potential concerns.

11.4.1.1 Immune Response

Uncontrolled immune responses can both limit the duration of expression of the transferred gene and cause direct injury to intraocular tissues. For these reasons, the benefit of gene therapy depends on immune tolerance to the vector and the gene transferred. Four independent clinical gene therapy trials for LCA have assessed cellular and humoural immune responses and safety in human subjects following subretinal delivery of AAV2

(Hauswirth et al. 2008; Maguire et al. 2008; Banin et al. 2010). Follow-up has surpassed 5 years, with no adverse sight-threatening inflammation reported to date (Simonelli et al. 2010; Testa et al. 2013; Jacobson et al. 2012). Furthermore bio-distribution studies have detected no systemic spread of AAV vector in the tears, saliva, serum, or semen, except for transient AAV detected in one subject in serum and tears for a few days after surgery. Furthermore, neutralising antibodies against rAAV2/2 were undetectable in the serum with the exception of two subjects with transient marginally increased titres (Hauswirth et al. 2008; Maguire et al. 2008) (for a detailed review, see Willett and Bennett 2013). Taken together, these data indicate a mild-adaptive humoural immune responses and an acceptable safety profile of AAV ocular gene therapy in humans.

11.4.1.2 Oncogenesis

Since the first gene therapy trial for x-linked severe combined immunodeficiency (X-SCID) reported iatrogenic acute lymphoblastic leukaemia after the ex vivo retroviral transduction of bone marrow cells (Hacein-Bey-Abina et al. 2003), oncogenesis has been a major concern in the field. Ectopic integration of vector DNA into the host genome has the theoretical potential to promote oncogenesis by upregulating endogenous proto-oncogenes as a consequence of promoter/enhancer sequences in the vector genes, or by disrupting tumour-suppressor genes. In contrast to retroviral vectors, which promote chromosomal integration, rAAV vectors pose minimal risk of mutagenic effects. The vast majority of rAAV vector genomes remain episomal in the host cell nucleus (Schnepp et al. 2003) and integration, if it occurs at all, is typically passive, largely random and of low frequency (Flotte et al. 1994; Ponnazhagan et al. 1997). rAAV integration studies in the mouse demonstrate that vector DNA integration occurs mainly in transcription units (53–72 %) and rarely (3.5 %) near or within cancer-related genes (Nakai et al. 2003; 2005). In human cell culture models, rAAV integrated with a slight preference to transcription units, but no integration near cancer-related genes has been reported (Miller et al. 2005). The oncogenic potential of rAAV2 in non-dividing cells, such as the naturally quiescent non-dividing cells in the eye, is likely to be lower still. The intraocular delivery of rAAV2 in p53 tumour-suppressor-gene knockout mice, which are highly susceptible to intraocular tumour formation, results in no increased risk of intraocular tumours (Balaggan et al. 2012). Furthermore, clinical trials of ocular gene therapy have reported no safety concerns of tumourigenesis up to 5 years following subretinal rAAV vector administration. Taken together, these findings are evidence of the highly limited oncogenic potential of rAAV vectors following intraocular administration. However, long-term safety data from clinical trials still needs to be awaited to exclude with confidence the risk of rAAV-induced ocular malignant transformation.

11.4.1.3 Inference with Vasoprotection and Neuroprotection

Long-term suppression of VEGF in the treatment of neovascular eye disease may risk compromising its role in maintaining the health of normal choroidal and retinal vasculature, as well as that of retinal neurones. Experimental studies in mice demonstrate that VEGF secreted by the RPE is essential to maintain the choriocapillaris and for the neuroprotection of photoreceptors. Genetic inactivation of the soluble VEGF isoforms VEGF120 and VEGF164 in mice is associated with progressive choroidal atrophy followed by retinal degeneration (Saint-Geniez et al. 2009). Similarly, repeated systemic or intraocular injections of neutralising VEGF antibodies causes retinal ganglion cell degeneration in the adult rat (Nishijima et al. 2007) and systemic administration of adenoviruses containing sFLt1 (Ad-sFlt1) cause inner and outer nuclear layers degeneration (Saint-Geniez et al. 2008). These findings highlight the important role of endogenous VEGF in the maintenance and function of the adult retina and raise safety concerns of long-term VEGF suppression by gene therapy. Other studies, however, have challenged these findings and suggest that prolonged blockade of VEGF does not damage retinal neurons or vasculature in mice (Ueno et al.

2008; Pellissier et al. 2014). Furthermore, anti-VEGF gene therapy using AAV2.sFLT01 in cynomolgus monkeys caused no adverse effects on retinal vascular or electroretinal function for up to 1 year after intraocular administration (Maclachlan et al. 2011). Long-term follow-up data of the 2 ongoing anti-VEGF gene therapy trials in exudative AMD is expected to provide further data on the safety of sustained anti-VEGF therapy.

11.5 Future Directions

11.5.1 Choosing the Optimal Vector System

11.5.1.1 Cell-Specific Vector Systems

The optimal choice of a vector system depends on the desired target cells, the vector's safety profile, transfection efficiency, and the longevity of transgene expression. In the last few years, rAAV viral vectors have become the vector of choice because of their long-term expression (Lebherz et al. 2005), minimal immune response, and favourable safety profile (Simonelli et al. 2010). Initial studies have used mainly AAV2 serotypes, but ongoing research has identified new variants of AAV based on engineered variants or naturally occurring AAV serotypes (Klimczak et al. 2009). These refined AAV variants are expected to enable more specific targeting of angiogenic molecules to the cell population of interest, thereby reducing the risks for adverse effects. Transgene delivery can be made more specific by cell-specific promoter systems which restrict transgene expression to the cell population of interest. Inner retinal vascular disease, such as PDR and RVO, require transgene delivery to inner retinal cells, whereas outer retinal vascular disease such as neovascular AMD may benefit primarily from transgene expression in the photoreceptors and RPE. The former may be achieved by introducing the GFAP, CD44, or RLBP1 promoter in the vector, which have been reported to be cell specific for Müller cells (Prentice et al. 2011; Greenberg et al. 2007; Esumi et al. 2004). As Müller cells are one of the major sources for VEGF production upon inner retinal hypoxia

(Watkins et al. 2013), this approach may enable specific suppression of VEGF production in the affected cells and thereby reduce any potential side-effects associated with VEGF inhibition in other cell types. On the other hand, cell-specific gene therapy to suppress CNV may be achieved by using photoreceptor-specific promoters such as human rhodopsin kinase (Khani et al. 2007) or RPE-specific promoters such as RPE65 or VMD2 (Esumi et al. 2004).

11.5.1.2 Regulation of Transgene Expression

Long-term uncontrolled constitutive transgene expression may in certain circumstances be undesirable, for example, where this might undermine physiological functions essential for retinal and vascular homeostasis in the mature retina. Pharmacologically inducible promoter systems offer an attractive strategy to regulate transgene expression temporally in response to the systemic delivery of an appropriate drug, i.e. mifepristone, ecdysone, doxycycline, or rapamycin. Preclinical studies have demonstrated promising results of inducible and long-term transgene expression in the retina following subretinal delivery of doxy-cyclin- or rapamycin-inducible AAV2 vector systems (Auricchio et al. 2002a; Lebherz et al. 2005; Folliot et al. 2003; McGee Sanftner et al. 2001). However, this approach depends on accurate dosing and regular clinical observation for adverse effects and is limited by inefficient drug penetration across the blood–retina barrier.

An alternative attractive approach is to couple transgene expression with a tissue-responsive promoter which drives transgene expression dependent on the local tissue environment, for example, tissue hypoxia, a central factor in the development of neovascular eye disease (Lange et al. 2011; Stefansson et al. 2011). This can be achieved by utilising the hypoxia-response element (HRE), a specific enhancer present in a number of angiogenic genes. Under hypoxic conditions, the activated hypoxia-inducible factor-1 binds to the HRE sequence and drives the expression of VEGF, EPO, and other hypoxia-regulated molecules. Hypoxia-inducible transgene expres-

sion systems have been applied to various ischaemic disease models including tumours, the ischaemic myocardium, stroke, and injured spinal cord (Kim et al. 2009). In the eye, delivery of rAAV expressing GFP under an HRE promoter results in transgene expression at sites of laser-induced CNV in mice, but not elsewhere (Bainbridge et al. 2003). Recently, this approach was combined with a cell-specific promoter system, demonstrating that an HRE-RPE65-GFP vector system led to strong transgene expression in hypoxic RPE cells, but it elicited no transgene expression in other hypoxic cell types or in normoxic cultured RPE cells (Dougherty et al. 2008). Similarly, a hypoxia-regulated, retinal glial cell-specific AAV vector was used successfully in the OIR mouse model leading to cell-specific transgene expression in hypoxic Müller cells in vivo (Prentice et al. 2011). These auto-initiated gene therapy approaches offer an attractive and intelligent way to achieve expression of angiostatic proteins for early intervention in neo-vascularisation, when it is most sensitive to inhibition.

11.5.1.3 Non-viral Gene Therapy

Because of the limited payload capacity and potential immunogenicity and oncogenicity of viral vector systems, there is a persistent need to refine and develop alternative gene delivery strategies. Non-viral gene transfer has historically been limited by short-lived and inefficient gene expression compared with viral vectors. Liposomes delivered topically and intravitreally have displayed poor transfection efficacy in the retina and RPE, attributed to the inner limiting membrane and blood–retina barrier that restricts passage of liposomes (Masuda et al. 1996). Subretinal delivery of liposomes demonstrated better results with varying degrees of expression and longevity (Hangai et al. 1996). Recent advances however have overcome some of these limitations through the use of refined liposomes, microparticles, or nanoparticles, which enhance nucleic acid stability and promote their cellular internalisation. Subretinal delivery of compacted DNA nanoparticles was reported to transfect nearly all RPE- and photoreceptor cells and produced expression levels almost equal to those of rhodopsin without provoking any immune responses in rodents (Farjo et al. 2006). Furthermore, adjunctive techniques such as electric current (electroporation or iontophoresis), high hydrostatic pressure, or ultrasound (sonophoresis) are now being evaluated to enhance nuclcic-acid delivery to cells (Andrieu-Soler et al. 2006). Electroporation of plasmids after subretinal administration in neonatal mice is associated with efficient transfection of RPE and photoreceptor cells and can mediate protection against retinal degeneration (Chen and Cepko 2009). Similarly, efficient and prolonged RPE transfection can be achieved in the adult rat after electroporation of subretinal plasmids containing specific RPE promoters (Kachi et al. 2006). Electroporation of sFlt-1 into the ciliary muscle can mediate a sustained reduction in VEGF levels and reduced vascular leakage in laser-induced CNV in rats (El Sanharawi et al. 2013). Taken together, these non-viral vector systems and adjunct techniques may offer efficient, long-term, and safe transfection of the retina and RPE that can be considered for future clinical application.

11.6 Conclusions

Although considerable progress has been made in our understanding and treatment of neovascular eye disease, there is a significant unmet need for the means to deliver angiostatic molecules to the retina in a sustained way. Gene therapy for neovascular eye disease is an emerging strategy that may prove to be safe, efficacious, fast-acting, and long-lasting following a single intraocular injection. Vector-mediated expression offers the additional potential advantage of regulated expression in response to exogenous or endogenous cues. Given the impact of anti-VEGF antibody treatment in neovascular eye disease and the encouraging findings of preclinical angio-

static gene therapy studies, further clinical trials are currently investigating the safety and efficacy of vectors expressing molecules that target the VEGF pathway and others that overexpress Endostatin and Angiostatin in neovascular AMD. These clinical trials are expected to provide valuable information regarding the efficacy and safety of angiostatic gene therapy in ncovascular eye disease. Although gene therapy appears acceptably safe in preclinical models, care needs to be taken with regard to long-term safety and efficacy of ocular gene therapy. Potential adverse effects such as oncogenesis, neuronal toxicity, and immune responses need to be excluded before gene therapy can become a routine therapy for neovascular eye disease. To address the possibility of local or systemic adverse effects, novel strategies can restrict transgene expression to the desired cell population by cell-specific promoters and viral tropisms. The incorporation of regulatable, pharmacological, or tissue-responsive elements into the vector construct can provide additional safety by preventing or reducing uncontrolled transgene expression. In this way, sites of active neovascularisation may be effectively targeted while minimising inappropriate expression elsewhere, or during periods of angiogenic inactivity. Finally, next-generation AAV vectors are expected to enable more rapid onset of expression and more efficient transduction of retinal cells following intravitreal vector delivery, which is potentially safer than subretinal delivery. These developments may be combined to offer the possibility of a cell-specific, regulatable, efficient, and safe transgene expression system that can provide lasting protection of sight in neovascular eye disease.

Compliance with Ethical Requirements The authors declare no competing financial interests.

No human or animal studies were performed by the authors for this chapter.

References

Adhi M, Cashman SM, Kumar-Singh R. Adeno-associated virus mediated delivery of a non-membrane targeted human soluble CD59 attenuates some aspects of diabetic retinopathy in mice. PLoS One. 2013;8(10): 79661.

Ali RR, Reichel MB, Byrnes AP, Stephens CJ, Thrasher AJ, Baker D, Hunt DM, Bhattacharya SS. Co-injection of adenovirus expressing CTLA4-Ig prolongs adeno-virally mediated lacZ reporter gene expression in the mouse retina. Gene Ther. 1998;5(11):1561–5.

Andrieu-Soler C, Bejjani R-A, de Bizemont T, Normand N, BenEzra D, Behar-Cohen F. Ocular gene therapy: a review of nonviral strategies. Mol Vis. 2006;12: 1334–47.

Askou AL, Pournaras J-AC, Pihlmann M, Svalgaard JD, Arsenijevic Y, Kostic C, Bek T, Dagnaes-Hansen F, Mikkelsen JG, Jensen TG, Corydon TJ. Reduction of choroidal neovascularization in mice by adeno-associated virus-delivered anti-vascular endothelial growth factor short hairpin RNA. J Gene Med. 2012;14(11):632–41.

Auricchio A, Rivera VM, Clackson T, O'Connor EE, Maguire AM, Tolentino MJ, Bennett J, Wilson JM. Pharmacological regulation of protein expression from adeno-associated viral vectors in the eye. Mol Ther. 2002a;6(2):238–42.

Auricchio A, Behling KC, Maguire AM, O'Connor EM, Bennett J, Wilson JM, Tolentino MJ. Inhibition of retinal neovascularization by intraocular viral-mediated delivery of anti-angiogenic agents. Mol Ther. 2002b; 6(4):490–4.

Bainbridge JW, Stephens C, Parsley K, Demaison C, Halfyard A, Thrasher AJ, Ali RR. In vivo gene transfer to the mouse eye using an HIV-based lentiviral vector; efficient long-term transduction of corneal endothelium and retinal pigment epithelium. Gene Ther. 2001;8(21):1665–8.

Bainbridge JWB, Mistry A, De Alwis M, Paleolog E, Baker A, Thrasher AJ, Ali RR. Inhibition of retinal neovascularisation by gene transfer of soluble VEGF receptor sFlt-1. Gene Ther. 2002;9(5):320–6.

Bainbridge JW, Mistry A, Binley K, De AM, Thrasher AJ, Naylor S, Ali RR. Hypoxia-regulated transgene expression in experimental retinal and choroidal neovascularization. Gene Ther. 2003;10(0969–7128):1049–54.

Bainbridge JWB, Smith AJ, Barker SS, Robbie S, Henderson R, Balaggan K, Viswanathan A, Holder GE, Stockman A, Tyler N, Petersen-Jones S, Bhattacharya SS, Thrasher AJ, Fitzke FW, Carter BJ, Rubin GS, Moore AT, Ali RR. Effect of gene therapy on visual function in Leber's congenital amaurosis. N Engl J Med. 2008;358(21):2231–9.

Balaggan KS, Binley K, Esapa M, Iqball S, Askham Z, Kan O, Tschernutter M, Bainbridge JWB, Naylor S, Ali RR. Stable and efficient intraocular gene transfer using pseudotyped EIAV lentiviral vectors. J Gene Med. 2006a;8(3):275–85.

Balaggan KS, Binley K, Esapa M, MacLaren RE, Iqball S, Duran Y, Pearson RA, Kan O, Barker SE, Smith AJ, Bainbridge JW, Naylor S, Ali RR. EIAV vector-mediated delivery of endostatin or angiostatin inhibits angiogenesis and vascular hyperpermeability in experimental CNV. Gene Ther. 2006b; 13(0969–7128):1153–65.

Balaggan KS, Duran Y, Georgiadis A, Thaung C, Barker SE, Buch PK, MacNeil A, Robbie S, Bainbridge JWB, Smith AJ, Ali RR. Absence of ocular malignant transformation after sub-retinal delivery of rAAV2/2 or integrating lentiviral vectors in p53-deficient mice. Gene Ther. 2012;19(2):182–8.

Banin E, Bandah-Rozenfeld D, Obolensky A, Cideciyan AV, Aleman TS, Marks-Ohana D, Sela M, Boye S, Sumaroka A, Roman AJ, Schwartz SB, Hauswirth WW, Jacobson SG, Hemo I, Sharon D. Molecular anthropology meets genetic medicine to treat blindness in the North African Jewish population: human gene therapy initiated in Israel. Hum Gene Ther. 2010;21(12):1749–57.

Bennett J, Wilson J, Sun D, Forbes B, Maguire A. Adenovirus vector-mediated in vivo gene transfer into adult murine retina. Invest Ophthalmol Vis Sci. 1994;35(5):2535–42.

Bennett J, Pakola S, Zeng Y, Maguire A. Humoral response after administration of E1-deleted adenoviruses: immune privilege of the subretinal space. Hum Gene Ther. 1996;7(14):1763–9.

Buch PK, Bainbridge JW, Ali RR. AAV-mediated gene therapy for retinal disorders: from mouse to man. Gene Ther. 2008;15(11):849–57.

Campochiaro PA, Nguyen QD, Shah SM, Klein ML, Holz E, Frank RN, Saperstein DA, Gupta A, Stout JT, Macko J, DiBartolomeo R, Wei LL. Adenoviral vector-delivered pigment epithelium-derived factor for neovascular age-related macular degeneration: results of a phase I clinical trial. Hum Gene Ther. 2006;17(2):167–76.

Cao W, Tombran-Tink J, Elias R, Sezate S, Mrazek D, McGinnis JF. In vivo protection of photoreceptors from light damage by pigment epithelium-derived factor. Invest Ophthalmol Vis Sci. 2001;42(7):1646–52.

Cashman SM, Bowman L, Christofferson J, Kumar-Singh R. Inhibition of choroidal neovascularization by adenovirus-mediated delivery of short hairpin RNAs targeting VEGF as a potential therapy for AMD. Invest Ophthalmol Vis Sci. 2006;47(8):3496–504.

Cashman SM, Ramo K, Kumar-Singh R. A non membrane-targeted human soluble CD59 attenuates choroidal neovascularization in a model of age related macular degeneration. PLoS One. 2011;6(4): e19078.

Chen B, Cepko CL. HDAC4 regulates neuronal survival in normal and diseased retinas. Science. 2009; 323(5911):256–9.

Deng W-T, Yan Z, Dinculescu A, Pang J, Teusner JT, Cortez NG, Berns KI, Hauswirth WW. Adeno-associated virus-mediated expression of vascular endothelial growth factor peptides inhibits retinal neovascularization in a mouse model of oxygen-induced retinopathy. Hum Gene Ther. 2005;16(11):1247–54.

Dougherty CJ, Smith GW, Dorey CK, Prentice HM, Webster KA, Blanks JC. Robust hypoxia-selective regulation of a retinal pigment epithelium-specific adeno-associated virus vector. Mol Vis. 2008;14:471–80.

El Sanharawi M, Touchard E, Benard R, Bigey P, Escriou V, Mehanna C, Naud M-C, Berdugo M, Jeanny J-C, Behar-Cohen F. Long-term efficacy of ciliary muscle gene transfer of three sFlt-1 variants in a rat model of laser-induced choroidal neovascularization. Gene Ther. 2013;20(11):1093–103.

Esumi N, Oshima Y, Li Y, Campochiaro PA, Zack DJ. Analysis of the VMD2 promoter and implication of E-box binding factors in its regulation. J Biol Chem. 2004;279(18):19064–73.

Farjo R, Skaggs J, Quiambao AB, Cooper MJ, Naash MI. Efficient non-viral ocular gene transfer with compacted DNA nanoparticles. PLoS One. 2006;1(1):e38.

Flotte TR, Afione SA, Zeitlin PL. Adeno-associated virus vector gene expression occurs in nondividing cells in the absence of vector DNA integration. Am J Respir Cell Mol Biol. 1994;11(5):517–21.

Folliot S, Briot D, Conrath H, Provost N, Cherel Y, Moullier P, Rolling F. Sustained tetracycline-regulated transgene expression in vivo in rat retinal ganglion cells using a single type 2 adeno-associated viral vector. J Gene Med. 2003;5(6):493–501.

Forrester JV, Xu H. Good news-bad news: the Yin and Yang of immune privilege in the eye. Front Immunol. 2012;3:338.

Friedmann T. A brief history of gene therapy. Nat Genet. 1992;2(2):93–8.

Gehlbach P, Demetriades AM, Yamamoto S, Deering T, Duh EJ, Yang HS, Cingolani C, Lai H, Wei L, Campochiaro PA. Periocular injection of an adenoviral vector encoding pigment epithelium-derived factor inhibits choroidal neovascularization. Gene Ther. 2003;10(8):637–46.

Greenberg KP, Geller SF, Schaffer DV, Flannery JG. Targeted transgene expression in Muller glia of normal and diseased retinas using lentiviral vectors. Invest Ophthalmol Vis Sci. 2007;48(4):1844–52.

Hacein-Bey-Abina S, Von Kalle C, Schmidt M, McCormack MP, Wulffraat N, Leboulch P, Lim A, Osborne CS, Pawliuk R, Morillon E, Sorensen R, Forster A, Fraser P, Cohen JI, de Saint Basile G, Alexander I, Wintergerst U, Frebourg T, Aurias A, Stoppa-Lyonnet D, Romana S, Radford-Weiss I, Gross F, Valensi F, Delabesse E, Macintyre E, Sigaux F, Soulier J, Leiva LE, Wissler M, Prinz C, Rabbitts TH, Le Deist F, Fischer A, Cavazzana-Calvo M. LMO2-associated clonal T cell proliferation in two patients after gene therapy for SCID-X1. Science. 2003;302(5644):415–9.

Hangai M, Kaneda Y, Tanihara H, Honda Y. In vivo gene transfer into the retina mediated by a novel liposome system. Invest Ophthalmol Vis Sci. 1996;37(13):2678–85.

Haurigot V, Villacampa P, Ribera A, Bosch A, Ramos D, Ruberte J, Bosch F. Long-term retinal PEDF overexpression prevents neovascularization in a murine adult model of retinopathy. PLoS One. 2012;7(7):e41511.

Hauswirth WW, Aleman TS, Kaushal S, Cideciyan AV, Schwartz SB, Wang L, Conlon TJ, Boye SL, Flotte TR, Byrne BJ, Jacobson SG. Treatment of Leber congenital amaurosis due to RPE65 mutations by ocular subretinal injection of adeno-associated virus gene vector: short-term results of a phase I trial. Hum Gene Ther. 2008;19(10):979–90.

Holekamp NM, Bouck N, Volpert O. Pigment epithelium-derived factor is deficient in the vitreous of patients with choroidal neovascularization due to age-related macular degeneration. Am J Ophthalmol. 2002; 134(2):220–7.

Honda M, Sakamoto T, Ishibashi T, Inomata H, Ueno H. Experimental subretinal neovascularization is inhibited by adenovirus-mediated soluble VEGF/flt-1 receptor gene transfection: a role of VEGF and possible treatment for SRN in age-related macular degeneration. Gene Ther. 2000;7(11):978–85.

Igarashi T, Miyake K, Kato K, Watanabe A, Ishizaki M, Ohara K, Shimada T. Lentivirus-mediated expression of angiostatin efficiently inhibits neovascularization in a murine proliferative retinopathy model. Gene Ther. 2003;10(3):219–26.

Igarashi T, Miyake K, Masuda I, Takahashi H, Shimada T. Adeno-associated vector (type 8)-mediated expression of soluble Flt-1 efficiently inhibits neovascularization in a murine choroidal neovascularization model. Hum Gene Ther. 2010;21(5):631–7.

Igarashi T, Miyake N, Fujimoto C, Yaguchi C, Iijima O, Shimada T, Takahashi H, Miyake K. Adeno-associated virus type 8 vector-mediated expression of siRNA targeting vascular endothelial growth factor efficiently inhibits neovascularization in a murine choroidal neovascularization model. Mol Vis. 2014;20:488–96.

Jacobson SG, Cideciyan AV, Ratnakaram R, Heon E, Schwartz SB, Roman AJ, Peden MC, Aleman TS, Boye SL, Sumaroka A, Conlon TJ, Calcedo R, Pang J-J, Erger KE, Olivares MB, Mullins CL, Swider M, Kaushal S, Feuer WJ, Iannaccone A, Fishman GA, Stone EM, Byrne BJ, Hauswirth WW. Gene therapy for Leber congenital amaurosis caused by RPE65 mutations: safety and efficacy in 15 children and adults followed up to 3 years. Arch Ophthalmol. 2012;130(1):9–24.

Jiang Y, Wang H, Culp D, Yang Z, Fotheringham L, Flannery J, Hammond S, Kafri T, Hartnett ME. Targeting Müller cell-derived VEGF164 to reduce intravitreal neovascularization in the rat model of retinopathy of prematurity. Invest Ophthalmol Vis Sci. 2014;55(2):824–31.

Kachi S, Esumi N, Zack DJ, Campochiaro PA. Sustained expression after nonviral ocular gene transfer using mammalian promoters. Gene Ther. 2006;13(9): 798–804.

Khani SC, Pawlyk BS, Bulgakov OV, Kasperek E, Young JE, Adamian M, Sun X, Smith AJ, Ali RR, Li T. AAV-mediated expression targeting of rod and cone photoreceptors with a human rhodopsin kinase promoter. Invest Ophthalmol Vis Sci. 2007;48(9):3954–61.

Kim HA, Mahato RI, Lee M. Hypoxia-specific gene expression for ischemic disease gene therapy. Adv Drug Deliv Rev. 2009;61(7–8):614–22.

Klimczak RR, Koerber JT, Dalkara D, Flannery JG, Schaffer DV. A novel adeno-associated viral variant for efficient and selective intravitreal transduction of rat Müller cells. PLoS One. 2009;4(10):e7467.

Koerber JT, Klimczak R, Jang J-H, Dalkara D, Flannery JG, Schaffer DV. Molecular evolution of adeno-associated virus for enhanced glial gene delivery. Mol Ther. 2009;17(12):2088–95.

Lai CC, Wu WC, Chen SL, Xiao X, Tsai TC, Huan SJ, Chen TL, Tsai RJ, Tsao YP. Suppression of choroidal neovascularization by adeno-associated virus vector expressing angiostatin. Invest Ophthalmol Vis Sci. 2001;42(10):2401–7.

Lai C-M, Shen W-Y, Brankov M, Lai YKY, Barnett NL, Lee S-Y, Yeo IYS, Mathur R, Ho JES, Pineda P, Barathi A, Ang C-L, Constable IJ, Rakoczy EP. Long-term evaluation of AAV-mediated sFlt-1 gene therapy for ocular neovascularization in mice and monkeys. Mol Ther. 2005;12(4):659–68.

Lai C-M, Estcourt MJ, Wikstrom M, Himbeck RP, Barnett NL, Brankov M, Tee LBG, Dunlop SA, Degli-Esposti MA, Rakoczy EP. rAAV.sFlt-1 gene therapy achieves lasting reversal of retinal neovascularization in the absence of a strong immune response to the viral vector. Invest Ophthalmol Vis Sci. 2009;50(9):4279–87.

Lamartina S, Cimino M, Roscilli G, Dammassa E, Lazzaro D, Rota R, Ciliberto G, Toniatti C. Helper-dependent adenovirus for the gene therapy of proliferative retinopathies: stable gene transfer, regulated gene expression and therapeutic efficacy. J Gene Med. 2007;9(10):862–74.

Lange CA, Stavrakas P, Luhmann UF, de Silva DJ, Ali RR, Gregor ZJ, Bainbridge JW. Intraocular oxygen distribution in advanced proliferative diabetic retinopathy. Am J Ophthalmol. 2011;152(1879–1891):406–12.

Lebherz C, Auricchio A, Maguire AM, Rivera VM, Tang W, Grant RL, Clackson T, Bennett J, Wilson JM. Long-term inducible gene expression in the eye via adeno-associated virus gene transfer in nonhuman primates. Hum Gene Ther. 2005;16(2):178–86.

Lukason M, DuFresne E, Rubin H, Pechan P, Li Q, Kim I, Kiss S, Flaxel C, Collins M, Miller J, Hauswirth W, Maclachlan T, Wadsworth S, Scaria A. Inhibition of choroidal neovascularization in a nonhuman primate model by intravitreal administration of an AAV2 vector expressing a novel anti-VEGF molecule. Mol Ther. 2011;19(2):260–5.

Maclachlan TK, Lukason M, Collins M, Munger R, Isenberger E, Rogers C, Malatos S, Dufresne E, Morris J, Calcedo R, Veres G, Scaria A, Andrews L, Wadsworth S. Preclinical safety evaluation of AAV2-sFLT01—a gene therapy for age-related macular degeneration. Mol Ther. 2011;19(2):326–34.

MacLaren RE, Groppe M, Barnard AR, Cottriall CL, Tolmachova T, Seymour L, Clark KR, During MJ, Cremers FPM, Black GCM, Lotery AJ, Downes SM, Webster AR, Seabra MC. Retinal gene therapy in

patients with choroideremia: initial findings from a phase 1/2 clinical trial. Lancet. 2014;383(9923):1129–37.

Maguire AM, Simonelli F, Pierce EA, Pugh EN, Mingozzi F, Bennicelli J, Banfi S, Marshall KA, Testa F, Surace EM, Rossi S, Lyubarsky A, Arruda VR, Konkle B, Stone E, Sun J, Jacobs J, Dell'Osso L, Hertle R, Ma J, Redmond TM, Zhu X, Hauck B, Zelenaia O, Shindler KS, Maguire MG, Wright JF, Volpe NJ, McDonnell JW, Auricchio A, High KA, Bennett J. Safety and efficacy of gene transfer for Leber's congenital amaurosis. N Engl J Med. 2008;358(21):2240–8.

Mao Y, Kiss S, Boyer JL, Hackett NR, Qiu J, Carbone A, Mezey JG, Kaminsky SM, D'Amico DJ, Crystal RG. Persistent suppression of ocular neovascularization with intravitreal administration of AAVrh.10 coding for bevacizumab. Hum Gene Ther. 2011;22(12):1525–35.

Masuda I, Matsuo T, Yasuda T, Matsuo N. Gene transfer with liposomes to the intraocular tissues by different routes of administration. Invest Ophthalmol Vis Sci. 1996;37(9):1914–20.

McGee Sanftner LH, Rendahl KG, Quiroz D, Coyne M, Ladner M, Manning WC, Flannery JG. Recombinant AAV-mediated delivery of a tet-inducible reporter gene to the rat retina. Mol Ther. 2001;3(5 Pt 1):688–96.

Miller DG, Trobridge GD, Petek LM, Jacobs MA, Kaul R, Russell DW. Large-scale analysis of adeno-associated virus vector integration sites in normal human cells. J Virol. 2005;79(17):11434–42.

Mori K, Duh E, Gehlbach P, Ando A, Takahashi K, Pearlman J, Mori K, Yang HS, Zack DJ, Ettyreddy D, Brough DE, Wei LL, Campochiaro PA. Pigment epithelium-derived factor inhibits retinal and choroidal neovascularization. J Cell Physiol. 2001;188(2):253–63.

Mori K, Gehlbach P, Yamamoto S, Duh E, Zack DJ, Li Q, Berns KI, Raisler BJ, Hauswirth WW, Campochiaro PA. AAV-mediated gene transfer of pigment epithelium-derived factor inhibits choroidal neovascularization. Invest Ophthalmol Vis Sci. 2002;43(6):1994–2000.

Nakai H, Montini E, Fuess S, Storm TA, Grompe M, Kay MA. AAV serotype 2 vectors preferentially integrate into active genes in mice. Nat Genet. 2003;34(3):297–302.

Nakai H, Wu X, Fuess S, Storm TA, Munroe D, Montini E, Burgess SM, Grompe M, Kay MA. Large-scale molecular characterization of adeno-associated virus vector integration in mouse liver. J Virol. 2005;79(6):3606–14.

Nishijima K, Ng YS, Zhong L, Bradley J, Schubert W, Jo N, Akita J, Samuelsson SJ, Robinson GS, Adamis AP, Shima DT. Vascular endothelial growth factor-A is a survival factor for retinal neurons and a critical neuroprotectant during the adaptive response to ischemic injury. Am J Pathol. 2007;171(0002–9440):53–67.

O'Reilly MS, Boehm T, Shing Y, Fukai N, Vasios G, Lane WS, Flynn E, Birkhead JR, Olsen BR, Folkman J. Endostatin: an endogenous inhibitor of angiogenesis and tumor growth. Cell. 1997;88(2):277–85.

Pechan P, Rubin H, Lukason M, Ardinger J, DuFresne E, Hauswirth WW, Wadsworth SC, Scaria A. Novel anti-VEGF chimeric molecules delivered by AAV vectors for inhibition of retinal neovascularization. Gene Ther. 2009;16(1):10–6.

Pellissier LP, Hoek RM, Vos RM, Aartsen WM, Klimczak RR, Hoyng SA, Flannery JG, Wijnholds J. Specific tools for targeting and expression in Müller glial cells. Mol Ther Methods Clin Dev. 2014;1:14009.

Ponnazhagan S, Erikson D, Kearns WG, Zhou SZ, Nahreini P, Wang XS, Srivastava A. Lack of site-specific integration of the recombinant adeno-associated virus 2 genomes in human cells. Hum Gene Ther. 1997;8(3):275–84.

Prentice HM, Biswal MR, Dorey CK, Blanks JC. Hypoxia-regulated retinal glial cell-specific promoter for potential gene therapy in disease. Invest Ophthalmol Vis Sci. 2011;52(12):8562–70.

Raisler BJ, Berns KI, Grant MB, Beliaev D, Hauswirth WW. Adeno-associated virus type-2 expression of pigmented epithelium-derived factor or Kringles 1-3 of angiostatin reduce retinal neovascularization. Proc Natl Acad Sci U S A. 2002;99(13):8909–14.

Ramírez M, Wu Z, Moreno-Carranza B, Jeziorski MC, Arnold E, Díaz-Lezama N, Martínez de la Escalera G, Colosi P, Clapp C. Vasoinhibin gene transfer by adeno-associated virus type 2 protects against VEGF- and diabetes-induced retinal vasopermeability. Invest Ophthalmol Vis Sci. 2011;52(12):8944–50.

Rasmussen H, Chu KW, Campochiaro P, Gehlbach PL, Haller JA, Handa JT, Nguyen QD, Sung JU. Clinical protocol. An open-label, phase I, single administration, dose-escalation study of ADGVPEDF.11D (ADPEDF) in neovascular age-related macular degeneration (AMD). Hum Gene Ther. 2001; 12(16):2029–32.

Reichel MB, Ali RR, Thrasher AJ, Hunt DM, Bhattacharya SS, Baker D. Immune responses limit adenovirally mediated gene expression in the adult mouse eye. Gene Ther. 1998;5(8):1038–46.

Reichel MB, Hudde T, Ali RR, Wiedemann P. Gene transfer in ophthalmology. Ophthalmologe. 1999; 96(9):570–7.

Rofagha S, Bhisitkul RB, Boyer DS, Sadda SR, Zhang K, SEVEN-UP Study Group. Seven-year outcomes in ranibizumab-treated patients in ANCHOR, MARINA, and HORIZON: a multicenter cohort study (SEVEN-UP). Ophthalmology. 2013;120(11):2292–9.

Rota R, Riccioni T, Zaccarini M, Lamartina S, Gallo AD, Fusco A, Kovesdi I, Balestrazzi E, Abeni DC, Ali RR, Capogrossi MC. Marked inhibition of retinal neovascularization in rats following soluble-flt-1 gene transfer. J Gene Med. 2004;6(9):992–1002.

Saint-Geniez M, Maharaj ASR, Walshe TE, Tucker BA, Sekiyama E, Kurihara T, Darland DC, Young MJ, D'Amore PA. Endogenous VEGF is required for visual function: evidence for a survival role on Müller cells and photoreceptors. PLoS One. 2008;3(11):e3554.

Saint-Geniez M, Kurihara T, Sekiyama E, Maldonado AE, D'Amore PA. An essential role for RPE-derived soluble VEGF in the maintenance of the choriocapillaris. Proc Natl Acad Sci U S A. 2009;106(1091–6490):18751–6.

Saishin Y, Silva RL, Saishin Y, Kachi S, Aslam S, Gong YY, Lai H, Carrion M, Harris B, Hamilton M, Wei L, Campochiaro PA. Periocular gene transfer of pigment epithelium-derived factor inhibits choroidal neovascularization in a human-sized eye. Hum Gene Ther. 2005;16(4):473–8.

Salam A, Mathew R, Sivaprasad S. Treatment of proliferative diabetic retinopathy with anti-VEGF agents. Acta Ophthalmol. 2001;89(1755–3768):405–11.

Schnepp BC, Clark KR, Klemanski DL, Pacak CA, Johnson PR. Genetic fate of recombinant adeno-associated virus vector genomes in muscle. J Virol. 2003;77(6):3495–504.

Shen J, Yang X, Xiao W-H, Hackett SF, Sato Y, Campochiaro PA. Vasohibin is up-regulated by VEGF in the retina and suppresses VEGF receptor 2 and retinal neovascularization. FASEB J. 2006;20(6): 723–5.

Simonelli F, Maguire AM, Testa F, Pierce EA, Mingozzi F, Bennicelli JL, Rossi S, Marshall K, Banfi S, Surace EM, Sun J, Redmond TM, Zhu X, Shindler KS, Ying G-S, Ziviello C, Acerra C, Wright JF, McDonnell JW, High KA, Bennett J, Auricchio A. Gene therapy for Leber's congenital amaurosis is safe and effective through 1.5 years after vector administration. Mol Ther. 2010;18(3):643–50.

Spranger J, Hammes HP, Preissner KT, Schatz H, Pfeiffer AF. Release of the angiogenesis inhibitor angiostatin in patients with proliferative diabetic retinopathy: association with retinal photocoagulation. Diabetologia. 2000;43(0012–186X):1404–7.

Steele FR, Chader GJ, Johnson LV, Tombran-Tink J. Pigment epithelium-derived factor: neurotrophic activity and identification as a member of the serine protease inhibitor gene family. Proc Natl Acad Sci U S A. 1993;90(4):1526–30.

Stefansson E, Geirsdottir A, Sigurdsson H. Metabolic physiology in age related macular degeneration. Prog Retin Eye Res. 2011;30(1):72–80.

Takahashi T, Nakamura T, Hayashi A, Kamei M, Nakabayashi M, Okada AA, Tomita N, Kaneda Y, Tano Y. Inhibition of experimental choroidal neovascularization by overexpression of tissue inhibitor of metalloproteinases-3 in retinal pigment epithelium cells. Am J Ophthalmol. 2000;130(6):774–81.

Takahashi K, Saishin Y, Saishin Y, Silva RL, Oshima Y, Oshima S, Melia M, Paszkiet B, Zerby D, Kadan MJ, Liau G, Kaleko M, Connelly S, Luo T, Campochiaro PA. Intraocular expression of endostatin reduces VEGF-induced retinal vascular permeability, neovascularization, and retinal detachment. FASEB J. 2003;17(8):896–8.

Testa F, Maguire AM, Rossi S, Pierce EA, Melillo P, Marshall K, Banfi S, Surace EM, Sun J, Acerra C, Wright JF, Wellman J, High KA, Auricchio A, Bennett J, Simonelli F. Three-year follow-up after unilateral subretinal delivery of adeno-associated virus in patients with Leber congenital Amaurosis type 2. Ophthalmology. 2013;120(6):1283–91.

Ueno S, Pease ME, Wersinger DMB, Masuda T, Vinores SA, Licht T, Zack DJ, Quigley H, Keshet E, Campochiaro PA. Prolonged blockade of VEGF family members does not cause identifiable damage to retinal neurons or vessels. J Cell Physiol. 2008;217(1):13–22.

Wakusawa R, Abe T, Sato H, Sonoda H, Sato M, Mitsuda Y, Takakura T, Fukushima T, Onami H, Nagai N, Ishikawa Y, Nishida K, Sato Y. Suppression of choroidal neovascularization by vasohibin-1, a vascular endothelium-derived angiogenic inhibitor. Invest Ophthalmol Vis Sci. 2011;52(6):3272–80.

Wang H, Smith GW, Yang Z, Jiang Y, McCloskey M, Greenberg K, Geisen P, Culp WD, Flannery J, Kafri T, Hammond S, Hartnett ME. Short hairpin RNA-mediated knockdown of VEGFA in Müller cells reduces intravitreal neovascularization in a rat model of retinopathy of prematurity. Am J Pathol. 2013;183(3):964–74.

Watkins WM, McCollum GW, Savage SR, Capozzi ME, Penn JS, Morrison DG. Hypoxia-induced expression of VEGF splice variants and protein in four retinal cell types. Exp Eye Res. 2013;116:240–6.

Willett K, Bennett J. Immunology of AAV-mediated gene transfer in the eye. Front Immunol. 2013;4:261.

Wu Z, Yang H, Colosi P. Effect of genome size on AAV vector packaging. Mol Ther. 2010;18(1):80–6.

Zhang SX, Wang JJ, Gao G, Parke K, Ma J. Pigment epithelium-derived factor downregulates vascular endothelial growth factor (VEGF) expression and inhibits VEGF-VEGF receptor 2 binding in diabetic retinopathy. J Mol Endocrinol. 2006;37(1):1–12.

Zhang X, Das SK, Passi SF, Uehara H, Bohner A, Chen M, Tiem M, Archer B, Ambati BK. AAV2 delivery of Flt23k intraceptors inhibits murine choroidal neovascularization. Mol Ther. 2015;123(2):226–34.

Index

© Springer International Publishing Switzerland 2016
A. Stahl (ed.), *Anti-Angiogenic Therapy in Ophthalmology*,
Essentials in Ophthalmology, DOI 10.1007/978-3-319-24097-8